Quantitative Methods for Traditional Chinese Medicine Development

Chapman & Hall/CRC Biostatistics Series

Editor-in-Chief

Shein-Chung Chow, Ph.D., Professor, Department of Biostatistics and Bioinformatics, Duke University School of Medicine, Durham, North Carolina

Series Editors

Byron Jones, Biometrical Fellow, Statistical Methodology, Integrated Information Sciences, Novartis Pharma AG, Basel, Switzerland

Jen-pei Liu, Professor, Division of Biometry, Department of Agronomy, National Taiwan University, Taipei, Taiwan

Karl E. Peace, Georgia Cancer Coalition, Distinguished Cancer Scholar, Senior Research Scientist and Professor of Biostatistics, Jiann-Ping Hsu College of Public Health, Georgia Southern University, Statesboro, Georgia

Bruce W. Turnbull, Professor, School of Operations Research and Industrial Engineering, Cornell University, Ithaca, New York

Published Titles

Adaptive Design Methods in Clinical Trials, Second Edition
Shein-Chung Chow and Mark Chang

Adaptive Designs for Sequential Treatment Allocation
Alessandro Baldi Antognini and Alessandra Giovagnoli

Adaptive Design Theory and Implementation Using SAS and R, Second Edition
Mark Chang

Advanced Bayesian Methods for Medical Test Accuracy
Lyle D. Broemeling

Advances in Clinical Trial Biostatistics
Nancy L. Geller

Applied Meta-Analysis with R
Ding-Geng (Din) Chen and Karl E. Peace

Basic Statistics and Pharmaceutical Statistical Applications, Second Edition
James E. De Muth

Bayesian Adaptive Methods for Clinical Trials
Scott M. Berry, Bradley P. Carlin, J. Jack Lee, and Peter Muller

Bayesian Analysis Made Simple: An Excel GUI for WinBUGS
Phil Woodward

Bayesian Methods for Measures of Agreement
Lyle D. Broemeling

Bayesian Methods for Repeated Measures
Lyle D. Broemeling

Bayesian Methods in Epidemiology
Lyle D. Broemeling

Bayesian Methods in Health Economics
Gianluca Baio

Bayesian Missing Data Problems: EM, Data Augmentation and Noniterative Computation
Ming T. Tan, Guo-Liang Tian, and Kai Wang Ng

Published Titles

Bayesian Modeling in Bioinformatics
Dipak K. Dey, Samiran Ghosh,
and Bani K. Mallick

Benefit-Risk Assessment in Pharmaceutical Research and Development
Andreas Sashegyi, James Felli,
and Rebecca Noel

Biosimilars: Design and Analysis of Follow-on Biologics
Shein-Chung Chow

Biostatistics: A Computing Approach
Stewart J. Anderson

Causal Analysis in Biomedicine and Epidemiology: Based on Minimal Sufficient Causation
Mikel Aickin

Clinical and Statistical Considerations in Personalized Medicine
Claudio Carini, Sandeep Menon,
and Mark Chang

Clinical Trial Data Analysis using R
Ding-Geng (Din) Chen and
Karl E. Peace

Clinical Trial Methodology
Karl E. Peace and
Ding-Geng (Din) Chen

Computational Methods in Biomedical Research
Ravindra Khattree and
Dayanand N. Naik

Computational Pharmacokinetics
Anders Källén

Confidence Intervals for Proportions and Related Measures of Effect Size
Robert G. Newcombe

Controversial Statistical Issues in Clinical Trials
Shein-Chung Chow

Data Analysis with Competing Risks and Intermediate States
Ronald B. Geskus

Data and Safety Monitoring Committees in Clinical Trials
Jay Herson

Design and Analysis of Animal Studies in Pharmaceutical Development
Shein-Chung Chow and
Jen-pei Liu

Design and Analysis of Bioavailability and Bioequivalence Studies, Third Edition
Shein-Chung Chow and
Jen-pei Liu

Design and Analysis of Bridging Studies
Jen-pei Liu, Shein-Chung Chow,
and Chin-Fu Hsiao

Design and Analysis of Clinical Trials for Predictive Medicine
Shigeyuki Matsui, Marc Buyse,
and Richard Simon

Design and Analysis of Clinical Trials with Time-to-Event Endpoints
Karl E. Peace

Design and Analysis of Non-Inferiority Trials
Mark D. Rothmann, Brian L. Wiens,
and Ivan S. F. Chan

Difference Equations with Public Health Applications
Lemuel A. Moyé and
Asha Seth Kapadia

DNA Methylation Microarrays: Experimental Design and Statistical Analysis
Sun-Chong Wang and
Arturas Petronis

Published Titles

DNA Microarrays and Related Genomics Techniques: Design, Analysis, and Interpretation of Experiments
David B. Allison, Grier P. Page, T. Mark Beasley, and Jode W. Edwards

Dose Finding by the Continual Reassessment Method
Ying Kuen Cheung

Dynamical Biostatistical Models
Daniel Commenges and Hélène Jacqmin-Gadda

Elementary Bayesian Biostatistics
Lemuel A. Moyé

Empirical Likelihood Method in Survival Analysis
Mai Zhou

Exposure–Response Modeling: Methods and Practical Implementation
Jixian Wang

Frailty Models in Survival Analysis
Andreas Wienke

Generalized Linear Models: A Bayesian Perspective
Dipak K. Dey, Sujit K. Ghosh, and Bani K. Mallick

Handbook of Regression and Modeling: Applications for the Clinical and Pharmaceutical Industries
Daryl S. Paulson

Inference Principles for Biostatisticians
Ian C. Marschner

Interval-Censored Time-to-Event Data: Methods and Applications
Ding-Geng (Din) Chen, Jianguo Sun, and Karl E. Peace

Introductory Adaptive Trial Designs: A Practical Guide with R
Mark Chang

Joint Models for Longitudinal and Time-to-Event Data: With Applications in R
Dimitris Rizopoulos

Measures of Interobserver Agreement and Reliability, Second Edition
Mohamed M. Shoukri

Medical Biostatistics, Third Edition
A. Indrayan

Meta-Analysis in Medicine and Health Policy
Dalene Stangl and Donald A. Berry

Mixed Effects Models for the Population Approach: Models, Tasks, Methods and Tools
Marc Lavielle

Modeling to Inform Infectious Disease Control
Niels G. Becker

Modern Adaptive Randomized Clinical Trials: Statistical and Practical Aspects
Oleksandr Sverdlov

Monte Carlo Simulation for the Pharmaceutical Industry: Concepts, Algorithms, and Case Studies
Mark Chang

Multiple Testing Problems in Pharmaceutical Statistics
Alex Dmitrienko, Ajit C. Tamhane, and Frank Bretz

Noninferiority Testing in Clinical Trials: Issues and Challenges
Tie-Hua Ng

Published Titles

Optimal Design for Nonlinear Response Models
Valerii V. Fedorov and Sergei L. Leonov

Patient-Reported Outcomes: Measurement, Implementation and Interpretation
Joseph C. Cappelleri, Kelly H. Zou, Andrew G. Bushmakin, Jose Ma. J. Alvir, Demissie Alemayehu, and Tara Symonds

Quantitative Evaluation of Safety in Drug Development: Design, Analysis and Reporting
Qi Jiang and H. Amy Xia

Quantitative Methods for Traditional Chinese Medicine Development
Shein-Chung Chow

Randomized Clinical Trials of Nonpharmacological Treatments
Isabelle Boutron, Philippe Ravaud, and David Moher

Randomized Phase II Cancer Clinical Trials
Sin-Ho Jung

Sample Size Calculations for Clustered and Longitudinal Outcomes in Clinical Research
Chul Ahn, Moonseong Heo, and Song Zhang

Sample Size Calculations in Clinical Research, Second Edition
Shein-Chung Chow, Jun Shao, and Hansheng Wang

Statistical Analysis of Human Growth and Development
Yin Bun Cheung

Statistical Design and Analysis of Clinical Trials: Principles and Methods
Weichung Joe Shih and Joseph Aisner

Statistical Design and Analysis of Stability Studies
Shein-Chung Chow

Statistical Evaluation of Diagnostic Performance: Topics in ROC Analysis
Kelly H. Zou, Aiyi Liu, Andriy Bandos, Lucila Ohno-Machado, and Howard Rockette

Statistical Methods for Clinical Trials
Mark X. Norleans

Statistical Methods for Drug Safety
Robert D. Gibbons and Anup K. Amatya

Statistical Methods for Immunogenicity Assessment
Harry Yang, Jianchun Zhang, Binbing Yu, and Wei Zhao

Statistical Methods in Drug Combination Studies
Wei Zhao and Harry Yang

Statistics in Drug Research: Methodologies and Recent Developments
Shein-Chung Chow and Jun Shao

Statistics in the Pharmaceutical Industry, Third Edition
Ralph Buncher and Jia-Yeong Tsay

Survival Analysis in Medicine and Genetics
Jialiang Li and Shuangge Ma

Theory of Drug Development
Eric B. Holmgren

Translational Medicine: Strategies and Statistical Methods
Dennis Cosmatos and Shein-Chung Chow

Chapman & Hall/CRC Biostatistics Series

Quantitative Methods for Traditional Chinese Medicine Development

Shein-Chung Chow

Duke University School of Medicine
Durham, North Carolina, USA

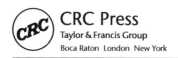

CRC Press is an imprint of the
Taylor & Francis Group, an **informa** business

A CHAPMAN & HALL BOOK

CRC Press
Taylor & Francis Group
6000 Broken Sound Parkway NW, Suite 300
Boca Raton, FL 33487-2742

First issued in paperback 2019

© 2016 by Taylor & Francis Group, LLC
CRC Press is an imprint of Taylor & Francis Group, an Informa business

No claim to original U.S. Government works

ISBN-13: 978-1-4822-3599-9 (hbk)
ISBN-13: 978-0-367-37738-0 (pbk)

This book contains information obtained from authentic and highly regarded sources. Reasonable efforts have been made to publish reliable data and information, but the author and publisher cannot assume responsibility for the validity of all materials or the consequences of their use. The authors and publishers have attempted to trace the copyright holders of all material reproduced in this publication and apologize to copyright holders if permission to publish in this form has not been obtained. If any copyright material has not been acknowledged please write and let us know so we may rectify in any future reprint.

Except as permitted under U.S. Copyright Law, no part of this book may be reprinted, reproduced, transmitted, or utilized in any form by any electronic, mechanical, or other means, now known or hereafter invented, including photocopying, microfilming, and recording, or in any information storage or retrieval system, without written permission from the publishers.

For permission to photocopy or use material electronically from this work, please access www.copyright. com (http://www.copyright.com/) or contact the Copyright Clearance Center, Inc. (CCC), 222 Rosewood Drive, Danvers, MA 01923, 978-750-8400. CCC is a not-for-profit organization that provides licenses and registration for a variety of users. For organizations that have been granted a photocopy license by the CCC, a separate system of payment has been arranged.

Trademark Notice: Product or corporate names may be trademarks or registered trademarks, and are used only for identification and explanation without intent to infringe.

Visit the Taylor & Francis Web site at
http://www.taylorandfrancis.com

and the CRC Press Web site at
http://www.crcpress.com

To my wife, Annpey

Contents

Preface..xxiii

1. Introduction..1
  1.1   Introduction 1
  1.2   What Is Traditional Chinese Medicine?..3
        1.2.1   Chinese Herbal Medicine 3
        1.2.2   Acupuncture...3
        1.2.3   Other TCM Therapies..4
        1.2.4   Botanical Drug Product 4
        1.2.5   Dietary Therapy 4
        1.2.6   Complementary and Alternative Medicine 4
        1.2.7   Remarks...5
  1.3   Fundamental Differences..6
        1.3.1   Medical Theory/Mechanism and Practice............................6
              1.3.1.1   Medical Theory and Mechanism 6
              1.3.1.2   Medical Practice 10
        1.3.2   Techniques of Diagnosis 10
               1.3.2.1   Objective versus Subjective Criteria
                      for Evaluability 11
        1.3.3   Treatment 11
               1.3.3.1   Single Active Ingredient versus Multiple
                      Components 12
               1.3.3.2   Fixed Dose versus Flexible Dose.........................12
        1.3.4   Remarks...13
  1.4   Basic Considerations for TCM Clinical Trials................................14
        1.4.1   Study Design 14
        1.4.2   Validation of Quantitative Instrument 14
        1.4.3   Clinical Endpoint...15
        1.4.4   Matching Placebo...16
        1.4.5   Sample Size Calculation..18
  1.5   Practical Issues of TCM Development 18
        1.5.1   Test for Consistency...19
        1.5.2   Stability Analysis 20
        1.5.3   Animal Studies...20
        1.5.4   Regulatory Requirements...21
        1.5.5   Indication and Label...22
  1.6   Globalization of TCM...22
        1.6.1   Consortium for Globalization of Chinese Medicine 22
        1.6.2   Remarks...23
  1.7   Aim and Scope of the Book 25

xi

2. Global Pharmaceutical Development 27
  2.1   Introduction 27
  2.2   Pharmaceutical Development Process 28
        2.2.1 Nonclinical Development 29
        2.2.2 Preclinical Development 30
        2.2.3 Clinical Development 30
  2.3   Regulatory Requirements 33
        2.3.1 Regulatory Process in the United States 33
        2.3.2 International Conference on Harmonization 35
        2.3.3 Remarks 37
  2.4   Practical Issues in Drug Development 37
        2.4.1 Multiregional Clinical Trials 39
        2.4.2 Bridging Studies 40
        2.4.3 Adaptive Design Methods in Clinical Trials 41
        2.4.4 Remarks 42
        2.4.5 Microdosing Approach 42
        2.4.6 Remarks 43
  2.5   Modernization of TCM Development 43
        2.5.1 Individualized Treatment 44
        2.5.2 Combinational Treatment 44
        2.5.3 Effective Treatment 45
  2.6   Concluding Remarks 45

3. Regulations on Traditional Chinese Medicine 49
  3.1   Introduction 49
  3.2   Regulations on TCM in China 51
        3.2.1 Background 51
        3.2.2 Regulations 51
                3.2.2.1 Regulatory Approval Process 51
                3.2.2.2 Drug Categories 52
                3.2.2.3 Documentation for Applications for New
                          Drugs 52
                3.2.2.4 Pharmacological Requirements 53
                3.2.2.5 Clinical Trials 54
                3.2.2.6 Raw Materials 55
                3.2.2.7 Manufacturing 55
                3.2.2.8 Quality Control 55
                3.2.2.9 Remarks 56
  3.3   Regulations on Herbal Products in Europe 56
        3.3.1 German Regulations on Herbal Products 57
                3.3.1.1 Herbal Medicines Market 57
                3.3.1.2 Legal Status 58
                3.3.1.3 Requirements for Marketing Authorizations
                          for Herbal Remedies 58
        3.3.2 Harmonization on Herbal Products in EU 59

3.4	Regulations on Herbal Products as Dietary Supplements in the United States	59
	3.4.1 Regulations for Dietary Supplements	59
	3.4.2 Quality Issue	60
	3.4.3 Safety Concern	61
	3.4.4 Remarks	61
3.5	Regulations on Herbal Products as Drug Products in the United States	61
	3.5.1 Botanical Drug Products	61
	3.5.2 Regulations on Botanical Products	62
	3.5.3 Current Review Process for Botanical Products	63
	3.5.4 Botanical Products versus Chemical Drugs	65
	3.5.4.1 Purification and Identification	65
	3.5.4.2 Test and Control	65
	3.5.4.3 Individualized Treatments	67
	3.5.4.4 Toxicity	68
	3.5.4.5 Prior Human Experience	68
	3.5.4.6 Priority	68
3.6	Conclusions	69

4. Reference Standards and Product Specifications 71

4.1	Introduction	71
4.2	Reference Standards	72
	4.2.1 Chinese Pharmacopoeia	72
	4.2.2 PDR for Herbal Medicines	74
	4.2.3 European Pharmacopoeia	76
	4.2.4 Remarks	77
4.3	Product Specifications	77
	4.3.1 Testing Procedure	78
	4.3.2 Sampling Plan and Acceptance Criteria	78
	4.3.2.1 Potency Testing	79
	4.3.2.2 Content Uniformity Testing	79
	4.3.2.3 Dissolution Testing	80
	4.3.2.4 Disintegration Testing	80
	4.3.3 Product Specification	81
	4.3.3.1 In-House Specifications	81
	4.3.3.2 Release Targets	82
	4.3.3.3 Remarks	83
	4.3.4 Probability of Passing USP Tests	84
4.4	Product Characterization	87
	4.4.1 Fixed-Dose Combination	87
	4.4.2 Multiple-Dose Combinations	89
	4.4.3 Global Superiority of Combination Drug	91
	4.4.4 Method of Response Surface	96
	4.4.5 Remarks	97

xiv

| 4.5 | Practical Issues | 98 |
| 4.6 | Concluding Remarks | 98 |

5. QOL-Like Quantitative Instrument for Evaluation of TCM 101

5.1	Introduction	101
5.2	QOL Assessment	102
5.3	Performance Characteristics	104
	5.3.1 Validity	104
	5.3.2 Reliability	106
	5.3.3 Reproducibility	108
5.4	Responsiveness and Sensitivity	108
	5.4.1 Statistical Model	109
	5.4.2 Precision Index	111
	5.4.3 Power Index	113
	5.4.4 Sample Size Determination	114
5.5	Utility Analysis and Calibration	116
	5.5.1 Utility Analysis	116
	5.5.2 Calibration	117
5.6	QOL-Like Instrument for Evaluation of TCM	118
	5.6.1 Remarks	121
5.7	Parallel Assessments	124
5.8	Concluding Remarks	129

6. Factor Analysis and Principal Component Analysis 131

6.1	Introduction	131
6.2	Factor Analysis	132
	6.2.1 Statistical Model	133
	6.2.2 Parameter Estimation	133
	6.2.3 Number of Factors	134
	6.2.4 An Example	135
6.3	Principal Component Analysis	136
	6.3.1 Singular Value Decomposition	139
	6.3.2 Principal Components	139
	6.3.3 Interpretation of Principal Components	140
6.4	Application of QOL in Hypertensive Patients	142
	6.4.1 Background	142
	6.4.2 Development of QOL Instrument	142
	6.4.2.1 Principal Component Analysis	143
	6.4.2.2 Factor Analysis	146
	6.4.3 Analysis Results	147
6.5	Concluding Remarks	149

7. Statistical Validation of Chinese Diagnostic Procedures 151

| 7.1 | Introduction | 151 |

Contents   **xv**

7.2	Chinese Diagnostic Procedure	152
7.3	Proposed Study Design	154
7.4	Calibration of Chinese Diagnostic Procedure	156
7.5	Validation of Chinese Diagnostic Procedure	157
	7.5.1 Validity	157
	7.5.2 Reliability	159
	7.5.3 Ruggedness	160
7.6	A Numerical Example	161
7.7	Concluding Remarks	167

8. Statistical Test for Consistency 171

8.1	Introduction	171
8.2	Consistency Index	172
8.3	Statistical Quality Control for Consistency	175
	8.3.1 Acceptance Criteria	176
	8.3.2 Sampling Plan	176
	8.3.3 Testing Procedure	179
	8.3.4 Strategy for Statistical Quality Control	179
	8.3.5 An Example	181
8.4	Tolerance Region Approach	183
	8.4.1 A Multivariate Random Effects Model	183
	8.4.2 An Example	187
8.5	Concluding Remarks	188

9. Statistical Process for Quality Control/Assurance 191

9.1	Introduction	191
9.2	Statistical Model	192
9.3	Assessing Consistency for QC/QA	195
	9.3.1 Sample Size Determination	195
	9.3.2 Hypotheses Testing	197
9.4	An Example	204
9.5	Discussion	208
9.6	Appendix: Proof of Theorem	209
	9.6.1 Appendix I. Proof of Lemma 9.1	209
	9.6.2 Appendix II. Proof of Lemma 9.2	212

10. Bioavailability and Bioequivalence 219

10.1	Introduction	219
10.2	What Is Bioavailability/Bioequivalence?	220
10.3	Bioequivalence Assessment for Generic Approval	222
	10.3.1 Basic Considerations	222
	10.3.1.1 Sample Size	222
	10.3.1.2 Subject Selection	223

10.3.1.3 Washout 223
10.3.1.4 Blood Sampling 223
10.3.1.5 IR Product versus CR Products 224
10.3.2 Study Design 224
10.3.3 Statistical Methods 225
10.3.4 Limitations of Average Bioequivalence 226
10.4 Drug Interchangeability 226
10.4.1 Drug Prescribability and Drug Switchability 227
10.4.2 Population and Individual Bioequivalence 227
10.4.3 A Review of the FDA Guidance on Population/
Individual Bioequivalence 229
10.4.3.1 Aggregated Criteria versus Disaggregated
Criteria 230
10.4.3.2 Masking Effect 231
10.4.3.3 Power and Sample Size Determination 231
10.4.3.4 Two-Stage Test Procedure 231
10.4.3.5 Replicated Crossover Design 232
10.4.3.6 Outlier Detection 232
10.5 Controversial Issues 233
10.5.1 Fundamental Bioequivalence Assumption 233
10.5.2 One-Size-Fits-All Criterion 234
10.5.3 Issues Related to Log Transformation 235
10.6 Frequently Asked Questions 238
10.6.1 What If We Pass Raw Data Model but Fail
Log-Transformed Data Model? 238
10.6.2 What If We Pass AUC but Fail C_{max}? 239
10.6.3 What If We Fail by a Relatively Small Margin? 240
10.6.4 Can We Still Assess Bioequivalence
If There Is a Significant Sequence Effect? 240
10.6.5 What Should We Do When We Have Almost Identical
Means but Still Fail to Meet the Bioequivalence
Criterion? 241
10.6.6 Power and Sample Size Calculation based on Raw
Data Model and Log-Transformed Model
Are Different 241
10.6.7 Adjustment for Multiplicity 242
10.7 Other Applications 242
10.7.1 Medical Devices 242
10.7.2 Follow-On Biologics 243
10.7.2.1 Fundamental Differences 243
10.7.2.2 Approval Pathway of Biosimilars 244
10.7.2.3 Biosimilarity 245
10.7.2.4 Interchangeability 245
10.7.2.5 Scientific Factors and Practical Issues 246
10.8 Concluding Remarks 247

Contents

xvii

11. Population Pharmacokinetics 249
  11.1 Introduction 249
  11.2 Regulatory Requirements 251
    11.2.1 Population PK Analysis 251
    11.2.2 Study Design 252
    11.2.3 Population PK Model Development/Validation 252
    11.2.4 Missing Data and Outlier 253
    11.2.5 Timing for Application 253
  11.3 Population PK Modeling.. 254
    11.3.1 Traditional Two-Stage Method 254
    11.3.2 Nonlinear Mixed Effects Modeling Approach 255
      11.3.2.1 First-Order Method 255
      11.3.2.2 An Example 257
      11.3.2.3 Other Approximations 259
      11.3.2.4 Bayesian Approach 260
  11.4 Design of Population PK.. 261
    11.4.1 Population Fisher's Information Matrix Approach......... 262
    11.4.2 Informative Block Randomized Approach 263
    11.4.3 Remarks.. 264
  11.5 An Example... 265
  11.6 Discussion 273
    11.6.1 Study Protocol 273
    11.6.2 Concerns and Challenges 273
    11.6.3 PK/PD.. 274
    11.6.4 Computer Simulation 275
    11.6.5 Software Applications................................. 275

12. Experience of Generic Drug Products with Multiple Components ... 277
  12.1 Introduction 277
  12.2 *In Vivo* Single Fasting Bioequivalence Study 279
    12.2.1 Study Design 279
    12.2.2 Sample Size 281
    12.2.3 Remarks.. 286
    12.2.4 Multiplicity of Studies and Ingredients.......... 286
    12.2.5 Baseline Adjustment................................... 287
    12.2.6 Logarithmic Transformation versus the Presence of a Significant First-Order Carryover Effect.......... 288
  12.3 *In Vivo* Drug Release Testing................................. 288
  12.4 Issues on FDA Conjugated Estrogen Bioequivalence Guidance ... 290
  12.5 Concluding Remarks 292

13. Stability Analysis for Drug Products with Multiple Components 295
  13.1 Introduction 295
  13.2 Regulatory Requirements 296
    13.2.1 FDA Stability Guidelines 296

xviii   *Contents*

               13.2.1.1 Batch Sampling Consideration 296
               13.2.1.2 Container (Closure) and Drug Product
                          Sampling.. 297
               13.2.1.3 Sampling Time Considerations 297
       13.2.2 ICH Guidelines for Stability 297
       13.2.3 Remarks.. 299
               13.2.3.1 Minimum Duration of Stability Testing 299
               13.2.3.2 Minimum Number of Batches Required
                          for Stability Testing 300
               13.2.3.3 Definition of Room Temperature 300
               13.2.3.4 Extension of Shelf Life 301
               13.2.3.5 Least Stable Batch 301
               13.2.3.6 Least Protective Packaging 301
               13.2.3.7 Replicates.. 301
               13.2.3.8 General Principles 302
  13.3 Statistical Model and Methods 302
       13.3.1 Statistical Model.. 302
       13.3.2 Statistical Methods 303
               13.3.2.1 Fixed Batches Approach..................................... 303
               13.3.2.2 Random Batches Approach................................. 304
               13.3.2.3 Remarks 306
       13.3.3 Two-Phase Shelf-Life Estimation.................................... 306
               13.3.3.1 First-Phase Shelf Life 307
               13.3.3.2 Case of Equal Second Phase Slopes.................. 309
               13.3.3.3 Determination of a Single Two-Phase
                          Shelf-Life Label... 310
               13.3.3.4 General Case of Unequal Second-Phase
                          Slopes 311
  13.4 Stability Designs 312
       13.4.1 Basic Matrix 2/3 on Time Design 312
       13.4.2 Matrix 2/3 on Time Design with Multiple Packages 313
       13.4.3 Matrix 2/3 on Time Design with Multiple Packages
              and Multiple Strengths 313
       13.4.4 Matrix 1/3 on Time Design 314
       13.4.5 Matrix on Batch-by-Strength-by-Package
              Combinations 314
       13.4.6 Uniform Matrix Design 315
       13.4.7 Comparison of Designs... 315
  13.5 Stability Analysis for Drug Products with Multiple Active
      Components.. 316
       13.5.1 Basic Idea.. 316
       13.5.2 Models and Assumptions.. 317
       13.5.3 Shelf-Life Determination 318
       13.5.4 An Example 319
       13.5.5 Discussion... 320

Contents xix

13.6 Stability Analysis with Discrete Responses 321
13.6.1 Remarks 324
13.7 Concluding Remarks 324

14. Case Studies 327
14.1 Introduction 327
14.2 Nonclinical Quality by Design 328
14.2.1 Concept of Quality by Design 328
14.2.2 Statistical Method for QbD 329
14.2.3 Case Study of QbD 332
14.3 Successful TCM Clinical Cases 336
14.3.1 Case 1: Power of Chinese Herbal Medicine 336
14.3.2 Case 2: Chinese Herbal Medicine Alleviates Eczema,
Allergies, and Stress 337
14.3.3 Case 3: Chinese Herbal Medicine Helps Upper
Respiratory Infection with Vertigo 338
14.3.4 Case 4: Chinese Herbal Medicine Cures Acute
Constipation 339
14.3.5 Remarks 340
14.4 Case Studies of Chinese Herbal Medicines 340
14.4.1 TCM in Cancer Care 341
14.4.1.1 Study Selection and Data Extraction 341
14.4.1.2 TCM Intervention 341
14.4.1.3 Randomization 342
14.4.1.4 Blinding 342
14.4.1.5 Outcome Measurement 342
14.4.1.6 Significant Evidence 343
14.4.1.7 Overall Conclusion/Recommendation 343
14.4.1.8 Remarks 343
14.4.2 Case Study: Modeling of Hypertension Prescriptions ... 344
14.4.2.1 Herb Properties and Medical Practice 344
14.4.2.2 Least Squares Support Vector Machine 346
14.4.2.3 An Example 349
14.4.2.4 Remarks 350
14.4.3 Case Study: Acupuncture for Treating Diabetes 350
14.4.3.1 TCM Classification of Diabetes 350
14.4.3.2 Diagnosis and Treatment 350
14.4.3.3 Successful Examples 351
14.4.4 Case Study: Treatment for Multiple Sclerosis 353
14.4.4.1 Diseases 353
14.4.4.2 Chinese Herbal Therapy 353
14.4.4.3 Multiple Sclerosis Clinical Trial 354
14.4.4.4 Amyotrophic Lateral Sclerosis and
Progressive Spinal Muscular Atrophy
Studies 356

xx   *Contents*

              14.4.4.5 Case Study for Myasthenia Gravis 358
              14.4.4.6 Remarks 359
   14.5 Concluding Remarks 359

15. Current Issues and Recent Developments 361
   15.1 Introduction 361
   15.2 Critical Issues in TCM Development 362
       15.2.1 Intellectual Property 362
              15.2.1.1 Patentability Requirements................................362
              15.2.1.2 Complexities of Patent Application 363
       15.2.2 Variation in Raw Materials....................................364
              15.2.2.1 Utilization Ratio of Extracts...............................364
              15.2.2.2 Batch Mixing Optimization Model 364
              15.2.2.3 Remarks 366
       15.2.3 Component-to-Component Interactions..........................366
              15.2.3.1 Factorial Design..366
              15.2.3.2 Fractional Factorial Design 367
              15.2.3.3 Central Composite Design 368
              15.2.3.4 Remarks 368
       15.2.4 Animal Studies..369
       15.2.5 Matching Placebo in Clinical Trials 370
       15.2.6 Calibration of Study Endpoints 371
       15.2.7 Package Insert...372
       15.2.8 Transition from Experience-Based to Evidence-Based
             Clinical Practice..372
       15.2.9 Prescription versus Dietary Supplement..........................373
   15.3 Frequently Asked Questions from a Regulatory Perspective 373
       15.3.1 Are INDs Required for Clinical Studies of Botanical
             Products That Are Lawfully Marketed as Dietary
             Supplements in the United States? 373
       15.3.2 Are INDs Required for Clinical Studies on Marketed
             Dietary Supplements for Research Purposes Only?....... 374
       15.3.3 Is There Any Other Setting in Which an IND
             Is Not Required for the Botanical Study?.......................... 374
       15.3.4 May a Sponsor Submit an IND for a Phase 3 Study
             of a Botanical Product Not Previously Studied
             under an IND?.. 374
       15.3.5 For NDA Approvals of Botanical Drug Products,
             Must All Studies Be Carried Out under INDs?...............375
       15.3.6 It Appears That the Changes in Regulatory
             Approaches Described in the Guidance on Botanical
             Drug Products Concern Only IND Applications.
             How Will These Changes Be Applied to the NDA
             Requirements for Botanical Drugs? 375

15.3.7 Some Botanical Preparations Are Not Administered Orally, e.g., Intravenous, Topical, and Inhalation Products. How Are These Non-Oral Formulations Considered in the Guidance? 376

15.3.8 In Terms of IND Requirements and Regulatory Review by the Agency, Is There Any Difference between a Commercial Development Program and an Academic Research Project? 376

15.3.9 Intellectual Property Rights Are a Difficult Issue for Developing New Drugs from Well Known Botanical Preparations. How Does FDA Protect the Confidentiality of a Sponsor's Submission? What Kind of IND/NDA Data May FDA Release without Prior Permission from the Sponsor? 376

15.3.10 How Does FDA Ensure That the New Botanical Drug Products Guidance Will Be Implemented Consistently across the Different New Drug Review Divisions? 377

15.3.11 One of the Major Premises of the New Guidance Is That Because Many Botanical Products Have Been Used by a Large Population for a Long Period of Time, They Are Presumed to Be Safe Enough to Be Studied in Clinical Trials without First Undergoing Conventional Nonclinical Studies. What Kind of Documentation Should a Sponsor Submit to Demonstrate Prior Human Experience with the Sponsor's Product? 377

15.3.12 In Many Cases, Botanical Therapies Are Highly Individualized with Variations in Relative Contents of Multiple Plant Ingredients Tailored for Each Patient. Must a Sponsor Submit a Separate IND for Every Change in Composition, If Similar Patients Are Being Treated for the Same Indication? 377

15.3.13 Many Medicinal Plants with Therapeutical Potential Are Quite Toxic. Does the New Guidance Address the Study of Such Botanicals? 377

15.3.14 There Is a Concern That If a Botanical Is Being Studied under an IND or Is Approved as a New Drug in an NDA, Its Subsequent Status as a Dietary Supplement May Be Jeopardized. Is This True? 378

15.3.15 What Is FDA's Advice on the Initial Approach for Sponsors Not Familiar with New Drug Development and Regulatory Processes? 378

15.3.16 The Guidance States That the Submission of an NDA for a Drug Derived from Plants Taken from the Wild Is an Extraordinary Circumstance Requiring the Submission of an Environmental Assessment (EA) under Section 25.21. Are Plants Maintained in Their Native Setting on Private Land Considered Wild?.........379

15.3.17 Is a Drug Made with a Commercially Available Crude Extract Viewed the Same as a Drug Derived from Plants Taken from the Wild for Purposes of Determining the Need for an EA? 379

15.3.18 What Is the GMP Status of Botanical Raw Materials (Starting Materials) in Terms of Compliance and Inspection? 379

15.3.19 Will FDA Assign the Same Level of Priority to Botanical Drug Products as to Other Drug with Respect to Meeting with IND Sponsors and NDA Applicants? 380

15.4 Recent Developments 380

15.4.1 Development of Diagnostic Checklist 380

15.4.1.1 Criticisms of Chinese Diagnostic Procedures...380

15.4.1.2 Objective Diagnostic Checklist 381

15.4.1.3 Remarks...382

15.4.2 Unified Approach for Assessing Health Profile.............382

15.4.3 Bridging Traditional Chinese Medicine 384

15.5 Concluding Remarks 384

References 387

Index 405

Preface

In recent years, as more and more innovative drug products are going off patent, the search for new medicines that can treat critical and/or life-threatening diseases has become the center of attention of many pharmaceutical companies and research organizations such as the US National Institutes of Health (NIH). This leads to the study of promising traditional Chinese (herbal) medicines (TCM), especially for those intended for treating critical and/or life-threatening diseases such as cancer. A TCM is defined as a Chinese herbal medicine developed for treating patients with certain diseases as diagnosed by the four Chinese major techniques of inspection, auscultation and olfaction, interrogation, and pulse taking and palpation based on traditional Chinese medical theory of global dynamic balance among the functions/activities of all organs of the body. The development of promising TCMs will benefit patients with critical or life-threatening diseases by providing an alternative for treatment and hopefully for cure. The development of promising TCMs will also enhance the search for personalized medicine because it focuses on the minimization of intrasubject variability for achieving the optimal therapeutic effect within individuals. The development of new treatments (focusing on efficacy) in conjunction with TCMs (focusing on the reduction/release of toxicity) has been the direction of future clinical research for treating critical or life-threatening diseases of many pharmaceutical companies and clinical research organizations.

Unlike evidence-based clinical research and development of a Western medicine (WM), clinical research and development of a TCM are usually experience-based with anticipated evaluator-to-evaluator variability due to subjective evaluation of the treatment under investigation. The use of TCM in humans for treating various diseases has a history of more than several thousand years, although not much convincing scientific documentation is available regarding clinical evidence of safety and efficacy. In the past several decades, regulatory agencies of both China and Taiwan have debated which direction TCM should take—Westernization or modernization. The Westernization of TCM refers to the adoption of the typical (Western) process of pharmaceutical/clinical research and development for scientific evaluation of the safety and effectiveness of the TCM products, while the modernization of TCM is to evaluate the safety and effectiveness of TCM the Chinese way (i.e., different sets of regulatory requirements and evaluation criteria may be applied) scientifically. Although both China and Taiwan do attempt to build up an environment for the modernization of TCM, they seem to adopt the Westernization approach at this moment. In pursuit of advancing TCM through the modernization way or the Westernization approach to benefit patients who suffer from critical and/or life-threatening

xxiii

xxiv *Preface*

diseases, a consortium for globalization of Chinese medicine (CGCM) was formed in 2003.

The purpose of this book is not only to provide a comprehensive summary of innovative thinking of quantitative methods for development of TCMs but also to provide a useful desk reference to the principal investigators engaged in TCM research and development for achieving the ultimate goal of personalized medicine the Western way. This book is intended to be the first book entirely devoted to the design and analysis for development of TCM the Western way. It covers all of the statistical issues that may be encountered at various stages of pharmaceutical/clinical development of a TCM. It is our goal to provide a state-of-the-art examination of the subject area to scientists and researchers engaged in pharmaceutical/clinical research and development of TCMs, those in regulatory agencies such as the China Food and Drug Administration (CFDA) of China, Taiwan Food and Drug Administration (TFDA) of Taiwan, and the US Food and Drug Administration (FDA), who have to make decisions in the review and approval process of TCM regulatory submissions, and to biostatisticians who provide the statistical support to the assessment of clinical safety and effectiveness of TCMs and related issues regarding quality control/assurance and test for consistency in manufacturing processes for TCMs. It is my hope that this book can serve as a bridge among the pharmaceutical industry, regulatory agencies, and academia.

This book consists of 15 chapters. The scope covers scientific/statistical issues that are commonly encountered in studies conducted at various stages of pharmaceutical/clinical research and development of TCMs. In Chapter 1, some background regarding fundamental differences between WMs and TCMs and practical issues that are commonly encountered during the development of TCMs have been discussed. In Chapter 2, the process of global pharmaceutical development of Western medicines is outlined. The feasibility of the process for modernization of TCM is also discussed. Chapter 3 summarizes regulatory requirements for the development of TCMs worldwide including Asian Pacific Region (e.g., China), Europe (e.g., Germany), and the United States. Also included in this chapter is a review of recent published FDA draft guidances on botanical drug products. Chapter 4 discusses the establishment of reference standards and product specifications for drug products and substances according to Pharmacopeia (e.g., USP and European Pharmacopeia). Commonly used QOL-like instruments for assessment of TCMs are described in Chapter 5. Chapter 6 outlines factor analysis and principal components analysis approaches for drug products with multiple components (or combinational drug products). Statistical validations of Chinese diagnostic procedures are discussed in Chapter 7. Chapter 8 discusses a general approach for testing consistency in terms of a proposed consistency index. Statistical processes for quality control/assurance including sampling plan, acceptance criteria, and testing procedure are introduced in Chapter 9. Bioavailability/bioequivalence and population pharmacokinetics

Preface

are reviewed in Chapters 10 and 11, respectively. Chapter 12 reviews regulatory experience for a bioequivalence review of generic drug products with multiple components such as Conjugated Estrogen USP. Stability analysis for drug products with multiple components is given in Chapter 13. Chapter 14 discusses some case studies of TCM clinical research and development. Chapter 15 provides a summary of current issues and recent developments.

From Taylor & Francis, I would like to thank David Grubbs for providing me the opportunity to work on this book project. I wish to thank colleagues from Duke University School of Medicine and many friends from academia, the pharmaceutical industry, and regulatory agencies from Taiwan, China, the United States, and the European Community for their support and discussions during the preparation of this book.

Finally, the views expressed are those of the author and not necessarily those of Duke University School of Medicine. I am solely responsible for the contents and errors of this book. Any comments and suggestions will be very much appreciated.

Shein-Chung Chow, PhD
Duke University School of Medicine
Durham, North Carolina, USA

1

Introduction

1.1 Introduction

In recent years, as more and more innovative drug products are going off patent, the search for new medicines that can treat critical and/or life-threatening diseases has become the center of attention of many major pharmaceutical companies and research organizations such as the United States (US) National Institutes of Health (NIH). This leads to the study of the potential use of promising traditional Chinese herbal medicines, especially for those intended for treating critical and/or life-threatening diseases such as cancer. In the Chinese community, most people consider traditional Chinese medicine (TCM) a Chinese herbal medicine, which was developed for treating patients with certain diseases as diagnosed by the four traditional Chinese diagnostic techniques of inspection, auscultation and olfaction, interrogation, and pulse taking and palpation (Table 1.1). Certain diseases are diagnosed based on traditional Chinese medical theory of *global dynamic balance* among the functions/activities of all organs of the body. Unlike (objective) evidence-based clinical research and development of a Western medicine (WM), clinical research and development of a TCM is considered experience-based with anticipated large evaluator-to-evaluator (i.e., Chinese doctor-to-Chinese doctor) variability due to subjective evaluation of the disease under study. The use of TCM in humans for treating various diseases has a history of several thousands of years, although not much convincing scientific documentation regarding clinical evidence of safety and efficacy of existing TCMs is available.

In the past several decades, regulatory agencies of both China and Taiwan have debated which direction TCM should take—Westernization or modernization. The Westernization of TCM refers to the adoption of the typical (Western) process of pharmaceutical/clinical research and development for scientific evaluation of the safety and effectiveness of the TCM products under investigation, while the modernization of TCM is to evaluate the safety and effectiveness of TCM *the Chinese way* (i.e., different sets of regulatory requirements and evaluation criteria may be applied) scientifically. Although both China and Taiwan do attempt to build up an environment

TABLE 1.1

Four Major Techniques in English and Chinese

Four Major Techniques	四診
1. Inspection	望
2. Auscultation and olfaction	聞
3. Interrogation	問
4. Pulse taking and palpation	切

for the modernization of TCM, they seem to adopt the Westernization approach. In pursuit of advancing the TCM through the modernization way or the Westernization approach to benefit patients who suffer from critical and/or life-threatening diseases, a consortium for globalization of Chinese medicine (Consortium for Globalization of Chinese Medicine) was formed in 2003.

In practice, it is a concern whether a TCM can be scientifically evaluated the Western way because of some fundamental differences between a WM and a TCM. These fundamental differences include, but are not limited to, differences in formulation and drug administration, medical theory/practice, diagnostic procedure, and criteria for evaluation. Under these differences, it is of interest to the investigators regarding how to design and conduct a scientifically valid (i.e., an adequate and well-controlled) clinical trial for evaluation of the clinical safety and efficacy of the TCM under investigation. In addition, it is also of particular interest to the investigators as to how to translate an observed significant difference detected by the Chinese diagnostic procedure to a clinically meaningful difference based on some well-established clinical study endpoint. The purpose of this chapter is not only to provide a comprehensive overview of the pharmaceutical/clinical research and development of TCMs but also to provide some basic considerations regarding practical issues that are commonly encountered during the process of pharmaceutical/clinical research and development of TCMs the Western way.

In the next section, the definition of TCM in a broader sense is given. Section 1.3 provides some fundamental differences between a WM and a TCM, which have an impact on the Westernization of TCM. Section 1.4 provides some basic considerations for TCM clinical trials. Some practical issues that are commonly encountered during the process of pharmaceutical/clinical research and development of a TCM are reviewed in Section 1.5. Section 1.6 introduces the organization of the Consortium for Globalization of Chinese Medicine and its recent development. The aims and scope of the book are given in the last section of this chapter.

Introduction

1.2 What Is Traditional Chinese Medicine?

Traditional Chinese medicine (TCM) originated in ancient China and has evolved over thousands of years. TCM usually refers to a broad range of Chinese medicine practice including various forms of herbal medicine, acupuncture, massage (*Tui Na*), exercise (*Qi Gong*), and dietary therapy, which are briefly described below.

1.2.1 Chinese Herbal Medicine

The Chinese *Materia Medica* (a pharmacological reference book used by TCM practitioners) contains hundreds of medicinal substances (primarily plants but also includes some minerals and animal products) classified by their perceived action in the body. Different parts of plants such as the leaves, roots, stems, flowers, and seeds are used. Usually, herbs are combined in formulas and given as teas, capsules, tinctures, or powders. Chinese herbal medicine has also been studied for a wide range of conditions. Most of the research has been done in China. Although there is evidence that herbs may be effective for some conditions, most studies have been methodologically flawed, and additional, better designed research is needed before any valid, reliable, and convincing conclusions can be drawn. Note that Chinese herbal medicine has been studied and commonly used for a wide range of conditions such as cancer, heart disease, diabetes, and HIV/AIDS. Some case studies are discussed in Chapter 14.

1.2.2 Acupuncture

Acupuncture involves the insertion of extremely thin needles through the skin at strategic points on the body. According to Chinese medical theory, acupuncture is a technique for balancing the flow of energy or life force. By stimulating specific points on the body, practitioners can remove blockages in the flow of *Qi*. Many Western practitioners, however, view the acupuncture points as places to stimulate nerves, muscles, and connective tissue. This stimulation appears to boost the activity of body's natural painkillers and increase blood flow. Acupuncture is considered a key component of TCM, which is most commonly used to treat pain. Acupuncture research has produced a large body of scientific evidence. Many studies suggest that it may be useful for a number of different conditions, but additional rigorous research for scientific evidence is still needed. Note that acupuncture has been used and studied for a wide range of conditions such as back pain, chemotherapy-induced nausea, depression, and osteoarthritis. In general, acupuncture is considered safe when performed by an *experienced* practitioner using sterile needles.

1.2.3 Other TCM Therapies

Other TCM therapies include, but are not limited to, (1) moxibustion (burning moxa—a cone or stick of dried, usually mugwort—on or near the skin, sometimes in conjunction with acupuncture), (2) cupping (applying a heated cup to the skin to create a slight suction), (3) Chinese massage, and (4) mind–body therapies such as *Qi Gong* and *Tai Chi*. In many cases, these TCM therapies are found useful for a number of different conditions. However, no scientific documentation regarding clinical evidence of safety and efficacy of these therapies is available. Thus, additional rigorous research for scientific evidence is still needed.

1.2.4 Botanical Drug Product

A botanical drug product is intended for use in the diagnosis, cure, mitigation, treatment, or prevention of disease in humans (FDA 2004). A botanical drug product consists of vegetable materials, which may include plant materials, algae, macroscopic fungi, or combinations thereof. A botanical drug product may be available as (but not limited to) a solution (e.g., tea), powder, tablet, capsule, elixir, topical, or injection. Botanical drug products often have unique features, for example, complex mixtures, lack of a distinct active ingredient, and substantial prior human use. Fermentation products and highly purified or chemically modified botanical substances are not considered botanical drug products.

1.2.5 Dietary Therapy

The US Food and Drug Administration (FDA) regulations for dietary supplements (including manufactured herbal products) are not the same as those for prescription or over-the-counter drugs. In general, the regulations for dietary supplements are less strict. Some Chinese herbal treatments may be safe, but others may not be. There have been reports of products being contaminated with drugs, toxins, or heavy metals or not containing the listed ingredients. Some of the herbs are very powerful, can interact with drugs, and may have serious side effects. For example, the Chinese herb ephedra (*Ma Huang*) has been linked to serious health complications, including heart attack and stroke. In 2004, the FDA banned the sale of ephedra-containing dietary supplements used for weight loss and performance enhancement, but the ban does not apply to TCM remedies or herbal teas.

1.2.6 Complementary and Alternative Medicine

In the United States, TCM is considered part of complementary and alternative medicine (CAM). The National Center for Complementary and Alternative Medicine (NCCAM) defines CAM as a group of diverse medical and health

Introduction 5

care systems, practices, and products that are not generally considered part of conventional medicine. Conventional medicine (also called Western or allopathic medicine) is medicine as practiced by holders of medical doctor (MD) and doctor of osteopathic medicine (DOM) degrees and by allied health professionals, such as physical therapists, psychologists, and registered nurses. The boundaries between CAM and conventional medicine are not absolute, and specific CAM practices may, over time, become widely accepted.

Complementary medicine refers to use of CAM together with conventional medicine, such as using acupuncture in addition to usual care to help lessen pain. Most CAM use by Americans is complementary. Alternative medicine, on the other hand, refers to CAM use in place of conventional medicine. Integrative medicine combines treatments from conventional medicine and CAM for which there is some high-quality evidence of safety and effectiveness. Thus, it is also known as integrated medicine.

1.2.7 Remarks

Herbal remedies and acupuncture are the treatments most commonly used by TCM practitioners. Other TCM practices include cupping, mind-body therapy, and dietary therapy. The TCM view of how the human body works, what causes illness, and how to treat illness is different from concepts. Although TCM is used by the American public, scientific evidence of its effectiveness is, for the most part, limited. Acupuncture has the largest body of evidence and is considered safe if practiced correctly. Some Chinese herbal remedies may be safe, but others may not be. TCM is typically delivered by a practitioner. Before using TCM, ask about the practitioner's qualifications, including training and licensure. Tell all your health care providers about any complementary and alternative practices you use. Give them a full picture of what you do to manage your health. This will help ensure coordinated and safe care.

A botanical drug product is considered a TCM. A botanical drug's special features require consideration and adjustment during the FDA review process. Thus, FDA issued a *Guidance for Industry-Botanical Drug Products* to take into consideration these features and to facilitate development of new therapies from botanical sources (FDA 2004). The Botanical Guidance applies to only botanical products intended to be developed and used as drugs.

CAM practices are often grouped into broad categories, such as natural products, mind and body medicine, and manipulative and body-based practices. Mind and body practices focus on the interactions among the brain, mind, body, and behavior, with the intent to use the mind to affect physical functioning and promote health, while manipulative and body-based practices focus primarily on the structures and systems of the body, including the bones and joints, soft tissues, and circulatory and lymphatic systems. Although these categories are not formally defined, they are useful for discussing CAM practices. Some CAM practices may fit into more than one category.

1.3 Fundamental Differences

The process for pharmaceutical/clinical research and development of WM is well established, and yet it is a lengthy and costly process (Chow and Liu 2013). This lengthy and costly process is necessary to ensure the efficacy, safety, purity, quality, stability, and reproducibility of the drug product under investigation. For pharmaceutical/clinical research and development of a TCM the Western way, one may consider directly applying this well-established process to the development of a TCM under investigation. However, this process may not be feasible owing to some fundamental differences between a TCM and a WM, which are summarized in Table 1.2. These fundamental differences in terms of (1) medical theory/mechanism and practice, (2) techniques of diagnosis, and (3) treatment are briefly described in the subsequent subsections.

1.3.1 Medical Theory/Mechanism and Practice

1.3.1.1 Medical Theory and Mechanism

TCM is a 3000-year-old holistic medical system encircling the entire scope of human experience. It combines the use of Chinese herbal medicines, acupuncture, massage, and therapeutic exercise such as *Qi Gong* (the practice of internal *air*) and *Tai Chi* for both treatment and prevention of disease. With its unique theories of etiology, diagnostic systems, and abundant historical literature, TCM itself consists of Chinese culture and philosophy, clinical practice experience, and the use of many medical herbs.

Chinese doctors believe a TCM function in the body is based on the eight principles (Table 1.3), five-element theory (Table 1.4), five *Zang* and six *Fu* (Table 1.5), and information regarding channels and collaterals. Eight principles consist of *Yin* and *Yang* (i.e., negative and positive) (see also, Table 1.6), cold and hot, external and internal, and *Shi* and *Xu* (i.e., weak and strong).

TABLE 1.2

Fundamental Differences between a WM and a TCM

Description	Western Medicine	Traditional Chinese Medicine
Active ingredient	Single	Multiple
Dose	Fixed	Flexible
Diagnostic procedure	Objective; validated	Subjective; not validated
Therapeutic index	Well-established	Not well-established
Medical mechanism	Specific organs	Global dynamic balance/harmony among organs
Medical perception	Evidence-based	Experience-based
Statistics	Population	Individual

Introduction 7

TABLE 1.3

Eight Principles

Eight Principles	八綱
Yin (negative)	陰
Yang (positive)	陽
Cold	寒
Hot	熱
External	表
Internal	裏
Weak	虛
Strong	實

TABLE 1.4

Five Elements in English and Chinese

Five Elements	五行
Metal	金
Wood	木
Water	水
Fire	火
Earth	土

TABLE 1.5

Five Zang and Six Fu in English and Chinese

Five Zang	五臟
Heart	心
Lung	肺
Spleen	脾
Liver	肝
Kidney	腎
Six Fu	六腑
Gall bladder	膽
Stomach	胃
Large intestine	大腸
Small intestine	小腸
Urinary bladder	膀胱
Three cavities (chest, epiastrium, hypogastrium)	三焦 (上焦: 橫隔以上 中焦: 橫隔到肚臍 下焦: 肚臍以下)

TABLE 1.6

Examples of Yang and Yin

English		Chinese	
Yang	Yin	陽	陰
Sun	Moon	日	月
Sky	Ground	天	地
Day time	Night	晝	夜
Hot	Cold	熱	寒
Left	Right	左	右
Up	Down	上	下
Spring	Autumn	春	秋
Summer	Winter	夏	冬
Six Fu	Five Zang	六腑	五臟
Strong	Weak	強壯	虛弱

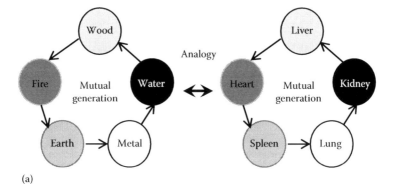

(a)

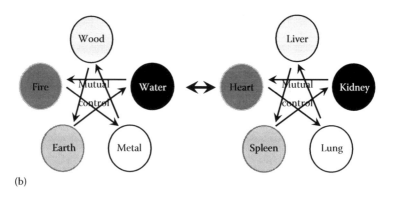

(b)

FIGURE 1.1
Relationships between the five elements. (a) Mutual generation and (b) mutual control.

Introduction 9

The eight principles help Chinese doctors to differentiate syndrome patterns. For instance, people with *Yin* will develop disease in a negative, passive, and cool way (e.g., diarrhea and back pain), while people with *Yang* will develop disease in an aggressive, active, progressive, and warm way (e.g., dry eyes, tinnitus, and night sweats). The five elements (earth, metal, water, wood, and fire) correspond to particular organs in the human body. Each element operates in harmony with the others. Figure 1.1 illustrates the operation relationships between the five elements.

The five *Zang* (or *Yin* organs) include heart (including the pericardium), lung, spleen, liver, and kidney, while the six *Fu* (or *Yang* organs) include gall bladder, stomach, large intestine, small intestine, urinary bladder, and three cavities (i.e., chest, epiastrium, and hypogastrium). *Zang* organs can manufacture and store fundamental substances. These substances are then transformed and transported by *Fu* organs. TCM treatments involve a thorough understanding of the clinical manifestations of *Zang Fu* organ imbalance and knowledge of appropriate acupuncture points and herbal therapy to rebalance or maintain the balance of the organs. The channels and collaterals are the representation of the organs of the body. They are responsible for conducting the flow of energy and blood through the entire body.

The elements of TCM can also help describe the etiology of disease including six exogenous factors (i.e., wind, cold, summer, dampness, dryness, and fire), seven emotional factors (i.e., anger, joy, worry, grief, anxiety, fear, and fright), and other pathogenic factors (Table 1.7). Once all of the information

TABLE 1.7

Exogenous Factors and Seven Emotional Factors in English and Chinese

Six Exogenous Factors	外在因素(六淫)
Wind	風
Cold	寒
Summer	暑
Dampness	濕
Dryness	燥
Fire	火
Seven Emotional Factors	內在因素(七情)
Angry	怒
Joy	喜
Worry	憂
Grief	悲
Anxiety	思
Fear	恐
Fright	驚

are collected and processed into a logical and workable diagnosis, the traditional Chinese medical doctor can determine the treatment approach.

Under the medical theory and mechanism described above, Chinese doctors believe that all of the organs within a healthy subject should reach the so-called *global dynamic balance or harmony* among organs. Once the global balance is broken at certain sites such as heart, liver, or kidney, some signs and symptoms then appear to reflect the imbalance at these sites. An experienced Chinese doctor usually assesses the causes of global imbalance before a TCM with flexible doses is prescribed to fix the problem. This approach is sometimes referred to as a personalized (or individualized) medicine approach.

1.3.1.2 Medical Practice

Different medical perceptions regarding signs and symptoms of certain diseases could lead to a different diagnosis and treatment for the diseases under study. For example, the signs and symptoms of type 2 diabetic subjects could be classified as the disease of *thirsty reduction* by Chinese doctors. The disease of type 2 diabetes is not recognized by Chinese medical literature, although they have the same signs and symptoms as the reduction of thirsty. This difference in medical perception and practice has an impact on the diagnosis and treatment of the disease.

In addition, we tend to see therapeutic effect of WMs sooner than TCMs. TCMs are often considered for patients who have chronic diseases or non-life-threatening diseases. For critical and/or life-threatening diseases such as cancer or stroke, TCMs are often used as the second or third line treatment with no other alternative treatments. In many cases such as patients with later phases of cancer, TCMs are often used in conjunction with WMs without the knowledge of the primary care physicians.

1.3.2 Techniques of Diagnosis

As indicated earlier, the Chinese diagnostic procedure for patients with certain diseases consists of four major techniques, namely, inspection, auscultation and olfaction, interrogation, and pulse taking and palpation (see also Table 1.1). All these diagnostic techniques aim mainly at providing an objective basis for differentiation of syndromes by collecting symptoms and signs from the patient. Inspection involves observing the patient's general appearance (strong or weak, fat or thin), mind, complexion (skin color), five sense organs (eye, ear, nose, lip, and tongue), secretions, and excretions. Auscultation involves listening to the voice, expression, respiration, vomit, and cough. Olfaction involves smelling the breath and body odor. Interrogation involves asking questions about specific symptoms and the general condition including history of the present disease, past history, personal life history, and

Introduction 11

family history. Pulse taking and palpation can help to judge the location and nature of a disease according to changes in the pulse.

The Chinese diagnostic procedure of inspection, auscultation and olfaction, interrogation, and pulse taking and palpation is subjective, with large between-rater variability (i.e., variability from one Chinese doctor to another). This subjectivity and variability will have an impact not only on the patient's evaluability but also the prescribability of TCM, which will be further discussed below.

1.3.2.1 Objective versus Subjective Criteria for Evaluability

For evaluation of a WM, objective criteria based on some well-established clinical study endpoints are usually considered. For example, response rate (i.e., complete response plus partial response based on tumor size) is considered a valid clinical endpoint for evaluating clinical efficacy of oncology drug products. Unlike WMs, Chinese diagnostic procedure for evaluation of a TCM is very subjective. The use of a subjective Chinese diagnostic procedure has raised the following issues. First, it is a concern whether the subjective Chinese diagnostic procedure can accurately and reliably evaluate clinical efficacy and safety of the TCM under investigation. Thus, it is suggested that the subjective Chinese diagnostic procedure should be validated in terms of its accuracy, precision, and ruggedness before it can be used in TCM clinical trials. A validated Chinese diagnostic procedure should be able to detect a clinically significant difference if the difference truly exists. On the other hand, it is not desirable to wrongly detect a difference when there is no difference.

In clinical trials, evaluation is usually based on some validated tools (instruments) such as laboratory tests. Test results are then evaluated against some normal ranges for abnormality. Thus, it is suggested that the Chinese diagnostic procedure must be validated in terms of validity and reliability, and its false positive and false negative rates, before it can be used for evaluation of clinical efficacy and safety of the TCM under investigation.

1.3.3 Treatment

TCM prescriptions typically consist of a combination of several components. The combination is usually determined based on the medical theory of global dynamic balance (or harmony) among organs and the observations from the Chinese diagnostic procedure. The use of Chinese diagnostic procedure is to find out what caused the imbalance among these organs. The treatment is to restore the balance among these organs. Thus, the dose and treatment duration are flexible in order to achieve the balance. This concept leads to the concept of so-called personalized (or individualized) medicine, which minimizes intrasubject variability.

1.3.3.1 Single Active Ingredient versus Multiple Components

Most WMs contain a single active ingredient. After drug discovery, an appropriate formulation (or dosage form) is necessarily developed so that the drug can be delivered to the site action in an efficient way. At the same time, an assay is necessarily developed to quantitate the potency of the drug. The drug is then tested on animals for toxicity and humans (healthy volunteers) for pharmacological activities. Unlike the WMs, TCMs usually consist of multiple components with certain relative proportions among the components. As a result, the typical approach for evaluation of single active ingredient for WM is not applicable.

In practice, one may suggest evaluating the TCM component by component. However, this is not feasible due to the following difficulties. First, in practice, analytical methods for quantitation of individual components are often not tractable. Thus, the pharmacological activities of these components are not known. It should be noted that the component that comprises the major proportion of the TCM may not be the most active component. On the other hand, the component that has the least proportion of the TCM may be the most active component of the TCM. In practice, it is not known which relative proportions among these components can lead to the optimal therapeutic effect of the TCM. In addition, the relative component-to-component and/or component by food interactions are usually unknown, which may have an impact on the evaluation of clinical efficacy and safety of the TCM.

1.3.3.2 Fixed Dose versus Flexible Dose

Most WMs are usually administered in a fixed dose (say a 10 mg tablet or capsule). On the other hand, because a TCM consists of multiple components with possible varied relative proportions among the components, a Chinese doctor usually prescribes the TCM with different relative proportions of the multiple components based on the signs and symptoms of the patient according to his/her best judgment following a subjective evaluation based on the Chinese diagnostic procedure. Thus, unlike a WM that is prescribed as a fixed dose, a TCM is often prescribed as an individualized flexible dose.

The approach of WM with a fixed dose is a population approach to minimize the between subject (or intersubject) variability, while the approach to TCM with an individualized flexible dose is to minimize the variability within each individual. In practice, it is a concern whether an individual flexible dose is compatible with a Western evaluation of the TCM. An individualized flexible dose depends heavily upon the Chinese doctor's subjective judgement, which may vary from one Chinese doctor to another. As a result, although an individualized flexible dose does minimize intrasubject variability, the variability from one Chinese doctor to another (i.e., the doctor-to-doctor or rater-to-rater variability) could be huge and hence non-negligible.

Introduction 13

1.3.4 Remarks

For the research and development of a TCM, before a TCM clinical trial is conducted, the following questions are necessarily asked:

1. Will the TCM clinical trial be conducted by Chinese doctors alone, Western clinicians alone, Western clinicians who have some background of Chinese herbal medicine alone, or both Chinese doctors and Western clinicians?
2. Will traditional Chinese diagnostic and/or trial procedures be used throughout the TCM clinical trial?
3. Upon approval, is the TCM intended for use by Chinese doctors or Western clinicians?

With respect to the first two questions, if the TCM clinical trial is to be conducted by Chinese doctors alone, the following questions arise. First, should the Chinese diagnostic procedure be validated in order to provide an accurate and reliable assessment of the TCM? In addition, it is of interest to determine how an observed difference obtained from the Chinese diagnostic procedure can be translated to the clinical endpoint commonly used in similar WM clinical trials with the same indication. These two questions can be addressed statistically by the calibration and validation of the Chinese diagnostic procedure with respect to some well-established clinical endpoints for evaluation of Western medicines. If the TCM clinical trial is to be conducted by Western clinicians or Western clinicians who have some background of Chinese herbal medicine, the standards and consistency of clinical results as compared to those WM clinical trials are ensured. However, the good characteristics of TCM may be lost during the process when the TCM clinical trials are conducted. On the other hand, if the TCM clinical trial is to be conducted by both Chinese doctors and Western clinicians, the difference in medical practice and/or possible disagreement regarding the diagnosis, treatment, and evaluation are major concerns.

For the third question, if the TCM is intended for use of Chinese doctors, but it is conducted by Western clinicians, the difference in perception regarding how to prescribe the TCM is of great concern. The preparation of a package insert based on the clinical data could be a major issue not only to the sponsor but also to regulatory authorities. Similar comments apply to the situation where the TCM is intended for use of Western clinicians, but the trial is conducted by Chinese doctors.

As a result, it is suggested that the intention of use (i.e., labeling for the indication) be clearly evaluated when planning a TCM clinical trial. In other words, the sponsor needs to determine whether the TCM is intended for use of Western clinician only, Chinese doctors only, or both Western clinicians and Chinese doctors at the planning stage of a TCM clinical trial for an adequate package insert of the target diseases under study.

1.4 Basic Considerations for TCM Clinical Trials

In this section, we describe some basic considerations that are necessary to ensure success of a TCM clinical trial.

1.4.1 Study Design

To demonstrate clinical efficacy and safety of a TCM under investigation, like WMs, it is suggested that a randomized parallel-group, placebo-controlled clinical trial be conducted. However, it may not be ethical if the disease under study is critical and/or life-threatening provided that a WM is available. Alternatively, a randomized placebo-control crossover clinical trial or a parallel-group design consisting of three arms (i.e., the TCM under study, a WM as an active control, and a placebo) is recommended. The three-arm, parallel-group design allows the establishment of noninferiority/equivalence of the TCM as compared to the active control (WM) and the demonstration of the superiority of the TCM with respect to the placebo. One of the advantages of a crossover clinical trial is that a comparison within each individual can be made, although it will take a longer time to complete the study. Although a crossover design requires a smaller sample size as compared to a parallel-group design, there are some limitations for the use of crossover design. First, baselines prior to dosing may not be the same. Second, when a significant sequence effect is observed, we would not be able to isolate the effects of period effect, carryover effect, and subject-by-treatment effect that are confounded to one another.

In many cases, factorial designs are used to evaluate the impact of specific components (with respect to the therapeutic effect) by fixing some of the components. For example, we may consider a parallel-group design comparing two treatment groups (one group is treated with the TCM with a specific component and the other group is treated with the TCM without the specific component). The design of this kind may be useful to identify the most active component of the TCM with respect to the diseases under study. However, it does not address the possible drug-to-drug interactions among the components.

1.4.2 Validation of Quantitative Instrument

In TCM medical practice, a Chinese doctor usually collects information from the patient with a certain disease through the four subjective diagnostic procedures as described in the previous section. The purpose of these subjective approaches is to collect information on various aspects of the disease under study such as signs, symptoms, patient's performance, and functional activities, so a quantitative instrument with a large number of questions/items is necessary and helpful. For a simple analysis and an easy interpretation,

Introduction   15

these questions are usually grouped to form subscales, composite scores (domains), or overall score. The items (or subscales) in each subscale (or composite score) are correlated. As a result, the structure of responses to a quantitative instrument is multidimensional, complex, and correlated. As mentioned above, a standardized quantitative tool (instrument) is necessary to reduce variability from one Chinese doctor to another (prior to conducting a clinical trial).

Guilford (1954) discussed several methods such as Cronbach's α for measuring the reliability of internal consistency of a quantitative instrument. Guyatt et al. (1989) indicated that a quantitative instrument should be validated in terms of its validity, reproducibility, and responsiveness. Hollenberg et al. (1991) discussed several methods for validation of a quantitative instrument, such as consensual validation, construct validation, and criterion-related validation. There is, however, no gold standard as to how a quantitative instrument should be validated. In this paper, we will focus on the validation of a quantitative instrument in terms of validity, reliability (or reproducibility), and responsiveness (see, e.g., Chow and Ki 1994, 1996). As indicated by Chow and Shao (2002), the validity of a quantitative instrument is the extent to which the instrument measures what it is designed to measure. It is a measure of bias of the instrument. The bias of a quantitative instrument reflects the accuracy of the instrument. The reliability of a quantitative instrument measures the variability of the instrument, which directly relates to the precision of the instrument. On the other hand, the responsiveness of a quantitative instrument is usually referred to as the ability of the instrument to detect a difference of clinical significance within a treatment.

Hsiao et al. (2009) considered a specific design for calibration/validation of the Chinese diagnostic procedure. In their proposed study design, qualified subjects are randomly assigned to receive either a TCM or a WM. Each patient will be evaluated by a Chinese doctor and a Western clinician independently, regardless which treatment group he/she is in. As a result, there are four groups of data, namely, (1) patients who receive TCM and are evaluated by a Chinese doctor, (2) patients who receive TCM but are evaluated by a Western clinician, (3) patients who receive WM but are evaluated by a Chinese doctor, and (4) patients who receive WM and are evaluated by a Western clinician. Groups 3 and 4 are used to establish a standard curve for calibration between the TCM and the WM. Groups 1 and 2 are then used to validate the Chinese diagnostic procedure based on the established standard curve.

1.4.3 Clinical Endpoint

Unlike WMs, the primary study endpoints for assessment of safety and effectiveness of a TCM are usually assessed subjectively by a quantitative instrument by experienced Chinese doctors. Although the quantitative instrument

16   *Quantitative Methods for Traditional Chinese Medicine Development*

is developed by the community of Chinese doctors and is considered a gold standard for assessment of safety and effectiveness of the TCM under investigation, it may not be accepted by the Western clinicians owing to fundamental differences in medical theory, perception, and practice. In practice, it is very difficult for a Western clinician to conceptually understand the clinical meaning of the difference detected by the subjective Chinese quantitative instrument. Consequently, whether the subjective quantitative instrument can accurately and reliably assess the safety and effectiveness of the TCM is always a concern to Western clinicians.

As an example, for assessment of safety and efficacy of a drug product for treatment of ischemic stroke, a commonly considered primary clinical endpoint is the functional status assessed by the so-called Barthel index. The Barthel index is an ordinal scale used to measure performance in activities of daily living, which was introduced by Mahoney and Barthel (1965). The Barthel index is a weighted functional assessment scoring technique composed of 10 items with a minimum total score of 0 (functional incompetence) and a maximum total score of 100 (functional competence) (Table 1.8). The Barthel index is a weighted scale measuring performance in self-care and mobility, which is widely accepted in ischemic stroke clinical trials. A patient may be considered a responder if his/her Barthel index is greater than or equal to 60. On the other hand, Chinese doctors usually consider a quantitative instrument developed by the Chinese medical community as the standard diagnostic procedure for assessment of ischemic stroke. The standard quantitative instrument is composed of six domains, which capture different information regarding patient performance, functional activities, and signs, symptoms, and status of the disease. Note that more details regarding the development of a quantitative instrument for evaluation of TCMs are provided in Chapter 5.

In practice, it is of interest to both Western clinicians and Chinese doctors how an observed clinically meaningful difference by the Chinese quantitative instrument can be translated to that of the primary study endpoint assessed by the Barthel index. To reduce the fundamental differences in medical theory/perception and practice, it is suggested that the subjective Chinese quantitative instrument be calibrated and validated with respect to that of the clinical endpoint assessed by the Barthel index before it can be used in TCM ischemic stroke clinical trials.

1.4.4 Matching Placebo

In clinical development, double-blind, placebo-control randomized clinical trials are often conducted for evaluation of the safety and effectiveness of a test treatment under investigation. To maintain blindness, a matching placebo should be identical to the active drug in all aspects of, size, color, coating, taste, texture, shape, and order except that it contains no active ingredient. In clinical trials, as advanced techniques are available for formulation, a matching

Introduction

TABLE 1.8

Barthel Index for Stroke

Item	Activity	Possible Score	Description
1	Feeding	0–10	0 = unable 5 = needs help cutting, spreading butter, etc., or requires modified diet 10 = independent
2	Bathing	0–5	0 = dependent 5 = independent (or in shower)
3	Grooming	0–5	0 = needs to help with personal care 5 = independent face/hair/teeth/shaving (implements provided)
4	Dressing	0–10	0 = dependent 5 = needs help but can do about half unaided 10 = independent (including buttons, zips, laces, etc.)
5	Bowels	0–10	0 = incontinent (or needs to be given enemas) 5 = occasional accident 10 = continent
6	Bladder	0–10	0 = incontinent, or catheterized and unable to manage alone 5 = occasional accident 10 = continent
7	Toilet use	0–10	0 = dependent 5 = needs some help, but can do something alone 10 = independent (on and off, dressing, wiping)
8	Transfers	0–15	0 = unable, no sitting balance 5 = major help (one or two people, physical), can sit 10 = minor help (verbal or physical) 15 = independent
9	Mobility	0–15	0 = immobile or <50 yards 5 = wheelchair independent, including corners, >50 yards 10 = walks with help of one person (verbal or physical) >50 yards 15 = independent (but may use any aid; for example, stick) >50 yards
10	Stairs	0–10	0 = unable 5 = needs help (verbal, physical, carrying aid) 10 = independent

Note: Total possible score (0–100).

placebo is not difficult to make because most Western medicines contain a single active ingredient. Unlike Western medicines, TCMs usually consist of a number of components, which often have different tastes. In TCM clinical trials, the TCM under investigation is often encapsulated. However, the test treatment will be easily unblinded if either the patient or Chinese doctor breaks the capsule. As a result, the preparation of matching placebo in TCM clinical trials plays an important role for the success of the TCM clinical trials.

1.4.5 Sample Size Calculation

In clinical trials, sample size is usually selected to achieve a desired power for detecting a clinically meaningful difference in one of the primary study endpoints for the intended indication of the treatment under investigation (see, e.g., Chow et al. 2002b). As a result, sample size calculation depends on the primary study endpoint and the clinically meaningful difference that one would like to detect. Different primary study endpoints may result in very different sample sizes.

For illustration purposes, consider the example concerning a TCM for treatment of ischemic stroke, which was developed with more than 30 years clinical experience with humans. Suppose a sponsor would like to conduct a clinical trial to scientifically evaluate the safety and efficacy of the TCM the Western way as compared to an active control (e.g., aspirin). Thus, the intended clinical trial is a double-blind, parallel-group, placebo-control, randomized trial. The primary clinical endpoint is the response rate (a patient is considered a responder if his/her Barthel index is greater than or equal to 60) based on the functional status assessed by the Barthel index. Sample size calculation is performed based on the response rate after 4 weeks of treatment under the hypotheses of testing for superiority. As a result, a sample size of 150 patients per treatment group is required for achieving an 80 percent power for establishment of superiority of the TCM over the active control agent. Alternatively, we may consider the quantitative instrument developed by experienced Chinese doctors as the primary study endpoint for sample size calculation. On the basis of a pilot study, about 65 percent (79 out of 122) of ischemic stroke patients were diagnosed by one domain of the quantitative instrument. A patient is considered a responder if his/her domain score is greater than or equal to 7. On the basis of this primary study endpoint, a sample size of 90 per treatment group is required to achieve an 80 percent power for establishment of superiority.

The difference in sample size leads to the question of whether the use of the primary endpoint of response rate based on one domain of the Chinese quantitative instrument could provide substantial evidence of safety and effectiveness of the TCM under investigation.

1.5 Practical Issues of TCM Development

Although TCM has a long history of being used in humans, no scientifically valid documentation is available. As indicated by the U.S. FDA, substantial evidence regarding safety and effectiveness of the test treatment under investigation can only be obtained by conducting adequate and well-controlled

Introduction 19

clinical trials. However, before the test treatment under investigation can be used in humans, sufficient information regarding chemistry, manufacturing, and control (CMC), clinical pharmacology, and toxicology must be provided (see, e.g., Chow and Liu 1995). Because most TCMs consist of multiple components with unknown pharmacological activities, valid information regarding CMC, clinical pharmacology, and toxicology is difficult to obtain. In what follows, these difficulties are briefly described.

1.5.1 Test for Consistency

As mentioned above, unlike most WMs, TCMs usually consist of a number of components, which are extracted from herbal samples. The herbal samples are normally dried at 60°C to a constant weight, followed by grinding in a mortar and storing in a desiccator. For water-soluble substances, an appropriate amount of water is first added to the dried material and boiled for about one hour. For alcohol soluble substances, 60 percent ethanol is added and the mixture is extracted at 60°C for one hour in an ultrasonic bath. After cooling to room temperature, the extract can be cleared by filtration through a net or centrifugation at 12,000 g for 10 min at 20°C, and the supernatant is used for further applications. The pharmacological activities, interactions, and relative proportions of these components are usually unknown. In practice, TCM is usually prescribed subjectively by an experienced Chinese doctor. As a result, the actual dose received by each individual varies depending on the signs and symptoms as perceived by the Chinese doctor. Although the purpose of this medical practice is to reduce the within-subject (or intrasubject) variability, it could also introduce non-negligible variability such as variations from component to component and from rater to rater (a Chinese doctor to another). Consequently, reproducibility or consistency of clinical results is questionable. Thus, how to ensure the reproducibility or consistency of the observed clinical results has become a great concern to regulatory agencies in the review and approval process. It is also a great concern to the sponsor of the manufacturing process. To address the question of reproducibility or consistency, a valid statistical quality control process on the raw materials and final product is suggested.

Tse et al. (2006) proposed a statistical quality control (QC) method to assess a proposed consistency index of raw materials, which are from different resources and/or final product, which may be manufactured at different sites. The consistency index is defined as the probability that the ratio of the characteristics (e.g., extract) of the most active component among the multiple components of a TCM from two different sites (locations) is within a limit of consistency. The consistency index closest to 1 indicates that the components from the two sites or locations are almost identical. The idea for testing consistency is to construct a 95 percent confidence interval for the proposed consistency index under a sampling plan. If the constructed 95 percent confidence lower limit is greater than a pre-specified QC lower limit, then we claim that the raw materials or final product have passed the QC and hence can be released for further process or use. Otherwise, the raw materials and/or final product should be rejected.

It should be noted that Tse et al. (2006) only focused on single (i.e., the most active) component, assuming that the most active component can be quantitatively identified among the multiple active components. Lu et al. (2007) extended the results to the case of two correlative components following a similar idea. Various sampling plans are obtained for various combinations of study parameters to reflect real practice in quality control of traditional Chinese medicine. More information can be found in Chapter 8.

1.5.2 Stability Analysis

Most regulatory agencies require that the expiration dating period (or shelf-life) of a drug product must be indicated in the immediate container label before it can be released for use. To fulfill this requirement, stability studies are usually conducted in order to characterize the degradation of the drug product. For drug products with a single active ingredient, statistical methods for determination of drug shelf-life are well established (e.g., FDA 1987; ICH 1993). However, regulatory requirements for estimation of drug shelf-life for drug products with multiple components are not available.

Following the concept of estimating shelf-life for drug products with a single active ingredient, two approaches are worth considering. First, we may (conservatively) consider the *minimum* of the shelf-lives obtained from each component of the drug product. This approach is conservative and yet may not be feasible due to the fact that (1) not all of the components of a TCM can be accurately and reliably quantitated, and (2) the resultant shelf-life may be too short to be useful (see, e.g., Pong and Raghavarao 2002). Alternatively, we may consider a two-stage approach for determination of drug shelf-life. At the first stage, an attempt should be made to identify the most active component(s) whenever possible. A shelf-life can then be obtained based on the method suggested in the FDA and ICH guidelines. At the second stage, the obtained shelf-life is adjusted on the basis of the relationship and/or interactions of the most active ingredient(s) and other components.

As an alternative, Chow and Shao (2007) proposed a statistical method for determining the shelf-life of a TCM following a similar idea suggested by the FDA, assuming that the components are linear combinations of some factors. More details regarding this method and various study designs for stability studies are given in Chapter 13.

1.5.3 Animal Studies

The purpose of animal studies is not only to study possible toxicity in animals but also to suggest an appropriate dose for use in humans, assuming

Introduction 21

that the established animal model is predictive of the human model. For a newly developed drug product, animal studies are necessary. However, for some well-known TCMs, which have been used in humans for years and have a very mild toxicity profile, it is questionable whether animal studies are necessary. It is suggested that all components of TCMs as described in *Chinese Pharmacopoeia* (CP) be classified into several categories depending on their potential toxicities and/or safety profiles as a basis for regulatory requirements for animal studies. In other words, for some well-known TCM components such as Ginseng, animal studies for testing toxicity may be waived depending on past experience of human use, although health risks or side effects following the proper administration of designated therapeutic dosages were not recorded in human use. Note that the German regulatory authority's herbal watchdog agency, commonly called Commission E, has conducted an intensive assessment of the peer-reviewed literature on some 300 common botanicals with respect to the quality of the clinical evidence and the uses for which the herb can be reasonably considered effective (PDR 1998).

1.5.4 Regulatory Requirements

Although the use of TCMs in humans has a long history, there have been no regulatory requirements regarding the assessment of safety and effectiveness of the TCMs until recently. For example, both regulatory authorities of China and Taiwan have published guidelines/guidance for clinical development of TCMs (see, e.g., MOPH 2002; DOH 2004a,b). In addition, the US Food and Drug Administration (FDA) also published guidance for botanical drug products (FDA 2004). These regulatory requirements for TCM research and development, especially for clinical development are very similar to well-established guidelines/guidances for pharmaceutical research and development for Western medicines. It is a concern whether these regulatory requirements and the corresponding statistical methods are feasible for research and development of TCM, based on the fact that there are so many fundamental differences in medical practice, drug administration, and diagnostic procedure. As a result, it is suggested that current regulatory requirements and the corresponding statistical methods should be modified in order to reflect these fundamental differences.

It is strongly recommended that regulatory requirements for the development, review, and approval process for Premarin® (conjugated estrogens tablets, USP) be consulted because Premarin is a WM consisting of multiple components that is similar to a TCM (FDA 1991; Liu and Chow 1996). Premarin, which contains multiple components of estrone, equilin, 17-dihydroequilin, 17α-estradiol, and 17β-dihydroequilin, is intended for treatment of moderate to severe vasomotor symptoms associated with the menopause. The experience with Premarin is helpful in developing appropriate guidelines/guidance for TCM drug products with multiple components.

1.5.5 Indication and Label

As indicated earlier, it is very important to clarify the intention for the use of a TCM (by Chinese doctors alone, Western clinicians alone, or both Chinese doctors and Western clinicians) once it is approved by the regulatory agencies. If a TCM is intended for use by Chinese doctors alone, the clinical trials conducted for obtaining substantial evidence should reflect medical theory of TCM and medical practice of Chinese doctors. The label should provide sufficient information as to how to prescribe the TCM the Chinese way. On the other hand, if the TCM under investigation is intended for use by Western clinicians alone, patients under study should be evaluated using clinical study endpoints for safety and efficacy the Western way. Consequently, the label should provide sufficient information for prescribing the TCM the Western way. If the TCM is intended for both Western clinicians and Chinese doctors, patients are necessarily evaluated by both Western clinical study endpoints and Chinese diagnostic procedures (e.g., some standardized quantitative instrument) provided that the Chinese diagnostic procedure has been calibrated and validated against the well-established Western clinical endpoint. In this case, there is a clear understanding how an observed difference by Chinese diagnostic procedure can be translated to a clinical effect that is familiar to Western clinicians, and vice versa.

1.6 Globalization of TCM

1.6.1 Consortium for Globalization of Chinese Medicine

As indicated earlier, in pursuit of advancing the TCM to benefit patients who suffer from critical and/or life-threatening diseases, a Consortium for Globalization of Chinese Medicine (CGCM) was formed at the University of Hong Kong in 2003. The goals of the consortium are multifold. First, it is to provide an environment for development of platform technologies required for advancing Chinese herbal medicine by joint efforts. Second, it is to facilitate interaction and collaboration among different institutes in advancing Chinese herbal medicine by information sharing. Third, it is to promote high-quality research and development of Chinese medicine internationally. In addition, it is to assist industry and regulatory agencies worldwide in (1) methodology development in TCM research and development and (2) guidance/guidelines development for evaluation and approval of TCM regulatory submissions. More details can be found at http://www .tcmedicine.org.

The CGCM aims at establishing a network among researchers from academia, industry, and regulatory agencies under an academic collaboration arrangement focusing on two main areas. The first area is for the development

Introduction 23

of a centralized database of Chinese medicine complete with formulations, botanical ingredients, and phytochemical substances along with associated biological information on traditional and modern therapeutic indication, clinical information, animal pharmacology, biochemical activities, toxicities, and manufacturing information. The other area of focus is for the standardization and adoption of a modern quality control platform for chemical and biological fingerprinting of botanical drugs for scientific and regulatory purposes. The Consortium had 13 institutional members since it was funded in 2003. As of August 2005, it has grown to 32 institutional members worldwide including Columbia University and Yale University in the United States.

To achieve the goal of globalization of Chinese medicine, the CGCM has established six working groups including (1) quality control, (2) informatics, (3) herbal resources, (4) clinical, (5) external affairs and industrial liaison, and (6) intellectual property. The Quality Control Working Group is to develop strategy and appropriate methodology including acceptance criteria, sampling plan, and testing procedure for assuring consistency of raw materials, in-process materials, and final products in post-approval manufacturing processes. The Informatics Working Group is to investigate possible biomarkers such as PK/PD markers or genomic markers for efficacy and safety in traditional Chinese medicine clinical trials. The Working Group for Herbal Resources is not only to identify resources of Chinese herbs worldwide, but also to determine potential differences in the same species of herbs. The External Affairs and Industrial Liaison Working Group is seeking collaboration in TCM research and development with the pharmaceutical industry and/or research organizations such as the National Institutes of Health (NIH) of the United States of America. The Working Group for Intellectual Property is to develop strategies for patent protection. The efforts of the six working groups will lead to advances in TCM research and development in the 21st century. However, it is also strongly suggested that a working group regarding regulatory requirements for review and approval of TCM be established to assist the sponsors to bring their promising (efficacious and safe) TCM products to the marketplace. The Working Group for Regulatory Affairs should be a collaborative team that includes regulatory agencies from Taiwan, China, the United States, Europe (such as Germany), and Japan for harmonized regulatory requirements.

1.6.2 Remarks

As indicated earlier, a TCM is defined as a Chinese herbal medicine developed for treating patients with certain diseases as diagnosed by the four major techniques of inspection, auscultation and olfaction, interrogation, and pulse taking and palpation based on traditional Chinese medical theory of global balance among the functions/activities of all organs of the body. When conducting a TCM clinical trial, it is suggested that the fundamental differences between a WM and a TCM, as described in Section 1.2, should be evaluated carefully for a valid and unbiased assessment of the safety and effectiveness of the TCM under investigation.

One of the key issues in TCM research and development is to clarify the difference between Westernization of TCM and modernization of TCM. For Westernization of TCM, we follow regulatory requirements at critical stages of the process for pharmaceutical development including drug discovery, formulation, laboratory development, animal studies, clinical development, manufacturing process validation and quality control, regulatory submission, review, and process despite the fundamental differences between WM and TCM. For modernization of TCM, it is suggested that regulatory requirements should be modified in order to account for the fundamental differences between WM and TCM. In other words, we still ought to be able to see if TCM is really working with modified regulatory requirements using Western clinical trials as a standard for comparison.

In practice, it is recognized that WMs tend to achieve the therapeutic effect sooner than that of TCMs for critical and/or life-threatening diseases. TCMs are found to be useful for patients with chronic diseases or non-life-threatening diseases. In many cases, TCMs have been shown to be effective in reducing toxicities or improving safety profile for patients with critical and/or life-threatening diseases. As a strategy for TCM research and development, it is suggested that (1) TCM be used in conjunction with a well-established WM as a supplement to improve its safety profile and/or enhance therapeutic effect whenever possible, and (2) TCM should be considered as the second line or third line treatment for patients who fail to respond to the available treatments. However, some sponsors are interested in focusing on the development of TCM as a dietary supplement due to (1) the lack or ambiguity of regulatory requirements, (2) the lack of understanding of the medical theory/mechanism of TCM, (3) the confidentiality of nondisclosure of the multiple components, and (4) the lack of understanding of pharmacological activities of the multiple components of TCM.

Because TCM consists of multiple components that may be manufactured from different sites or locations, the post-approval consistency in quality of the final product is both a challenge to the sponsor and a concern to the regulatory authority. As a result, some post-approval tests, such as tests for content uniformity, weight variation, and/or dissolution and (manufacturing) process validation, must be performed for quality assurance before the approved TCM can be released for use.

Most recently, *Statistics in Medicine* (Vol. 31, No. 7, 2012) published a special issue on TCM development which covers a variety of topics in TCM development, these topics include discovering herbal functional groups (He et al. 2012), basic theory, diagnostic and therapeutic system (Hu and Liu 2012), assessing diagnostic accuracy in the absence of a gold standard (Wang and Zhou 2012), randomized clinical trials (Lao et al. 2012), model for syndrome evaluation (Li et al. 2012), issues of design and analysis of acupuncture trials (Ping et al. 2012), and statistical models for osteoporosis TCM trials (Zhou et al. 2012a,b).

1.7 Aim and Scope of the Book

This book is intended to be the first book entirely devoted to the design and analysis for development of TCM the Western way. It covers all of the statistical issues that may be encountered at various stages of pharmaceutical/clinical development of a TCM. It is our goal to provide a useful desk reference and the state-of-the-art examination of the subject area to scientists and researchers engaged in pharmaceutical/clinical research and development of TCMs, those in regulatory agencies such as the China Food and Drug Administration (CFDA) of China, Taiwan Food and Drug Administration (TFDA) of Taiwan, and the U.S. FDA, who have to make decisions in the review and approval process of TCM regulatory submissions, and to biostatisticians who provide the statistical support to the assessment of clinical safety and effectiveness of TCMs and related issues regarding quality control/assurance and test for consistency in manufacturing processes for TCMs. I hope that this book can serve as a bridge among the pharmaceutical industry, regulatory agencies, and academia.

This book consists of 15 chapters. The scope covers scientific/statistical issues that are commonly encountered in studies conducted at various stages of pharmaceutical/clinical research and development of TCMs. In this chapter, some background regarding fundamental differences between WMs and TCMs and practical issues that are commonly encountered during the development of TCMs have been discussed. In Chapter 2, the process of global pharmaceutical development of Western medicines is outlined. The feasibility of the process for modernization of TCM is also discussed. Chapter 3 summarizes regulatory requirements for the development of TCMs worldwide including Asian Pacific Region (e.g., China), Europe (e.g., Germany), and the United States. Also included in this chapter is a review of recent published FDA draft guidances on botanical drug products. Chapter 4 discusses the establishment of product specifications and reference standards for TCMs. Commonly used QOL-like instruments for assessment of TCMs are described in Chapter 5. Chapter 6 outlines factor analysis and principal components analysis approaches for drug products with multiple components (or combinational drug products). Statistical validations of Chinese diagnostic procedures are discussed in Chapter 7. Chapter 8 discusses a general approach for testing consistency in terms of proposed consistency index. A statistical process for quality control/assurance including sampling plan, acceptance criteria, and testing procedure is introduced in Chapter 9. Bioavailability and bioequivalence for generic approval and population pharmacokinetics are reviewed in Chapters 10 and 11, respectively. Chapter 12 reviews regulatory experience for bioequivalence review of generic drug products with multiple components such as Conjugated Estrogen USP. Stability analysis for drug products with multiple components is given in Chapter 13. Chapter 14 discusses some case studies of TCM clinical research and development. Chapter 15 provides a summary of current issues and recent developments.

For each chapter, whenever possible, examples are included to illustrate the described statistical methods for evaluation of clinical safety and efficacy of TCMs. In addition, if applicable, topics for future research are provided. All computations in this book are performed using SAS version 9.2 or higher. Other statistical packages such as R and S-plus can also be applied.

2

Global Pharmaceutical Development

2.1 Introduction

It is recognized that in the past decade the increasing spending on biomedical research does not reflect an increase in the success rate of pharmaceutical development. Woodcock (2004) pointed out that the causes of the situation include (1) a diminished margin for improvement that escalates the level of difficulty in proving drug benefits, (2) genomics and other new science have not yet reached their full potential, (3) mergers and other business arrangements have decreased candidates, (4) easy targets are the focus as chronic diseases are harder to study, (5) failure rates have not improved, and (6) rapidly escalating costs and complexity decrease willingness/ability to bring many candidates forward into the clinic. As the low success rate may be due to an inefficient go/no-go decision process based on limited (or insufficient) information available from studies conducted in early phase clinical development, it is suggested that from bench-to-bedside translational research such as biomarker studies and genomic-guide clinical studies be conducted in the early phase of pharmaceutical development with rigorous scientific/statistical justification to increase the probability of success of the development of the drug product under investigation.

For global pharmaceutical (drug) development, health regulatory authorities in different countries or regions have different requirements for approval of commercial use of the drug products. As a result, considerable resources had been spent by the pharmaceutical industry in the preparation of different documents for applications of the same pharmaceutical product to meet different regulatory requirements requested by different countries or regions. However, because of globalization of the pharmaceutical industry, arbitrary differences in regulations, increase in health care costs, need for reduction of time for patients to access new drugs and of experimental use of humans and animals without compromising safety, the necessity to standardize these similar yet different regulatory requirements has been recognized by both regulatory authorities and the pharmaceutical industry. Hence, the International Conference on Harmonization (ICH) of Technical Requirements for the Registration of Pharmaceuticals for Human Use was organized in 1990 to provide an opportunity for important initiatives to be developed by regulatory authorities as well as the industry association for the promotion of international harmonization of regulatory requirements.

For the development of traditional Chinese medicine (TCM), it is suggested the well-established scientific process of pharmaceutical development of Western medicines be considered, although there are fundamental differences in culture, medical theory/practice, and treatment between TCMs and Western medicines. As most of TCMs consist of multiple active and/or inactive components, the dose and treatment duration of TCM is often flexible depending on the observations collected from the four subjective Chinese diagnostic procedures. This individualized treatment has posed a major challenge to the modernization of TCM development in practice. In addition, an appropriate selection of relative proportions (ratios) of individual components for achieving optimal therapeutic effect is a critical issue for subjects in the target patient population, which is another challenge to the modernization of TCM development.

In the next section, an overview of the global pharmaceutical development process that is commonly considered by the pharmaceutical industry in the United States is provided. In Section 2.3, regulatory requirements for pharmaceutical development set by the U.S. Food and Drug Administration (FDA) and ICH are briefly described. Practical issues regarding global drug development are discussed in Section 2.4. Also included in Section 2.4 are discussions on future perspectives on potential use of adaptive design methods and a microdosing approach not only for shortening the development process but also for increasing the probability of success of the development process with the limited resources available. Section 2.5 provides Chinese perspectives regarding the modernization of TCM development. Some brief concluding remarks are given in the last section of this chapter.

2.2 Pharmaceutical Development Process

As pointed out by Chow and Shao (2002), the pharmaceutical development process is a lengthy and costly process to ensure the safety and efficacy of the drug products under investigation before they can be approved by the regulatory agencies for use in humans. This lengthy and costly development process is necessary to assure that the approved drug product will possess some good drug characteristics such as identity, purity, quality, strength, stability, and reproducibility. A typical pharmaceutical development process involves drug discovery, formulation, laboratory development, animal studies for toxicity, clinical development, and regulatory submission/review and approval. Pharmaceutical development is a continual process, which can be classified into three phases of development, namely, nonclinical development (e.g., drug

Global Pharmaceutical Development 29

discovery, formulation, laboratory development, scale-up, manufacturing process validation, stability, and quality control/assurance [ICH 1996; Chow 1997b; FDA 2001b]), preclinical development (e.g., animal studies for toxicity, bioavailability and bioequivalence studies, and pharmacokinetic and pharmacodynamic studies), and clinical development (e.g., phases I-III clinical trials for assessment of safety and efficacy). These phases may occur in sequential order or be overlapped during the development process. To provide a better understanding of the pharmaceutical development process, these critical phases of pharmaceutical development are briefly outlined below.

2.2.1 Nonclinical Development

Nonclinical development includes drug discovery, formulation, laboratory development such as analytical method development and validation, (manufacturing) process validation, stability, statistical quality control, and quality assurance (see, e.g., Chow and Liu 1995). Drug discovery usually consists of the phases of drug screening and drug lead optimization. At the drug screening phase, the mass compounds are screened to identify those that are active from those that are not. Lead optimization is a process of finding a compound with some advantages over related leads based on some physical, chemical, and/or pharmacological properties. In practice, the success rate for identifying a promising active compound is usually relatively low. As a result, there may be a few compounds that are identified as promising active compounds.

The purpose of formulation is to develop a dosage form (e.g., tablets or capsules) such that the drug can be delivered to the site of action efficiently. For laboratory development, an analytical method is necessarily developed to quantitate the potency (strength) of the drug product. Analytical method development and validation play an important role in quality control and quality assurance of the drug product. To ensure that a drug product will meet the US Pharmacopeia/National Formulary (USP/NF) (2000, 2012) standards for the identity, strength, quality, and purity of the drug product, a number of tests such as potency testing, weight variation testing, content uniformity testing, dissolution testing, and disintegration testing are usually performed at various stages of the manufacturing process. These tests are referred to as USP/NF tests. At the same time, stability studies are usually conducted to characterize the degradation of the drug product over time under appropriate storage conditions. Stability data can then be used to determine the drug expiration dating period (or drug shelf-life) as it is required by the regulatory agency to be indicated in the immediate label of the container.

After the drug product has been approved by the regulatory agency for use in humans, a scale-up program is usually carried out to ensure that a production batch can meet USP/NF standards for the identity, strength, quality, and purity of the drug before a batch of the product is released to the market. The purpose of a scale-up program is not only to identify, evaluate, and

30   *Quantitative Methods for Traditional Chinese Medicine Development*

optimize critical formulation and/or (manufacturing) process factors of the drug product but also to maximize or minimize excipient range. A successful scale-up program can result in an improvement in formulation/process or at least a recommendation on a revised procedure for formulation/process of the drug product. During the nonclinical development, the manufacturing process is necessarily validated in order to produce drug products with good drug characteristics such as identity, purity, strength, quality, stability, and reproducibility. Process validation is important in nonclinical development to ensure that the manufacturing process does what it purports to do.

2.2.2 Preclinical Development

The primary focus of preclinical development is to evaluate the safety of the drug product through *in vitro* assays and animal studies. In general, *in vitro* assays or animal toxicity studies are intended to alert the clinical investigators to the potential toxic effects associated with the investigational drugs so that those effects may be watched for during the clinical investigation. Preclinical testing involves dose selection, toxicological testing for toxicity and carcinogenicity, and animal pharmacokinetics. For selection of an appropriate dose, dose response (dose ranging) studies in animals are usually conducted to determine the effective dose, such as the median effective dose (ED_{50}). Preclinical development is critical in the pharmaceutical development process because it is not ethical to investigate certain toxicities such as the impairment of fertility, teratology, mutagenicity, and overdose in humans (Chow and Liu 1998, 2004). Animal models are then used as a surrogate for human testing under the assumption that they can be predictive of clinical outcomes in humans.

Following the administration of a drug, it is also important to study the rate and extent of absorption, the amount of drug in the blood stream, become available, and the elimination of the drug. For this purpose, a comparative bioavailability study in humans is usually conducted to characterize the profile of the blood or plasma concentration–time curve by means of several pharmacokinetic parameters such as area under the blood or plasma concentration–time curve (AUC), maximum concentration (C_{max}), and time to achieve maximum concentration (t_{max}). It should be noted that the identified compounds will have to pass the stages of nonclinical/preclinical development before they can be used in humans.

2.2.3 Clinical Development

Clinical development in the development of a pharmaceutical entity is to scientifically evaluate benefits (e.g., efficacy) and risks (e.g., safety) of promising pharmaceutical entities at a minimum cost and within a relatively short time frame. As indicated by Chow and Liu (2000, 2004, 2013), approximately 75 percent of pharmaceutical development is devoted to clinical development and regulatory registration. In a set of new regulations promulgated in 1987 and known as the IND Rewrite, the phases of clinical investigation adopted by the US FDA since the late 1970s is generally divided into three phases, see, e.g., Code of Federal Regulations (CFR), Part 312.21. These phases of clinical investigation are usually conducted sequentially but may overlap.

The primary objective of phase I is not only to determine the metabolism and pharmacological activities of the drug in humans, the side effects associated with increasing doses, and the early evidence on effectiveness but also to obtain sufficient information about the drug's pharmacokinetics and pharmacological effects to permit the design of well-controlled and scientifically valid phase II studies. The primary objectives of phase II studies are not only to first evaluate the effectiveness of a drug based on clinical endpoints for a particular indication or indications in patients with the disease or condition under study but also to determine the dosing ranges and doses for phase III studies and the common short-term side effects and risks associated with the drug. Note that some pharmaceutical companies further differentiate phase II into phases IIA and phase IIB. For example, clinical studies designed to evaluate dosing are referred to as phase IIA studies, while studies designed to determine the effectiveness of the drug are called phase IIB. In some cases, clinical studies based on clinical endpoints are considered phase IIB studies. The primary objectives of phase III studies are to (1) gather additional information about the effectiveness and safety needed to evaluate the overall benefit-risk relationship of the drug and (2) to provide an adequate basis for physician labeling. Note that studies conducted after regulatory submission before approval are generally referred to as phase IIIB studies.

In addition to the three phases of clinical development, many pharmaceutical companies consider studies performed after a drug is approved for marketing as phase IV studies. The purpose for conducting phase IV studies is to elucidate further the incidence of adverse reactions and determine the effect of a drug on morbidity or mortality. In addition, a phase IV trial may be conducted to study a patient population not previously studied such as children. In practice, phase IV studies are usually considered useful market-oriented comparison studies against competitor such as quality of life studies. As indicated by Chow and Shao (2002), in practice, it is estimated that about 8–10 × 1000 compounds screened may finally reach the phase of clinical development for human testing. The probability of success for those compounds that reach clinical development is relatively low. As a result, a thoughtful clinical development plan is necessary to ensure the success of the development of a promising pharmaceutical entity.

In practice, phases I/II are considered early phase clinical development, while phase III/IV are viewed as later phase clinical development. However, in the pharmaceutical industry, some pharmaceutical companies consider clinical studies up to phase IIA are early phase clinical development.

Phase I clinical investigation provides an initial introduction of an investigational new drug to humans. Phase I clinical investigation includes studies of drug metabolism, bioavailability, dose ranging, and multiple doses. Phase I studies usually involve 20–80 normal volunteer subjects or patients. In several therapeutic areas, patients with the diseases are subjects rather than healthy volunteers. This tradition is strongest in oncology because many cytotoxic agents cause damage to DNA. For similar reasons, many anti-AIDS drugs are not tested initially in healthy subjects. In neuropharmacology, some categories of drugs have an acclimatization or tolerance aspect, which makes them difficult to study in healthy subjects.

For phase I clinical investigation, FDA's review will focus on the assessment of safety. Therefore, extensive safety information such as detailed laboratory evaluations is usually collected at very extensive schedules. A typical phase I design for tolerability and safety is a dose escalation trial design in which successive groups (cohorts) of patients are given successively higher doses of the treatment until some of the patients in a cohort experience unacceptable side effects. In most phase I trials of this kind, there are three to six patients in each cohort. The starting dose at the first cohort is usually at a rather low dose. If unacceptable side effects are not seen in the first cohort, patients in the next cohort will receive a higher dose. This continues until a dose is reached at which it is too toxic for some patients (say one out of three). Then, the previous dose level is considered to be the maximum tolerable dose (MTD). It should be noted that MTD is usually the most effective dose, which is often chosen as the optimal dose for phase II studies in practice. Also, as indicated by the FDA, phase I studies are usually less detailed and more flexible than for subsequent phases, adaptive (flexible) designs are usually considered.

Phase II studies are the first controlled clinical studies of the drug under investigation. Phase II studies usually involve no more than several hundred patients. A commonly employed study design for a phase II study is a randomized, parallel group (either a placebo-control or an active-control) study. Patients will be randomly assigned to each of the treatment groups to receive the dose determined in the prior phase I study. Many phase II trials, however, are conducted in two stages. The idea is to stop the trial as soon as it can be known that the treatment is ineffective. On the other hand, we wish to continue the trial if the treatment has been shown to be effective. In a two-stage design, after a predetermined number of patients have been treated, the trial is paused and the response rate is evaluated. If the response rate is less than a pre-specified minimum goal (undesirable response rate), it is concluded that the treatment is not worth pursuing and the trial is stopped. Otherwise, the trial continues and additional patients will be enrolled to permit determination of the response rate for achieving desired accuracy with certain statistical power. It should be noted that if the trial has reached the second stage, it indicates that at least some of the patients are responding to the treatment though the response rate could still be low at the first stage.

In practice, it is not uncommon to combine a phase I and a phase II trial of the same treatment into a single protocol for clinical investigation of the

Global Pharmaceutical Development 33

treatment under study. A combined phase I and phase II study is usually referred to as a phase I/II study. As a result, the study objectives of the phase I/II study will include objectives from phase I and phase II parts. For example, in a phase I/II study, we may want to determine the MTD and at the same time to demonstrate its clinical efficacy. In this case, the determination of MTD (phase I) and demonstration of clinical efficacy (phase II) are the study objectives of the phase I/II trial. A typical trial design is to include two phases—the first phase is to determine the MTD and the second phase is to demonstrate clinical efficacy that follows immediately afterward. At the first trial phase, we could include several dose groups (say four dose groups). In each dose group, patients will be randomly assigned to receive the treatment and a placebo at a 4:1 ratio. As a result, a total of 40 subjects are required (10 subjects per dose group with 8 subjects in the treatment group and 2 subjects in the placebo group) for determination of the MTD. Once the MTD is identified, additional subjects will be recruited for demonstration of clinical efficacy at a selected optimal dose during the second phase of the study.

2.3 Regulatory Requirements

For marketing approval of pharmaceutical entities, the regulatory process and requirements vary from country (region) to country (region) (see, e.g., Zhang 1998). For example, the European Union (EU), Japan, and the United States have similar but different requirements as to the conduct of clinical trials and the submission, review, and approval of clinical results for pharmaceutical entities. For simplicity, we will focus on the regulatory process and requirements for the conduct, submission, review, and approval of clinical trials currently adopted in the United States.

2.3.1 Regulatory Process in the United States

For evaluation and marketing approval of drugs, biological products, and medical devices, sponsors are required to submit substantial evidence of effectiveness and safety accumulated from adequate and well-controlled clinical trials to Center for Drug Evaluation and Research (CDER), Center for Biologics Evaluation and Research (CBER), or Center for Devices and Radiological Health (CDRH) of the FDA, respectively. The current regulations for conducting clinical trials and the submission, review, and approval of clinical results for pharmaceutical entities in the United States can be found in CFR (e.g., see 21 CFR Parts 50, 56, 312, and 314). These regulations are developed based on the Federal Food, Drug, and Cosmetic (FD&C) Act passed in 1938. Table 2.1 summarizes the most relevant regulations with respect to clinical trials. These regulations cover not only pharmaceutical

TABLE 2.1

U.S. Codes of Federal Regulation for Approving Pharmaceutical Entities

CFR Number	Regulations
21 CFR 50	Protection of human subjects
21 CFR 54	Financial disclosure by clinical investigators
21 CFR 56	Institutional review boards (IRB)
21 CFR 312	Investigational New Drug Application (IND)
Subpart E	Treatment IND
21 CFR 314	Applications for FDA approval to market a new drug
Subpart C	Abbreviated applications
Subpart H	Accelerated approval
21 CFR 601	Establishment license and product license applications (ELA and PLA)
Subpart E	Accelerated approval
21 CFR 316	Orphan drugs
21 CFR 320	Bioavailability and bioequivalence requirements
21 CFR 330	Over-the-counter (OTC) human drugs
21 CFR 812	Investigational device exemptions (IDE)
21 CFR 814	Premarket approval of medical devices (PMA)
21 CFR 60	Patent term restoration
21 CFR 201	Labeling
21 CFR 202	Prescription drug advertising
21 CFR 203	Prescription drug marketing

entities such as drugs, biological products, and medical devices under investigation but also the welfare of participating subjects and the labeling and advertising of pharmaceutical products. It can be seen from Table 2.1 that pharmaceutical entities can be roughly divided into three categories based on the FD&C Act and hence the CFR. These categories include drug products, biological products, and medical devices. For the first category, a drug is as defined in the FD&C Act (21 U.S.C. 321) as an article that is (1) recognized in the US Pharmacopeia, official Homeopathic Pharmacopeia of the United States, or official National Formulary, or a supplement to any of them; (2) intended for use in the diagnosis, cure, mitigation, treatment, or prevention of disease in humans or other animals; or (3) intended to affect the structure or function of the body of humans or other animals. For the second category, a biological product is defined in the 1944 Biologics Act (46 U.S.C. 262) as a virus, therapeutic serum, toxin, antitoxin, bacterial or viral vaccine, blood, blood component or derivative, allergenic product, or analogous product, applicable to the prevention, treatment, or cure of disease or injuries in humans. Finally, a medical device is defined as an instrument, apparatus, implement, machine contrivance, implant, *in vitro* reagent, or other similar or related article, including any component, part, or accessory that—similar to a drug—is (1) recognized in the official National Formulary or the U.S.

Global Pharmaceutical Development 35

Pharmacopeia or any supplement in them; (2) intended for use in the diagnosis in humans or other animals; or (3) intended to affect the structure or function of the body of humans or other animals.

The CDER of the FDA has jurisdiction over administration of regulation and approval of pharmaceutical products classified as *drug*. These regulations include Investigational New Drug Application (IND) and New Drug Application (NDA) for new drugs, orphan drugs, and over-the-counter (OTC) human drugs and Abbreviated New Drug Application (ANDA) for generic drugs. On the other hand, the CBER is responsible for enforcing the regulations of biological products through processes such an Establishment License Application (ELA) or Product License Application (PLA). Administration of the regulations for medical devices belongs to the jurisdiction of the CDRH through Investigational Device Exemptions (IDE) and Premarket Approval of Medical Devices (PMA) and other means.

2.3.2 International Conference on Harmonization

Health regulatory authorities in different countries have different requirements for approval of commercial use of the drug products. As a result, considerable resources have been spent by the pharmaceutical industry in the preparation of different documents for applications of the same pharmaceutical product to meet different regulatory requirements requested by different countries or regions. However, because of globalization of the pharmaceutical industry, arbitrary differences in regulations, increase in health care costs, need for reduction of time for patients to access new drugs and of experimental use of humans and animals without compromising safety, the necessity to standardize these similar yet different regulatory requirements has been recognized by both regulatory authorities and pharmaceutical industry. Hence, the International Conference on Harmonization (ICH) of Technical Requirements for the Registration of Pharmaceuticals for Human Use was organized in 1990 to provide an opportunity for important initiatives to be developed by regulatory authorities as well as industry association for the promotion of international harmonization of regulatory requirements.

ICH was originally concerned with tripartite harmonization of technical requirements for the registration of pharmaceutical products among three regions: the European Union, Japan, and the United States. Basically, the ICH Steering Committee is the governing body consisting of six cosponsors: European Commission of the European Union, the European Federation of Pharmaceutical Industries' Associations (EFPIA), the Japanese Ministry of Health, Labor and Welfare (MHLW), the Japanese Pharmaceutical Manufacturers Association (JPMA), the CDER and CBER of the FDA, and the Pharmaceutical Research and Manufacturers of America (PhRMA). Each of its six cosponsors has two seats on the Steering Committee:

one from a regulatory authority and one from the pharmaceutical industry, from each of the three regions. The functions of the ICH steering committee include (1) determining policies and procedures, (2) selecting topics, (3) monitoring progress, and (4) overseeing preparation of biannual conferences. The ICH Steering Committee also includes observers from the World Health Organization, Health Canada, and the European Free Trade Area (EFTA). In addition, two seats of the ICH Steering Committee are given to the International Federation of Pharmaceutical Manufacturers Association (IFPMA), who hosts the ICH Secretariat at Geneva, Switzerland, and participates as a nonvoting member of the Steering Committee, which coordinates the preparation of documentation. The Global Cooperation Group (GCG) was formed as a subcommittee of the ICH Steering committee in 1999 in response to interest in the non-ICH regions. Currently, the GCG includes the following organizations and countries: Asia-Pacific Economic Cooperation (APEC), Association of Southeast Asian Nations (ASEAN), Pan American Network for Drug Regulatory Harmonization (PANDRH), Southern African Development Community (SADC), Australia, Brazil, China, Chinese Taipei, India, South Korea, Russia, and Singapore.

In order to harmonize technical procedures the ICH has issued a number of guidelines and draft guidelines. After the ICH Steering Committee selected the topics, the ICH guidelines were initiated by a concept paper and went through a five-step review process. A complete updated list of the ICH guidelines or draft guidelines can be found in its website: http://www.ich.org. As can be seen, these guidelines are not only for harmonization of design, conduct, analysis, and report for a single clinical trial but also for consensus in protecting and maintaining the scientific integrity of the entire clinical development plan of a pharmaceutical entity. Along this line, Chow (1997a) introduced the concept of *Good Statistics Practice* in drug development and regulatory approval process as the foundation of ICH GCP (see also, FDA 1988). The concepts and principles stated in the ICH clinical guidelines can be found in the works of ICH (1998, 2009) and Chow and Liu (2004).

Although the primary goals of the ICH are to harmonize the technical procedures and documents for regulatory submissions, some regulatory agencies still request the unique documentation specific to the regions. For example, the integrated summary of effectiveness (ISE) and integrated summary of safety (ISS) in the Summary of the Clinical and Statistical Section of an NDA are unique to the FDA. In addition, the FDA points out that section of *Summary of Clinical Efficacy* and section of *Summary of Clinical Safety* in Module 2 of ICH M4—Efficacy does not describe the needed level of detail for an ISE and ISS. In addition, these clinical summary sections of M2 are limited to only 400 pages, whereas a typical ISS alone often can be substantially larger. On the other hand, Module 5 is designed to contain more detailed in-depth analysis and has no space limitation. In addition, the FDA issued guidance on electronic formats using electronic common technical document (eCTD) specifications.

2.3.3 Remarks

Current FDA requirements for registration adherence to the principles of good clinical practices (GCPs), including adequate human subject protection is universally recognized as a critical requirement to the conduct of research involving human subjects. GCP is defined as a standard for the design, conduct, performance, monitoring, auditing, recording, analysis, and reporting of clinical trials in a way that provides assurance that the data and reported results are credible and accurate and that the rights, safety, and well-being of trial subjects are protected (FDA 1988; ICH 1998). Compliance with principles of GCP, as harmonized by FDA/ICH, is a significant regulatory challenge for global acceptance of clinical trials completed in Asia. Note that FDA/ICH guidance on GCP was developed with consideration of the current GCP practices of the European Union, Japan, and the United States, Australia, Canada, the Nordic countries, and the World Health Organization (WHO). Medical practices of Asian countries such as China, India, Taiwan, and Thailand were not harmonized.

Practical challenges in Asian clinical trials include (1) inexperience, (2) GCP training, (3) protocol execution/deviations (differentiating between medical practice and clinical research, documentation, and storage capabilities), (4) serious adverse event (SAE) reporting, (5) infrastructure and equipment (e.g., computers, software, scanners, faxes, refrigerators, freezers, and pumps), and (6) capabilities to produce eCTD formats vary or are not required. Regulatory challenges in trial execution in global pharmaceutical/clinical development in Asian Pacific Region are mostly GCP-related. These challenges include (1) protocol translation (e.g., language barriers), (2) investigator qualifications (e.g., documentation of training), (3) enrollment, (4) informed consent, (5) patient compliance, and (6) dropout rates and follow-ups. In addition, each Asian country's policies on protocol approvals, insurance regulations, import licenses, and a myriad of other factors can affect a sponsor's ability to establish and run clinical trial sites.

2.4 Practical Issues in Drug Development

On March 16, 2004, the FDA released a report addressing the recent slowdown in innovative medical therapies submitted to the FDA for approval, "Innovation/Stagnation: Challenge and Opportunity on the Critical Path to New Medical Products." The report describes the urgent need to modernize the medical product development process—the Critical Path—to make product development more predictable and less costly. Through this initiative, the FDA took the lead in the development of a national Critical Path Opportunities List, to bring concrete focus to these tasks. As a result, the

FDA released a Critical Path Opportunities List that outlines 76 initial projects to bridge the gap between the quick pace of new biomedical discoveries and the slower pace at which those discoveries are currently developed into therapies two years later. See, for example, http://www.fda.gov/oc/initiatives/criticalpath. The Critical Path Opportunities List consists of six broad topic areas of (1) development of biomarkers, (2) clinical trial designs, (3) bioinformatics, (4) manufacturing, (5) public health needs, and (6) pediatrics. As indicated in the Critical Path Opportunities Report, biomarker development and streamlining clinical trials are the two most important areas for improving medical product development. The streamlining of clinical trials calls for advancing innovative trial designs such as adaptive designs to improve innovation in clinical development. These 76 initial projects are the most pressing scientific and/or technical hurdles causing major delays and other problems in the drug, device, and/or biologic development process. Among these 76 initial projects, many of them involve early phase clinical development (i.e., phase I/II studies), which are critical to the success of the development of a pharmaceutical entity (i.e., drug, device, and/or biologic). Some commonly encountered practical issues that may cause major delays and/or failure of the development process are briefly outlined below.

Global drug development plays an important role in a scientific manner in pharmaceutical research (ICH 1997). However, the statistical work to draw a statistical inference with regard to translational medicine research is still in a preliminary stage. To provide a comprehensive understanding of statistical design and methodology commonly employed in global drug development, under the support of the Bureau of Pharmaceutical Affairs, Department of Health (DOH), Taiwan, National Health Research Institutes (NHRI), and Formosa Cancer Foundation organized one symposium on "Current Advanced Statistical Issues in Clinical Trials—Flexibility and Globalization" held on November 21, 2008, and a closed-door meeting on "Designs of Clinical Trials in New Drug Developments" held on November 22, 2008, in Taipei, Taiwan. As a result, a proposal for statistical guidance to multiregional trials was developed. This proposal is briefly described below.

Within the Asian region, each country may consider accepting all the data derived from other countries in the Asian region. For example, Taiwan accepts all Asian data. A study by Lin et al. (2001) found that the so-called *Taiwanese*, accounting for 91 percent of the total population in Taiwan, comprise Minnan and Hakka people who are closely related to the southern Han and are clustered with other southern Asian populations such as Thai and Malaysian in terms of HLA typing. Those who are the descendants of northern Han are separated from the southern Asian cluster and form a cluster with the other northern Asian populations such as Korean and Japanese. The Taiwanese regulatory authority, therefore, accepts data from trials conducted in Taiwan as well as in other Asian countries if those trials meet Taiwanese regulatory standards and were conducted in compliance with GCP requirements.

Global Pharmaceutical Development

2.4.1 Multiregional Clinical Trials

As indicated by Uesaka (2009), the primary objective of a multiregional bridging trial is to show the efficacy of a drug in all participating regions while also evaluating the possibility of applying the overall trial results to each region. To apply the overall results to a specific region, the results in that region should be consistent with either the overall results or the results from other regions. A typical approach is to show consistency among regions by demonstrating that there exists no treatment-by-region interaction. Recently, the Ministry of Health, Labor and Welfare (MHLW) of Japan published guidance on Basic Principles on Global Clinical Trials that outlines the basic concepts for planning and implementation of multiregional trials in a Q&A format. In this guidance, special consideration was placed on the determination of the number of Japanese subjects required in a multiregional trial. As indicated, the selected sample size should be able to establish the consistency of treatment effects between the Japanese group and the entire group.

To establish the consistency of the treatment effects between the Japanese group and the entire group, it is suggested that the selected size should satisfy

$$P\left(\frac{D_J}{D_{All}} > \rho\right) \geq 1 - \gamma, \tag{2.1}$$

where D_J and D_{All} are the treatment effects for the Japanese group and the entire group, respectively. Along this line, Quan et al. (2009) derived closed form formulas for the sample size calculation/allocation for normal, binary and survival endpoints. As an example, the formula for continuous endpoint assuming that $D_J = D_{NJ} = D_{All} = D$, where D_{NJ} is the treatment effect for the non-Japanese subjects, is given below.

$$N_J \geq \frac{z_{1-\gamma}^2 N}{(z_{1-\alpha/2} + z_{1-\beta})^2 (1-\rho)^2 + z_{1-\gamma}^2 (2\rho - \rho^2)}, \tag{2.2}$$

where N and N_J are the sample size for the entire group and the Japanese group. Note that the MHLW of Japan recommends that ρ should be chosen to be either 0.5 or greater and γ should be chosen to be either 0.8 or greater in Equation 2.1. As an example, if we choose $\rho = 0.5$, $\gamma = 0.8$, $\alpha = 0.05$, and $\beta = 0.9$, then $N_J/N = 0.224$. In other words, the sample size for the Japanese group has to be at least 22.4 percent of the overall sample size for the multiregional trial.

In practice, $1 - \rho$ is often considered a noninferiority margin. If ρ is chosen to be greater than 0.5, the Japanese sample size will increase substantially. It should be noted that the sample size formulas given by Quan et al. (2009) are

40 *Quantitative Methods for Traditional Chinese Medicine Development*

derived under the assumption that there is no difference in treatment effects for the Japanese group and non-Japanese group. In practice, it is expected that there is a difference in treatment effects due to ethnic difference. Thus, the formulas for sample size calculation/allocation derived by Quan et al. (2009) are necessarily modified in order to take into consideration the effect due to ethnic differences.

2.4.2 Bridging Studies

The aim of a multiregional trial is to show the efficacy of a drug in various global regions and concurrently to evaluate the possibility of applying the overall trial results to each region. Therefore, how to bridge the results of the multiregional trial to the "Asian region" is another important issue. As indicated earlier, the Japanese Ministry of Health, Labor and Welfare (MHLW) has published the *Basic Principles on Global Clinical Trials* guidance to promote Japan's participation in global development and international clinical study recently. It outlines the basic concepts for planning and implementing the multiregional trials in a Q&A format. Special consideration was placed on the establishment of the consistency of treatment effects between the Japanese group and the entire group. The same consistency criterion can also be used to examine whether the overall results from the multiregional trial can be applied to the Asian region.

Let D_{Asia} be the observed treatment effect for the Asian region and D_{All} the observed treatment effect from all regions. Given that the overall result is significant at α level, we will judge whether the treatment is effective in the Asian region by the following criterion:

$$D_{\text{Asia}} \geq \rho\, D_{\text{All}} \quad \text{for some } 0 < \rho < 1. \tag{2.3}$$

Other consistency criteria can be found in the work of Uesaka (2009) and Ko et al. (2010). Selection of the magnitude ρ of consistency trend may be critical. All differences in ethnic factors between the Asian region and other regions should be taken into account. The Japanese MHLW suggests that ρ be 0.5 or greater. However, the determination of ρ will be and should be different from product to product and from therapeutic area to therapeutic area. For example, in a multiregional liver cancer trial, the Asian region can definitely require a larger value of ρ because it will contribute more subjects than other regions.

In addition to the consistency criterion in Equation 2.3, the following criteria suggested by Uesaka (2009) and Ko et al. (2010) can also be used:

$$D_{\text{Asia}} \geq \rho\, D_C \quad \text{for some } 0 < \rho < 1;$$

$$\rho \leq D_{\text{Asia}}/D_{\text{All}} \leq 1/\rho \quad \text{for some } 0 < \rho < 1;$$

$$\rho \leq D_{\text{Asia}}/D_C \leq 1/\rho \quad \text{for some } 0 < \rho < 1;$$

Global Pharmaceutical Development 41

where D_C denotes the observed treatment effect from regions other than the Asian region. The first criterion is to assess whether the treatment effect in the Asian region is as large as that of the other regions, while the last two criteria are to assess the consistency of the treatment effect of the Asian region with overall regions or other regions.

2.4.3 Adaptive Design Methods in Clinical Trials

In recent years, the use of adaptive design methods has become very popular owing to its flexibility and efficiency for identifying any possible signal or trend of clinical benefits (preferably the optimal clinical benefits) with the limited resources available (see, e.g., Chow and Chang 2006; Pong and Chow 2010). In its recent draft guidance, the FDA defined an adaptive design clinical study as a study that includes a prospectively planned opportunity for modification of one or more specified aspects of the study design and hypotheses based on analysis of data (usually interim data) from subjects in the study. The FDA emphasizes that one of the major characteristics of an adaptive design is the prospectively planned opportunity. Changes should be made based on analysis of data (usually interim data). In the draft guidance, the FDA classifies adaptive designs as either well-understood designs or less well understood designs, depending on the nature of adaptations either blinded or unblinded (FDA 2010).

On the other hand, Chow et al. (2005) provided a broader definition of an adaptive design. They define an adaptive design of a clinical trial as a design that allows adaptations or modifications to some aspects (e.g., trial procedures and/or statistical methods) of the trial after its initiation without undermining the validity and integrity of the trial. Trial procedures are referred to as the eligibility criteria, study dose, treatment duration, study endpoints, laboratory testing procedures, diagnostic procedures, criteria for evaluability, and assessment of clinical responses. Statistical methods include randomization scheme, study design selection, study objectives/hypotheses, sample size calculation, data monitoring and interim analysis, statistical analysis plan, and/or methods for data analysis.

Depending on the types of adaptation or modification made, commonly employed adaptive design methods in clinical trials include, but are not limited to (1) a group sequential design, (2) a sample size reestimation (or an N-adjustable) design, (3) an adaptive seamless (e.g., phase I/II or phase II/III) design, (4) a drop-the-loser (or pick-the-winner) design, (5) an adaptive randomization design, (6) an adaptive dose finding (escalation) design, (7) a biomarker-adaptive design, (8) an adaptive treatment-switching design, (9) an adaptive-hypotheses design, and (10) any combinations of the above (see also, Chow and Chang 2006; Pong and Chow 2010).

In its draft guidance, the FDA classifies adaptive designs into categories of well-understood and less well-understood designs. For those less well-understood adaptive designs such as adaptive dose finding designs and two-stage phase I/II (or phase II/III) seamless adaptive designs, statistical methods are not well established and hence should be used with caution. In practice, misuse of adaptive design methods in clinical trials is a concern to both clinical scientists and regulatory agencies. It is suggested that the escalating momentum for the use of adaptive design methods in clinical trials be slowed in order to allow time for development of appropriate statistical methodologies.

2.4.4 Remarks

More and more clinical trials utilizing adaptive design methods have been conducted in global pharmaceutical (clinical) development since the publication of the FDA draft guidance on adaptive clinical trial designs in 2010. For those clinical trials utilizing less well understood adaptive designs, commonly asked questions from the FDA include the following: (1) How to control the overall type I error rate? (2) How to pool data collected before and after the adaptation for a combined analysis? (3) How to perform sample size estimation and/or sample size allocation (if a multiple-stage adaptive design is used)? and (4) How to determine safety and futility/efficacy boundaries if a group sequential design is used. The FDA does not have any objections to the use of adaptive design methods in clinical trials if the sponsor can (1) develop clinical strategy for preventing possible operational bias due to the application of adaptive design methods and (2) fully address the above questions.

2.4.5 Microdosing Approach

In pharmaceutical research and development, microdose studies are designed not only to evaluate pharmacokinetics or imaging of specific targets but also not to induce pharmacologic effects. Because of this, the risk to human subjects is very limited and information adequate to support the initiation of such limited human studies can be derived from limited nonclinical safety studies. A microdose is defined as less than 1/100th of the dose of a test substance calculated (based on animal data) to yield a pharmacologic effect of the test substance with a maximum dose of ≤ 100 µg. Owing to differences in molecular weights as compared to synthetic drugs, the maximum dose for protein products is ≤ 30 nmol.

As indicated in the FDA Exploratory IND 2006 guidance, it is suggested that preclinical and clinical approaches, as well as chemistry, manufacturing, and controls information, should be considered when planning exploratory studies in humans, including studies of closely related drugs or therapeutic biological products, under an investigational new drug (IND) application (21 CFR 312). Existing regulations allow a great deal of flexibility in the amount of data that needs to be submitted with an IND application, depending on the goals of the proposed investigation, the specific human testing proposed, and the expected risks.

The FDA currently accepts the use of extended single-dose toxicity studies in animals to support single-dose studies in humans. For microdose studies, a

Global Pharmaceutical Development

single mammalian species (both sexes) can be used if justified by *in vitro* metabolism data and by comparative data on *in vitro* pharmacodynamics effects. The route of exposure in animals should be by the intended clinical route. In these studies, animals should be observed for 14 days post-dosing with an interim necropsy, typically on day 2 and endpoints evaluated should include body weights. Because microdose studies involve only single exposures to microgram quantities of test materials and because such exposures are comparable to routine environmental exposures, routine generic toxicology testing is not needed. For similar reasons, safety pharmacology studies are also not recommended.

2.4.6 Remarks

The concept of the microdosing approach in pharmaceutical development is encouraging. As indicated by Burt (2011), the use of human microdosing in pharmaceutical development has the following benefits that (1) it takes just six months from lab bench to completion of clinical studies, (2) smarter lead candidate selection, (3) reduces expensive late stage attrition (i.e., kill ineffective compound early and cheap), (4) substantially reduced preclinical toxicology package compared to phase I, (5) only gram quantities of non-GMP drug (typically 10 g) are needed, (6) any route of administration is possible, including intravenous, (7) absolute oral bioavailability calculation, (8) drugs can be tested in sensitive populations; renally impaired patients, women of child-bearing age and cancer patients, and (9) reduces use of animals in research. However, there are statistical issues/concerns regarding the validity of the human microdosing approach in pharmaceutical development. These statistical issues include (1) the selection of microdose (e.g., "how to distinguish the effect due to microdose and the placebo effect?" and "how to select the initial dose and the dose range under study?"), (2) the selection of study endpoint (e.g., "should a clinical endpoint or a surrogate endpoint or a biomarker be used?" and "whether the surrogate or biomarker is predictive of clinical endpoint?"), (3) the determination of sample size (e.g., precision analysis or power analysis), and (4) model selection and validation (e.g., "how to handle inter- and intrasubject variabilities?" and "how to determine the impact of nonlinearity for the dose range under study?"). In addition, it is a concern that the extrapolation based on results from microdose to regular dose may not be reliable because the variability associated with the dose is usually proportional to the dose.

2.5 Modernization of TCM Development

As indicated in Chapter 1, there is a debate about how to achieve modernization of TCM development—either the Western way or the Chinese way? Both regulatory authorities of China and Taiwan seem to prefer the Westernization approach. In pursuit of advancing the TCM through the Westernization approach to benefit patients who suffer from critical and/or life-threatening diseases, the TCM development focuses on (1) individualized treatment for achieving optimal therapeutic effect, (2) combinational treatment as a supplemental treatment for reducing harmful toxicity and consequently improving tolerability and safety profile, and (3) effective TCM treatment by identifying the optimal ratios among individual components of TCM, which are briefly described below.

2.5.1 Individualized Treatment

TCM typically consists of several components. The combination is usually determined based on observations from the four Chinese diagnostic procedures under the medical theory of global dynamic balance (or harmony) among organs. The use of the four Chinese diagnostic procedures is to diagnose the possible causes for the imbalance among these organs. Individualized treatment is to minimize the intrasubject variability for achieving the optimal therapeutic effect by restoring the balance among these organs. Thus, the dose and treatment duration are flexible but different from subject to subject. The concept of individualized treatment leads to the innovative thinking of personalized medicine.

The concept of individualized treatment is widely accepted by the medical community for personalized medicine. However, it also posts a major challenge to the investigators for modernization of TCM development because the doses and treatment durations are different from subject to subject. Moreover, the determination of dose and treatment duration is made based on the four subjective Chinese diagnostic procedures, which may be conducted by inexperienced Chinese doctors. In this case, significant rater-to-rater variability is anticipated, which has a negative impact on the prescribed individualized treatment and consequently it may not achieve the optimal intended therapeutic effect.

2.5.2 Combinational Treatment

One of major challenges for the modernization of TCM development is the characterization of individual components of the TCMs. Most TCMs contain a number of individual components, among which, some may be efficacious and some may reduce toxicity on specific organs such as liver or kidney. In this case, the investigators may consider combinational treatment by combining some of the individual components of the TCM in conjunction with an active control agent (i.e., a drug product that has been approved by the regulatory agency and currently available in the marketplace) to treat a critical disease under study. As an example, suppose that a component A of a given TCM is found to be able to reduce the toxicity that induced by having

Global Pharmaceutical Development 45

drug B for treating a critical disease (e.g., cancer). In this case, drug B can achieve an efficacy study endpoint while component A can help in reducing toxicity of drug B and consequently improving the safety profile. The combinational treatment (Western drug for efficacy and TCM for toxicity) for treating critical diseases such as cancer and AIDS has become increasingly popular in recent years.

Note that the pharmacological activities of some individual components of a given TCM, and the relationships among these individual components, are usually unknown. In practice, the development of TCM is considered incomplete until all of the components can be fully characterized. This has been a major challenge and/or an obstacle for the modernization of TCM development.

2.5.3 Effective Treatment

Unlike Western medicines, TCMs do not have fixed doses. Flexible doses allow the Chinese doctor to prescribe effective treatment individually based on the observations obtained from the four subjective Chinese diagnostic procedures. For modernization of TCM development, it is not feasible to have effective treatment individually. For development of TCMs, several attempts are made to develop a fixed dose (i.e., fixed ratios among individual components) for the population rather than individuals. In this case, multilevel factorial design is usually considered to identify the best combination of individual components for the TCM under development.

2.6 Concluding Remarks

The development process of a promising compound is a lengthy and costly process. At the screening stage, many candidate compounds may be dropped owing to intolerable toxicity/safety or lack of efficacy based on preclinical data. In practice, it is most likely that only a handful of promising compounds can make it to the stage of clinical development. As a result, how to select the most promising compounds among these handfuls of compounds for continued clinical development has become a challenge to the clinical development team under possible resources/budget constraints. A wrong decision could lead to a total disaster for the sponsor (all of the efforts and investment has been wasted). The objective for assessment of the probability of success is multifold. First, it is to obtain accurate and reliable individual estimates of the probability of success at each stage and an overall estimate of the overall probability of success. Second, it is to obtain a lower confidence boundary of the overall probability of success. Third, it is to a perform a sensitivity analysis of the probability of success with respect to relatively changes in the early phase of clinical development versus the later phase of clinical development, assuming a fixed total resources/budget.

As indicated earlier, the pharmaceutical/clinical development process of a compound is a sequential process that consists of several phases of development such as pre-clinical phase and phases I-III of clinical development. At each phase of development, a go/no-go decision is necessarily made. As discussed in the previous section, the go/no-go decision is usually made at each phase of development either based on a subjective evaluation, the simple approach, or a decision-tree approach. In this section, we attempt to study the assessment of the probability of success of the development process.

Let S_1, S_2,..., and S_K denote stage 1, 2,..., and K of the development process of a pharmaceutical compound, respectively. Also, let p_1, p_2,..., and p_K be the probability of success at stage 1, 2,..., and K, respectively. Thus, the probability of success can be obtained as

$$P(\text{Success}) = P(S_1)P(S_2|S_1)\cdots P(S_K|S_{K-1}),$$

where $P(S_i)$ is defined as the probability of observing a positive result at the ith stage. That is,

$$P(S_i) = P(\text{positive}|T_i, n_i),$$

where a positive result is referred to as the rejection of the null hypothesis of no treatment difference at the α level of significance and there is an 80 percent power for correctly detecting a clinically important difference δ, in which n_i and T_i are the corresponding sample size and test statistic of the study conducted at the ith stage, where $i = 1, 2,...,K$. It should be noted that in practice, there may be more than one study conducted at the same stage. In other words, $n_i = n_{ij}$ and $T_i = T_{ij}$, where $j = 1, 2,..., J_i$. In this paper, for simplicity, we will consider the case where $J_i = 1$ for all i. For illustration purposes, Table 2.2 summarizes probabilities of success of pharmaceutical development of a promising compound with various scenarios of success at an early stage of pharmaceutical development.

TABLE 2.2

Probability of Success for Pharmaceutical Development

$P(S_1)$	$P(S_2|S_1)$	$P(S_3|S_2)$	$P(S_4|S_3)$	$P(S_4|S_3)$
0.5	0.9	0.9	0.9	0.365
0.6	0.9	0.9	0.9	0.437
0.7	0.9	0.9	0.9	0.510
0.8	0.9	0.9	0.9	0.583
0.9	0.9	0.9	0.9	0.656
0.95	0.9	0.9	0.9	0.693

Note: S_i indicates the ith stage of pharmaceutical development.

Global Pharmaceutical Development 47

As can be seen from Table 2.2, the probability of success at the early stage of clinical development is critical. If the probability of success at the early stage is less than 70 percent, we may have an overall probability of success of less than 50 percent; even the probabilities of success at subsequent stages of clinical development are as high as 90 percent.

Global drug development involves the conduct of global (multiregional or multinational) clinical trials and bridging studies. In practice, conducting global (multiregional or multinational) clinical trials often encounters practical issues, challenges, and difficulties due to differences in culture, medical practice, and regulatory review/approval process from region (country) to region (country). Conducting bridging studies is necessary in order to determine (1) whether or not patients at different regions (countries) will respond to the test treatment differently (e.g., owing to differences in ethnic factors) and (2) whether foreign (clinical) data can be extrapolated to the new region reliably with valid scientific/statistical justification. To ensure the success of global drug development, it is suggested that (1) regulatory requirements from different regions (countries) be harmonized and (2) innovative methodologies such as adaptive design methods and microdosing approach be used.

3

Regulations on Traditional Chinese Medicine

3.1 Introduction

Traditional Chinese medicine (TCM) is one of the oldest forms of medicine in the world. As indicated in Chapter 1, TCMs are fundamentally different from Western medicines. For example, As indicated in Chapter 1, most TCMs contain several active and/or inactive components whose pharmacological activities are usually unknown. Chinese medical theory believes in global dynamic balance or harmony among organs. Once the imbalance occurs, signs and symptoms of the specific organs will show that there are potential problems. The basic principle of TCM is to readjust and balance the elements in the human body so that the body will return to a normal and healthy level. Western medicine, on the other hand, is like a key to a lock. The mechanism and the compound are very clearly and precisely designed to hit the target (e.g., specific organ) to fix the problem. In practice, there are several blind areas (diseases) in Western medicines that might be solved by alternative medicine such as filterable virus, most chronic degenerative diseases (diabetes, hypertension, and kidney failure), most mental diseases (depression), most self-immune and allergy diseases (asthma, rheumatoid, and leukemia), and most kinds of cancer and stubborn dermal diseases (World Health Organization [WHO] 1998).

TCM has been shown to be effective in many diseases such as cancer, heart disease, diabetes, and HIV/AIDS. Its increasing use is evidence of alternatives to conventional medicines especially at terminal phases of critical diseases such as cancer. TCMs offer cost-effective approaches not only to managing and preventing complex chronic illness but also to providing hope (alternative treatment) to subjects with complex chronic and life-threatening diseases. Unlike Western medicines, TCM has been viewed as food or dietary supplements rather than drugs worldwide in the past several decades. In 1984, the Chinese government published the *Drug Administration Law of the People's Republic of China*, which put forth regulations for evaluation and approval of TCMs as drugs (see also MOPH 1992). Similarly, in the United States, the Federal Government regulates TCM through the Food

49

and Drug Administration (FDA) as foods rather than as drugs per old regulations, which have some limitations and are not appropriate. In order to meet the special properties of TCM, protect customers, provide incentives for research on TCM-based drug development, and benefit public health, the FDA released new guidance on a botanical drug in 2004 (FDA 2004). On October 31, 2006, the FDA approved the first ever submitted New Drug Application (NDA) for a botanical drug product, Polyphenon® E Ointment. (Veregen™) developed by a German biotech company MediGene AG. Veregen is intended for the treatment of external and perianal genital warts (Wall Street Journal 2007). The significant impact of this change in pharmaceutical industry is far reaching. It is expected to have more botanical drugs and tighter competition in the near future. TCM will certainly play a more important role and make greater contributions to health care of human beings.

There is mounting evidence that TCMs could produce tangible benefits for sufferers of diseases (e.g., everyone from menopausal women to cancer patients) that have confounded both Western and Eastern medicines. Intuitively, one may consider taking drug combinations that have been used for thousands of years and applying strict scientific tests to them to find out what makes them work. Then, distilling the active compound and making a pill. However, because traditional Chinese remedies have been used successfully for centuries, drugs developed from those formulas cannot be patented. Thus, no international drug behemoth is driving this research. Another daunting challenge is how to obtain approval from the US FDA. Until recently, the FDA required proof of how a certain medicine affects the body. That's easy with Western medicines. Most TCMs, however, are unable to prove to the FDA which ingredients do what. A Chinese herbal formula is a carefully balanced recipe of several different herbs. Each herb has its own specific functions. An herbal formula is even tailor-made to suit a particular patient.

As the Chinese government encourages global development of TCMs the Western way, it is suggested that the process of pharmaceutical development of Western medicines be followed in order to provide substantial evidence of safety and efficacy of the TCMs under investigation scientifically. The purpose of this chapter is to provide a summary of regulations on traditional Chinese herbal medicines published by the WHO, People's Republic of China, the European Union, and the United States.

In Section 3.2 regulations on TCM in China are briefly outlined. Also included in the discussion are recent regulations that were put into effect in 2003. Section 3.3 describes regulations on Chinese herbal medicine in Europe focusing on current regulations adopted in Germany. Regulations on TCM as food and dietary supplements and drugs in the United States are reviewed in Sections 3.4 and 3.5, respectively. Section 3.6 provides concluding remarks on harmonization of TCM regulations worldwide.

Regulations on Traditional Chinese Medicine

3.2 Regulations on TCM in China

3.2.1 Background

TCM has a long history of several thousand years. Discovery of medicinal materials in ancient times was closely related to the life and the labor of people and their natural living conditions. Chinese people discovered that many natural materials could be used to treat diseases, and great experience in this field has gradually been accumulated. The *Chinese Materia* is one of the best documented and most extensive sources, as well as the one that enjoys the most continued use, including more than 7000 species of medicinal plants.

In the past several decades, traditional Chinese medicine has developed steadily. As indicated by the WHO (1996, 1998), by the end of 1995, there were 2522 TCM hospitals with a total of 276,000 beds. Most of the general hospitals have a TCM department. There are 940 factories and plants for the manufacture of herbal medicines. The 1990 edition of the *Chinese Pharmacopeia* included 784 articles on traditional Chinese medicines and 509 articles on Chinese patent medicines. The monographs describe the source or the substances used, prescriptions, methods of preparation, identification, examination, extraction, effects, and main indications as well as methods of use, dosage, precautions, etc. (see, e.g., WHO 1996). Further information on herbal medicines is available in the new edition of the *Pharmacopoeia of the People's Republic of China* (Wang 1991).

3.2.2 Regulations

In China, herbal medicines are normally considered as medicinal products with special requirements for marketing. In 1984, the Ministry of Public Health (MOPH) was authorized to approve new drugs based on the *Drug Administration Law of the People's Republic of China*. New drugs are referred to as drugs that have not been produced previously in China or drugs for which a new indication, a change in the route of administration, or a change of dosage form is to be adopted. Any unit or individual engaged in the development, production, distribution, prescription, inspection, and surveillance of new drugs must adhere to the provisions of the document. The regulation includes general principles concerning new drugs, their classification, research, clinical trials, approval, and manufacture.

3.2.2.1 Regulatory Approval Process

According to the *Drug Administration Law of the People's Republic of China*, new drugs have to be examined in terms of quality, safety, and efficacy and approved (with respect to special labeling). After approval, a new drug certificate is granted with an approval number. The manufacturer or sponsor is then permitted to put the product on the market. This procedure reflects the respect in which traditional experiences are held, while modern scientific and technical knowledge is used in appraising the therapeutic effects and the quality of the modified traditional medicines and contributes administratively to the exploitation of traditional Chinese medicine (Wang 1991).

Article 3 of the *Drug Administration Law of the People's Republic of China* (MOPH 1984) states

> The State encourages the development of both modern and traditional drugs, the role of which in the prevention and treatment of diseases as well as in health care will be fully brought into play. The State protects the resources of wild herbal drugs and encourages domestic cultivation of herbal drugs.

3.2.2.2 Drug Categories

On the basis of the Amendment and Supplemental Regulation of Approval of New TCM Drugs, implemented September 1, 1992, new TCM drugs are classified into five categories (Table 3.1).

3.2.2.3 Documentation for Applications for New Drugs

On the basis of Article 21 of the Drug Administration Law, the clinical trial or clinical verification of a new drug should be sanctioned by the Ministry of Public Health or the health bureau of the province, autonomous region, or municipality. A new drug will be approved for clinical use and a license issued by the MOPH, if the clinical trial or clinical verification has been

TABLE 3.1

Classification of TCMs in China

Classification	Description
Category 1	Artificial imitations of TCM herbs; Newly discovered medicinal plants and their preparations; Single active principal extracted from TCM plant material and their preparations.
Category 2	Chinese medicinal herbal injections; Parts of TCM medicinal plants newly employed as a remedy and their preparations; Non-single components extracted from TCM and natural plants and their preparations; TCM materials obtained by artificial techniques in vivo and their preparations.
Category 3	New TCM preparations; Combined preparations of TCM and modern medicine in which TCM medicine is the main component; Cultivated material which traditionally is imported.
Category 4	New dosage forms or new routes of administration of TCM drug; Materials introduced from other parts of the country and those for cultivation instead of harvesting in the wild.
Category 5	TCM products with new and additional indications.

Regulations on Traditional Chinese Medicine 53

completed and an appraisal of its efficacy has been made. Pursuant to Articles 21 and 22 of the Drug Administration Law, on 1 July 1985, the Ministry of Public Health issued and implemented a regulation for the Approval of New Drugs. Several appendices provide detailed information on the application form, list of documents required, and technical requirements of toxicological and clinical studies on new modern drugs, and new TCM drugs (MOPH 1984).

In addition, all research on new medicines should provide data on toxicity, pharmacological properties, and clinical research, as well as detailed documentation on the quality of the medicinal material and the pharmaceutical form. For the five categories mentioned above, different requirements have to be fulfilled for the medicinal material as well as for their pharmaceutical preparation. Proprietary medicines included in the national pharmacopoeia and new medicines approved by the MOPH are exempted from clinical testing when only the dosage form is changed, such as from powder into gelatin capsules or from tablets into granular form infused with boiling water, without changes in the indications for cardinal symptoms or dosage.

The report on the medicinal material should contain the following items in applications for clinical research: purpose of research, previous experience or modern research data, source of material, cultivation, processing, properties, data based on Chinese pharmacology and experience, efficacy with respect to cardinal symptoms, pharmacological research data, acute toxicity tests, data on mutagenicity/carcinogenicity/reproductive toxicity (only for category 1), draft on quality standards, stability, and the proposed plan for clinical research. A separate application for production should include documentation on quality standards, stability tests, a summary of clinical studies, and packaging material.

The report on pharmaceutical preparation has to meet similar requirements to the report on medicinal material, depending on the drug category indicated in Table 3.1.

3.2.2.4 Pharmacological Requirements

Technical requirements for pharmacological studies are laid down in a special paragraph. The tests on major drug effects should be designed in such a way that the special characteristics of traditional Chinese medicine are taken into consideration. Two or more methods should be selected for research on the major drug actions, based on the effects of the new medicine on the complex of symptoms or the illness. For new medicines in categories 1, 2, and 3, this research should be sufficient to verify the major therapeutic functions and other important therapeutic effects. For new medicines in category 4, two (or more) tests on the major effects are required, or else well-documented material has to be submitted. For new medicines in category 5, only tests on the major effects of the medicine on *new* cardinal symptoms are required. Research on general pharmacology should be performed on

54   *Quantitative Methods for Traditional Chinese Medicine Development*

the nervous system, on the cardiovascular system, and on the respiratory system. Technical requirements for studies on toxicity are also laid down in a special paragraph. Here a difference is drawn between a clinical trial and a clinical verification. Clinical trials should be conducted for new medicines of categories 1, 2, and 3, and clinical verifications are required for new medicines of categories 4 and 5. Clinical trials are divided into three phases, but clinical verification does not have phases.

3.2.2.5 Clinical Trials

The purpose of a clinical trial phase I is to study the reaction and the tolerance of the human body to the new medicine and to find out the safe dosage. Medicines in categories 1 and 2 that have either toxic or incompatible compounds have to go through phase I of the clinical trial. For dosage determination, the dosage used in animal tests may be used as a reference. The purpose of phase II of a clinical trial is to obtain an accurate evaluation of the curative effects of the new medicine and its safety. In addition, a comparison has to be made between the new medicine and known drugs, so as to determine its advantages and disadvantages. Phase II consists of two parts, the first applies when the treatment is performed and the second when the treatment is expanded. The dosage used in the clinical trial should be based on pharmacodynamics tests made beforehand and clinical facts, or the results of phase I. For the selection of cases, there are strict standards on diagnosis, and the diagnosis is based on overall analyses of symptoms and signs, the course, nature and location of the illness, and the patient's physical condition, according to the basic theories of TCM. For the performance of a clinical trial, either the single- or the double-blind method may be used, according to need or the actual circumstances. When the curative effects are determined, four ratings are applicable: clinical recovery, significantly effective, effective, and noneffective. The evaluation of curative effects should be based on the clinical symptoms (symptoms and physical signs), objective standards for curative effects, and the ultimate results on the patient.

The objective of the clinical trial phase III is the further investigation of the safe use or effectiveness of the new medicine on the basis of the findings of phase II. The main purpose is to have clinical trials on a new medicine during its trial production or after it has been put on the market for a period of time. This is to make up for deficiencies in phase II, to observe further the curative effects and the nature of its effects on cardinal symptoms and adverse reactions.

Clinical verification is applicable for new medicines in categories 4 and 5, the purpose being to observe their curative effects, contraindications, and precautions. Different groups should be used for control and for comparison. For new medicines that have changed their dosage forms, the control should be same pharmaceutical form as the original form. For those medicines that

Regulations on Traditional Chinese Medicine

have additional curative effects, a known medicine with curative effects on the same illness should be selected as control.

The summary of the clinical trial should be objective and comprehensive and should be an accurate reflection of the whole process. The discussion in the final report should include a conclusion that is based on the outcome of the tests, the functions and effects on cardinal symptoms, the scope of application of the new medicine, its administration, the course of treatment, curative effects, safety, adverse reactions (including the measures to be taken), contraindications, and precautions. An objective evaluation on the characteristics of the new medicine should also be made.

3.2.2.6 Raw Materials

Technical requirements for studies on quality standards for Chinese medicinal material and medicines are also presented in the *Drug Administration Law of the People's Republic of China*. The source (i.e., original plant, part of the plant, harvesting conditions), properties, identification, test for impurities, assay, and processing all have to be described. The quality standards for Chinese medicines should include the prescription, the way of processing, the properties, the identification, the examination, and the assay in accordance with the general guidelines laid down in the pharmacopoeia. A further special paragraph describes the technical requirements for studies on stability and identifies which items have to be checked for which dosage form.

3.2.2.7 Manufacturing

Regarding the manufacturing of herbal medicines, Article 5 indicated that the manufacturer or sponsor should have sufficient staff with an adequate number of pharmacists or technical personnel with a title equivalent to or higher than associate engineer, and skilled workers adaptable to the scale of drug production. In addition, the preparation and slicing of raw plant materials should be performed by experienced pharmaceutical professionals familiar with the property of raw materials and registered with the health bureau above the county level to ensure that the processed medicinal plant materials are in compliance with the specifications of the Pharmacopoeia of the People's Republic of China or the processing norms stipulated by the health bureau of the province, autonomous region or municipality, see, Article 6 of MOPH (1984).

3.2.2.8 Quality Control

For the control of drug handling enterprises, Article 11 states that a drug handling enterprise should be established with an adequate number of pharmaceutical technicians adaptable to the scale of its business. However, enterprises engaged in the handling of modern drugs may be staffed with pharmaceutical

56 Quantitative Methods for Traditional Chinese Medicine Development

TABLE 3.2

Order of the State Council of the People's Republic of China

Chapter	Title	No. of Articles
I	General Provisions	7
II	Medical Institutions and Practitioners of Traditional Chinese Medicines	6
III	Education and Scientific Research on Traditional Chinese Medicines	11
IV	Guaranty Measures	7
V	Legal Liabilities	8

Note: The new regulations on TCM were adopted at the Third Executive Meeting of the State Council on April 2, 2003, and is promulgated and come into force on October 1, 2003.

professionals familiar with the property of drugs and registered with the health bureau above the county level, if pharmaceutical technicians are not available. Article 15 states that in the market of country fairs only the sale of medicinal plant materials is permitted, with certain exceptions.

3.2.2.9 Remarks

It should be noted that the MOPH of China has the authority to restrict or prohibit the exportation of medicinal plant materials and patent herbal medicines if they are in short supply in the domestic market (see, e.g., Article 29 of MOPH, 1984). In addition, the sale of medicinal plant materials newly discovered or introduced from abroad is not allowed unless it is approved by the health bureau of the province, autonomous region or municipality (see, Article 31 of MOPH, 1984).

In 2003, the Chinese government published new regulations *Order of the State Council of the People's Republic of China* to strengthen regulatory requirement for evaluation and approval of traditional Chinese medicines. The new regulations on TCM were adopted at the Third Executive Meeting of the State Council on April 2, 2003, and are promulgated and come into force on October 1, 2003. The new regulations contain five Chapters with 39 Articles (see Table 3.2).

3.3 Regulations on Herbal Products in Europe

Countries in the European Community (EC) including Austria, Belgium, Bulgaria, Estonia, Denmark, Finland, France, Germany, Greece, Hungary, Iceland, Ireland, Italy, the Netherlands, Norway, Portugal, Spain, Sweden, Switzerland, Turkey, and United Kingdom have similar but different

Regulations on Traditional Chinese Medicine 57

regulations on TCM. The EC has developed a comprehensive legislative network to facilitate the free movement of goods, capital, services, and persons in the EU. According to Directives 65/65/EEC (EC 1991) and 75/318/EEC (EC 1975a), pharmaceutical products require premarketing approval before gaining access to the market. Requirements for the documentation of quality, safety, and efficacy, the dossier, and expert reports are provided in Directive 91/507/EEC (EC 1991). Article 39 Para 2 of Directive 75/319/EEC (EC 1975b) obliged Member States to check all products on the market at that time, with a deadline of 12 years, to determine whether they met the requirements of these directives. Countries have taken different approaches in reviewing phytomedicines.

As indicated by Yang (2007), Europe accepted TCM earlier than the United States. For example, acupuncture has been popular in the continent for a century, and herbs are regarded as drugs and prescribed by physicians. In most European counties, acupuncture and herbal therapy are conducted mainly by Western medical doctors. In 2004, the governments of Italy and China signed agreements to intensify cooperation in the development and marketing of TCM, which faces difficulties entering the global market due to the lack of scientific evidence as to its safety and efficacy. The investments were increased in clinical studies and personnel exchanges to make TCM acceptable to public organizations and more patients in the West. In the same year, the European Union formed a new government panel to investigate the safety of herbal medicines. The Committee on Herbal Medicinal Products held its meetings every two months under new EU legislation designed to protect consumers. One of the goals of the panel is to harmonize regulation of the herbal product industry across the European Union. But so far, Germany and France are in advance in this field. Both countries have established their own complete effective regulatory systems specifically for TCM. For illustrative purposes, in what follows, we will focus on German regulations on TCM.

3.3.1 German Regulations on Herbal Products

3.3.1.1 Herbal Medicines Market

According to a report by Institut für Medizinische Statistik (IMS) (ESCOP 1990), the German herbal medicines market was worth US$ 1.7 billion in 1989, which was about 10 percent of the total pharmaceutical market in Germany. As indicated by a study conducted by the Allensbach Institute, about 58 percent of the German population had taken herbal remedies. The study also showed that over the years the number of younger people using natural medicines had increased significantly. The majority of the German population (85 percent) believe that the experience of physicians, practitioners, and patients should be accepted as a proof of the efficacy of natural medicines (AI 1989). In Germany, herbal medicines are available over-the-counter and on medical prescription through pharmacies. In principle, they are reimbursable under the health insurance system unless special criteria for exclusion apply. As indicated by Schwabe and Paffrath (1995), herbal medicines can be found among the 2000 most important drugs prescribed by medical doctors and reimbursed by health insurance.

3.3.1.2 Legal Status

In Germany, herbal medicines are considered as medicines. On January 1, 1978, the Second Medicines Act was enacted; this set new standards for herbal medicines. Under this regulation, proof of quality, safety, and efficacy become pre-requirements for the registration of medicines. The Medicines Act requires all member states to conduct review of all herbal medicines on the market to make sure that they are in accordance with the European Directive (Article 39 para 2 of Council Directive 75/319/EEC). The review of existing products was to establish *a priori* criteria for active ingredients that would be authorized. The review of herbal remedies is typically done by Commission E (a pluridisciplinary commission of experts consisting of pharmacists, pharmacologists, toxicologists, clinical pharmacologists, biostatisticians, medical doctors from hospitals, and general medical practitioners). Commission E is responsible for the evaluation of medicinal plants. The results (monographs) have been published in the Bundesanzeiger (Federal Gazette) since 1984, which cover most of the ingredients of industrially prepared herbal medicines on the market.

3.3.1.3 Requirements for Marketing Authorizations for Herbal Remedies

The Federal Institute for Drugs and Medical Devices, Bundesinstitut für Arzneimittel und Medizinprodukte (BfArM) is responsible for the assessment of medicines and the verification of submitted dossiers with respect to quality, safety, and efficacy. European Directives set forth criteria and guidelines for registration of herbal medicines. In practice, criteria and monographs developed by Commission E are widely used to document safety and efficacy of herbal remedies. Monographs developed by Commission E usually contain pharmacological, toxicological, and clinical information regarding quality, safety, and efficacy of herbal medicines. In addition, the monographs also include analytical test requirements and the texts for labels and package leaflets. Note that 279 monographs of standardized marketing authorizations (mainly for herbal teas) have been published. An applicant referring to such a monograph does not need to present any documentation to the BfArM.

In 1994, the fifth amendment of the German Medicines Act was passed and became effective. It not only provides a new procedure for proof of quality, safety, and efficacy but also widens the scope of existing legislation for products including herbal medicines already on the market. To assist the sponsors, the BfArM has compiled lists indicating which preparations are allowed

Regulations on Traditional Chinese Medicine 59

under this regulation and which traditional indications can be claimed. This new system may offer a legal possibility for a large number of preparations without sufficient scientific documentation as proof of efficacy to be re-registered under such a simplified procedure (see, e.g., Steinhoff 1993).

3.3.2 Harmonization on Herbal Products in EU

In the interest of harmonization of requirements across Member States within the European Community (EC), a system of mutual recognition of marketing authorization decisions has been installed (EC 1993). This system of mutual recognition indicates that an assessment by one national authority should be sufficient for subsequent registration in other Member States within EC. Under this system, the summary of product characteristics (SPC) approved by the first authority must be taken into account. If differences in evaluation occur between national authorities, a decision will be reached by an EC procedure. Note that there exist no uniform criteria regarding the assessment of safety and efficacy of herbal medicines but there is a guideline for quality of herbal remedies (EC 1989). The harmonization of scientific assessment is considered a precondition for adjustment of different marketing authorization decisions, particularly in the field of phytomedicines. As a result, the European Scientific Cooperative on Phytotherapy (ESCOP) was founded in 1989. The main objectives of ESCOP are to establish harmonized criteria for the assessment of phytomedicines and to support scientific research and to contribute to the acceptance of phytotherapy at a European level. In October 1990, the first five monographs were presented at a symposium in Brussels and were officially submitted to the Committee on Proprietary Medicinal Products (CPMP) of EC. Since then, the ESCOP continued preparing harmonized SPC proposals and completed 50 monographs by end of December 1996. Criteria for the selection of medicinal plants and the preparation of draft SPCs by the Scientific Committee are important for inclusion in the European Pharmacopoeia or a national pharmacopoeia. When a harmonized draft is regarded as finalized by the Scientific Committee, it is circulated to an independent Board of Supervising Editors. Members of this Board are scientists and experts from academia in European countries.

3.4 Regulations on Herbal Products as Dietary Supplements in the United States

3.4.1 Regulations for Dietary Supplements

In the United States, herbal and other dietary supplements are regulated as foods or nutraceuticals rather than drugs by the FDA. Nutraceutical is defined as any substance that may be considered as food or part of food that provides medical or health benefits, including the prevention and treatment of disease. This means that traditional Chinese herbal remedies do not have to meet the same standards as drugs and over-the-counter medications for proof of safety and effectiveness. In fact, the FDA cannot restrict the use of supplements unless substantial harm has been proven. It is highly imperative to have regulations for traditional Chinese herbal medicines or supplement. In 1997, per recommendation by Presidential Commission, the FDA was asked to convene an expert committee to review the wealth of information that already exists on botanicals and inform consumers and manufacturers about unsafe preparations.

FDA regulation of herbs falls into a somewhat gray area between food and drugs. Depending on their intended use, herbs and other products, such as vitamins and diet aids, might sometimes be considered foods, drugs, or both. However, herbs and herbal teas have been used for medicinal purposes for centuries. Many of today's most potent medicines, such as digitalis, morphine, and opium, are also derived from herbs. If an herbal tea makes a claim to prevent or cure a disease, FDA considers it to be a drug and regulates it as a drug product. This means the tea must be approved by FDA as safe and effective for its intended use.

In general, regulations on foods or dietary supplements are less strict than those on drugs (see, e.g., Abdel-Rahman et al. 2011). This can be demonstrated in two aspects specifically. First, unlike drug products, clinical studies in humans for evaluation of a supplement's safety are not required before the supplement is marketed. Second, the manufacturer does not have to prove that the supplement is effective. The manufacturer can indicate that the product addresses a nutrient deficiency, supports health, or reduces the risk of developing a health problem, However, if the manufacturer does make a claim, it must be followed by the statement that "This statement has not been evaluated by the Food and Drug Administration" and that "This product is not intended to diagnose, treat, cure, or prevent any disease."

3.4.2 Quality Issue

In practice, the FDA generally does not analyze the content of dietary supplements. Thus, the manufacturer is not required to prove quality of dietary supplements. However, manufacturers must meet the FDA's requirement for good manufacturing practice (GMP) for foods. GMPs describe conditions under which products must be prepared, packed, and stored.

Some manufacturers voluntarily follow the FDA's current good manufacturing practice (cGMP) for drugs, which are much stringent for quality control/assurance and consequently for product consistency. If the FDA finds a dietary supplement to be unsafe once it is on the market, only then can it take action against the manufacturer and/or distributor by issuing a warning or requiring the product to be removed from the marketplace. In March 2003, the

Regulations on Traditional Chinese Medicine 61

FDA published new proposed guidelines for supplements that would require manufacturers to avoid contaminating their products with other herbs, pesticides, heavy metals, or prescription drugs. The guidelines also require supplement labels to be accurate. The Federal Government also regulates supplement advertising, through the Federal Trade Commission. It requires that all information about supplements be truthful and not mislead consumers.

3.4.3 Safety Concern

Although herbs have been used as dietary supplements for years, quality and safety of herbal preparations could be a great concern. In late 1990s, several dozen Japanese died after taking a popular liver tonic called shosikoto, which had been certified by the national health insurance program, but its safety was never tested. In 2004, the May issue of "Consumer Reports" published a list of the 12 most dangerous supplements. Two traditional Chinese herbal products from China are categorized as absolutely dangerous due to their containing of aristolochic acid. Taking these two supplements could result in cancer, renal disease, or even death. Thus, it is suggested that these supplements should not be used. Herbal supplements can cause problems if they are not used correctly or if they are taken in large amounts. In some cases, people have experienced negative effects even though they followed the instructions on a supplement label.

3.4.4 Remarks

The manufacturer of a dietary supplement is responsible for ensuring the quality, safety, and effectiveness of the product before it can be sold in the market place. The FDA does not require testing of dietary supplements prior to marketing. However, while manufacturers are prohibited from selling dangerous products, the FDA can remove a product from the marketplace if the product is dangerous to public health. Furthermore, if in the labeling or marketing of a dietary supplement a claim is made that the product can diagnose, treat, cure, or prevent disease, the product is considered an unapproved new drug and hence it cannot be sold over-the-counter.

3.5 Regulations on Herbal Products as Drug Products in the United States

3.5.1 Botanical Drug Products

As indicated in the previous section, TCM is often considered as food or dietary supplements. In early 2000s, with the increasing demand, the FDA was under pressure to regulate the TCM as drugs rather than as foods. The FDA's old regulations require sponsors to identify exactly what kind of herbal ingredients can cure and prove their effectiveness. Owing to the complex nature of a typical herbal drug and the lack of knowledge of its active constituent(s), the requirements of old regulations may not be appropriate. Following European regulations for traditional Chinese herbal medicine and to meet the special properties of TCM, FDA lowered the hurdle by setting a new regulation specifically for botanical drug products including TCM.

FDA defines a botanical product as a finished, labeled product that contains vegetable matter, which may include plant materials, algae, or combinations of these. Depending in part on its intended use, a botanical product may be a food, drug, medical device, or cosmetic. Only when a botanical product is intended for use in diagnosing, mitigating, treating, curing, or preventing disease is it taken as a botanical drug product or botanical drug and subject to the new regulation as a drug. A botanical drug substance, on the other hand, is a drug substance derived from one or more plants, algae, or macroscopic fungi. It can be made from one or more botanical raw materials. A botanical drug substance does not include a highly purified or chemically modified substance derived from natural sources.

3.5.2 Regulations on Botanical Products

In 2004, the US FDA published guidance on botanical drug products, which explains when a botanical drug may be marketed under an over-the-counter drug monograph, when FDA regulations require approval for marketing of NDA, and when INDs for botanical products currently lawfully marketed as foods in the United States (FDA 2004). To provide a better understanding of the review process in the Center for Drug Evaluation and Research (CDER) for INDs and NDAs for botanical drug products, the CDER of FDA also published the Manual of Policies and Procedures (MAPP): Review of Botanical Drug Products, which describes the review process in CDER for INDs and NDAs for botanical drug products (MAPP 2004). The MAPP (2004) recommends that the guidance entitled *Guidance for Industry – INDs for Phase 2 and Phase 3 Studies, Chemistry, Manufacturing, and Controls Information* be consulted for preparing CMC information that would be submitted for phase 2 and phase 3 studies required for botanical drug product development conducted under INDs in the United States (FDA 2003c).

As indicated in the 2003 FDA guidance, similar to conventional drug development, the INDs for botanical drug products should include protocols, chemistry, manufacturing, and control (CMC), pharmacological and toxicology information, and previous human experience with the product (Table 3.3). Requirements for CMC and nonclinical safety assessment are given in Tables 3.4 and 3.5, respectively. Table 3.4 indicates that animal safety tests need to be performed. This requirement, however, refers to an acute animal toxicity test applied only to an injectable drug product. For matching

Regulations on Traditional Chinese Medicine

TABLE 3.3

Basic Format for IND for Botanical Drug Products

Cover sheet
Table of contents
Introductory statement and general investigational plan
Investigator's brochure
Protocols
Chemistry, manufacturing, and controls
Pharmacological and toxicology information
Previous human experience with the product

TABLE 3.4

CMC Requirements for INDs of Botanical Drug Products

Botanical raw material
Botanical drug substance and product
Animal safety test
Placebo
Labeling
Environmental assessment

TABLE 3.5

Requirements for Nonclinical Safety Assessment

Repeat-dose general toxicity studies
Nonclinical pharmacokinetic/toxicokinetic studies
Reproductive toxicology
Genotoxicity studies
Carcinogenicity studies
Special pharmacology/toxicology studies
Regulatory consideration

placebo, the FDA requires that the components of any placebo used must be described. For phase 3 clinical studies, the FDA requires that the following information that (1) description of product and documentation of human experience, (2) chemistry, manufacturing, and controls, (3) nonclinical safety assessment, (4) bioavailability and clinical pharmacology, and (5) clinical considerations must be provided. Figure 3.1 provides a summary for information required for an IND of botanical drug products.

3.5.3 Current Review Process for Botanical Products

Regulatory review of botanical submission includes CMC information review, clinical pharmacology/biopharmaceutics information review, nonclinical

64   *Quantitative Methods for Traditional Chinese Medicine Development*

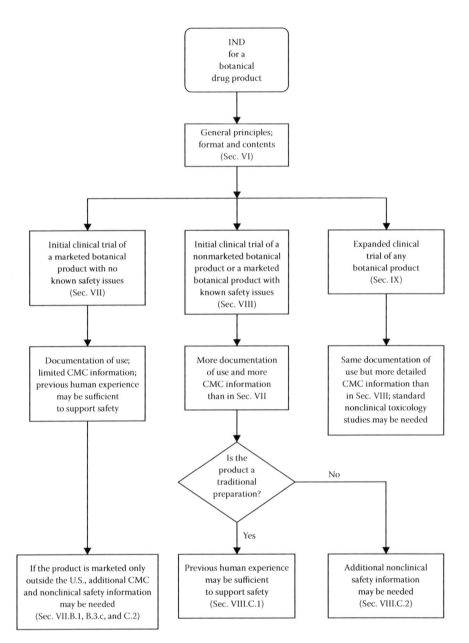

FIGURE 3.1
Information required for an IND of botanical drug products.

pharmacology and toxicology information review, and medical/statistical information review. For each botanical submission, the FDA establishes a botanical review team (BRT) to assist the review divisions for review of the botanical submission. The BRT review covers (1) biology of medicinal plant identification, potential misuse of related species, (2) pharmacology of the botanical product-activity/toxicology in old documents and new testings, (3) prior human experiences with the botanical product—past clinical use and relevance to current setting. The botanical team will perform pharmacognosy review throughout the IND and NDA process and a botanical-specific medical review. For issues related to specific applications, the botanical team will not have direct contact with the sponsors. However, the botanical team may respond directly to general inquiries related to botanical guidance and other relevant policies/procedures. Note that all communications will be transmitted through the review division. A flow chart that describes regulatory approaches for marketing botanical drug products is given in Figure 3.2.

3.5.4 Botanical Products versus Chemical Drugs

Although regulatory requirements for botanical products are similar to those for chemical drugs in principle, there are many differences in policy issues, which are summarized below.

3.5.4.1 Purification and Identification

Botanical drugs are derived from vegetable matter and are usually prepared as complex mixtures. Their chemical constituents are not always well defined. In many cases, the active constituent in a botanical drug is not identified nor is its biological activity well characterized. A new botanical drug (containing multiple chemical constituents) may qualify as a new chemical entity. Both purification and identification of the active ingredients in botanicals are optional and not required. In the initial stage of clinical studies of a botanical drug, it is generally not necessary to identify the active constituents or other biological markers or to have a chemical identification and assay for a particular constituent or marker. Identification by spectroscopic and/or chromatographic fingerprinting and strength by dry weight (weight minus water or solvents) can be acceptable alternatives.

3.5.4.2 Test and Control

Because of the complex nature of a typical botanical drug and the lack of knowledge of its active constituent(s), the FDA may rely on a combination of tests and controls to ensure the identity, purity, quality, strength, potency, and consistency of botanical drugs. These tests and controls include (1) multiple tests for drug substance and drug product (e.g., spectroscopic and/or

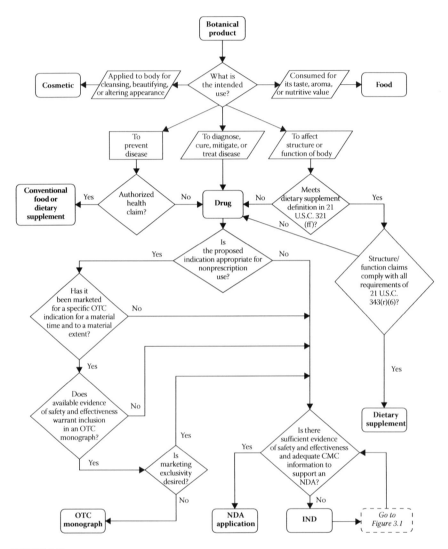

FIGURE 3.2
Regulatory approaches for marketing botanical drug products.

chromatographic fingerprints, chemical assay of characteristic markers, and biological assay), (2) raw material and process controls (e.g., strict quality controls for the botanical raw materials and adequate in-process controls), and (3) process validation (especially for the drug substance).

Raw material and environmental issue: because the botanical drug products are allowed to remain as complex mixtures, quality consistency is a more complicated issue than that of nonbotanicals. Plant materials used in the production of botanical drug products often are not completely

Regulations on Traditional Chinese Medicine

characterized and defined or are prone to contamination, deterioration, and variation in composition and properties. In many cases, the active constituent in a botanical drug is not identified nor is its biological activity well characterized. Therefore, in contrast to the situation with synthetic or highly purified drug products, it may be difficult to ensure the quality of a botanical drug by controlling only the corresponding drug substance and drug product. To ensure that a botanical drug product used in clinical trials is of consistently good quality and that sufficient information exists to meet the requirements, the sponsor should have, in addition to final product testing, appropriate quality controls for the botanical raw materials. It became necessary to extend the control of botanical drug substance and product to that of botanical raw material, and in some cases, to the agricultural aspects of growing/harvesting medicinal plants by following good agricultural and good collection practices for starting materials of herbal origin. The FDA encourages early consultation with the Agency on environment-related aspects of a requested action, especially one that involves harvesting a wild species to ensure that planning and decisions reflect environmental values, avoid delays later in the process, and avoid potential conflicts.

Bioavailability: because there could be more than one active constituent in a botanical drug or the active constituent may not be identified, it could be difficult or impossible to perform standard *in vivo* bioavailability and pharmacokinetic studies. If this is not possible, the bioavailability of a botanical drug could be based on clinical effects observed in well-controlled clinical trials. FDA may, for good cause, waive or defer the *in vivo* bioavailability study requirement if a waiver or deferral is compatible with the protection of the public health.

FDA does not require that all studies submitted in an NDA be conducted under an IND. Clinical studies need not necessarily be conducted under an IND (i.e., if they are carried out abroad). The clinical data generated from these studies conducted without an IND can be used to support an NDA if the studies were adequately designed and conducted under good clinical practices. However, although an IND is not required by law in all cases, the sponsor is encouraged to go through the IND process.

3.5.4.3 Individualized Treatments

In many cases, botanical therapies are highly individualized with variations in relative contents of multiple plant ingredients tailored for each patient. A sponsor may not submit a separate IND for every change in composition if similar patients are being treated for the same indication. Studies can be designed to take into account individualized treatments. Multiple formulations can be included in one IND if they are being studied under a single clinical trial. It is important that the IND provide the rationale for using multiple formulations and the criteria used to assign patients to different treatment regimens.

3.5.4.4 Toxicity

Many medicinal plants with therapeutic potential are quite toxic. Well-known examples of safety issues concerning botanicals include the nephrotoxicity associated with herbal preparations containing aristolochic acid and the hepatotoxicity associated with comfrey products containing pyrrolizidine alkaloid. Other examples include the cardiovascular and central nervous system effects associated with yohimbe and the hepatotoxicity associated with germander and chaparral. When the potential benefit of an investigational drug outweighs its risk in the intended patient population, clinical trials may be allowed to proceed under an IND.

3.5.4.5 Prior Human Experience

The Guidance also stipulates that because many botanicals have been used as medicine in alternative medical systems for a long time, prior human experience may substitute for animal toxicology studies in the preliminary safety evaluation of IND studies. How these human data, mostly not of modern scientific quality, can be useful to support an NDA application was not clearly described in the Guidance. The Agency recognizes that prior human experience with a botanical product can be documented in many different forms and sources, some of which may not meet the quality standards of modern scientific testing. The sponsor is encouraged to provide as much data as possible, and the review team for the botanical drug IND generally will accept all available information for regulatory consideration. The FDA will assess the quality of the submitted data on a case-by-case basis. It should be emphasized that, in reviewing botanical drugs, the Agency does not lower or raise the safety and efficacy standards for marketing approval that apply to purified chemical drugs.

3.5.4.6 Priority

The FDA treats botanical and purified chemical drugs the same. The FDA will assign the same level of priority to botanical drug products as to other drugs with respect to meeting with IND sponsors and NDA applicants. For clinical data to support marketing approval, there should be no difference between botanical and nonbotanical drugs. The Guidance also provides two flow charts for (1) the regulatory approaches for marketing botanical drug products and (2) the information to be provided in an IND for a botanical drug. The two flow charts are included in this chapter to elucidate the process of the new policy. With the release of the new FDA guidance and approval of first botanical drug, more and more botanical drugs are predicted to be developed and get into the approval process. In the near future, botanical drugs will be accepted by the mainstream medical field. The competition in the drug industry will be tighter.

3.6 Conclusions

Traditional chinese medicines (TCM) have worked well for centuries. The interest in using them is growing, and the research on them is increasing. The Western narrow scientific approach tends to miss the point of the ancient practices. Consequently, it has become a hurdle to the acceptance of TCM in the mainstream. The FDA's old regulations on drugs have some limitations and are not appropriate to regulate TCM as drugs. The FDA's recent release of new guidance and approval of the first botanical drug brings a significant impact in drug industry. More botanical drugs and tighter competition are expected. There is a potential role for some complementary medicine and natural health products in preparing us to meet the challenges of the 21st century. The FDA hired experts to enrich the education sector and have the new Botanicals Review Team (BTR) to perform pharmaceutical assessment. The team includes a team leader, pharmacologist, reviewer, and other experts. Now many companies are submitting applications of botanical drug products to the FDA and some drugs are into the clinical stage. Currently, about 250 botanicals have been approved into clinical trials. Most drugs are based on traditional Chinese medicine.

For too long, the natural health products industry has kept its distance from medical research and from clinical medical practice, focusing instead on the short-term marketing advantages derived from keeping herbal and nutritional remedies exempt from any FDA review of efficacy. A wiser approach should be for the natural products industry to work with medical research, including the FDA, so that consumers and medical practitioners could be warned about potential harm and assured that the claimed health benefits were really there. The public needs good science to sort the worthless and dangerous from the potentially helpful. Many scientists support efforts to investigate alternative therapies "provided that the research is held to rigorous scientific standards, is suitably peer-reviewed, and is fairly administered," as expressed by Nobel laureates Paul Berg, a Stanford University biochemist, and Jerome Friedman, a Massachusetts Institute of Technology physicist. However, Western pharmacology studies focus on identifying single compounds to treat diseases.

In early 1990s, the FDA started drafting of *Guidance for Industry: Botanical Drug Products*. The final version was released in June 2004. Currently, there are several botanical drugs, including cascara, psyllium, and sienna, that are included in the OTC drug review. On October 31, 2006, just about 2 years after the release of its new regulation, FDA approved the first ever submitted New Drug Application (NDA) for a botanical drug product, Polyphenon E Ointment. The approval for Polyphenon E Ointment has been made out to the name Veregen. The product is developed by a German biotech company MediGene AG and is indicated for the treatment of external and perianal genital warts. Orally administered green tea, catechins, or catechins-rich green tea extracts were reported to have several health benefits including anti-oxidative, chemo-preventive, anti-tumor, and other health protective activities. Although tea was considered a panacea for some, as a *Materia Medica* in TCM, tea is known to have side effects. Overdose of tea could cause sleeplessness or insomnia. MediGene AG tried a new way of using green tea. The clinical trial indicated that Veregen showed high and sustained efficacy with very few adverse events in the treatment of genital warts. The results come from an international phase III trial with more than 1000 patients in 15 countries medicated with Veregen. For the purpose of FDA approval, the safety and efficacy of Veregen were studied in two randomized, double-blind clinical studies on nearly 400 adults with external genital and anal warts.

The significance of this approval is that the active substance in Veregen is an extract from green tea leaves. Veregen is a relatively simple botanical derived from a single part of a single plant (green tea leaves), containing a class of well-studied chemical entities as the major active ingredients (catechins). Because of the unique nature of botanicals, the FDA finds it appropriate to apply regulatory policies that differ from those applied to synthetic, semisynthetic, or otherwise highly purified or chemically modified drugs. The major change in the new policy is that, for those who want to develop prescribed drugs from plant extracts, they only need to extract one effective material, and this extracted material may contain hundreds of compounds. There is no longer a need to indicate the effect of each single compound. The implementation of the new policy brought about a substantial growth in NDA submission of herbal drug products so that the FDA even set up a special office to receive such applications.

4

Reference Standards and Product Specifications

4.1 Introduction

As discussed in Chapter 1, most TCMs consist of a number of active and/ or inactive ingredients (components). These components may be extracted from natural resources such as plants. In practice, however, some components may not be able to be fully characterized even with advanced technology. Thus, many of their pharmacological activities may remain unknown. In this case, it is almost impossible to evaluate the effectiveness and safety of the TCM under investigation following the process of pharmaceutical development the Western way. For commonly used Chinese herbal medicines, the Pharmacopoeia of the People's Republic of China (*Chinese Pharmacopoeia*) is an official and authoritative compendium of Chinese herbal medicines. It covers almost all traditional Chinese herbal medicines and most Western medicines and preparations. It provides information on the standards of purity, description, test, dosage, precaution, storage, and strength for each herbal medicine. The herbal medicines included in the *Chinese Pharmacopoeia* are considered reference standards in TCM development. These reference standards are useful in establishing product specification in TCM development.

For a given TCM, although analytical methods and reference standards for individual components may be available in the Pharmacopoeia, the relative proportions of individual components toward the final product of TCM are usually unknown. Thus, analytical methods for quantitative assessment of these components are necessarily developed based on available reference standards. In most TCMs, the relative proportions of individual components may have an impact on the clinical outcomes (i.e., safety and efficacy). Thus, it is important not only to establish reference standards, specifications, and/ or relative proportions of individual components for achieving the optimal therapeutic effect but also to study the possible component-to-component interaction. In some cases, some of these individual components may not be relevant to the clinical efficacy but to reduce the incidence of adverse events

71

72 Quantitative Methods for Traditional Chinese Medicine Development

for tolerability. To address these questions, a factorial design for combinational drug products at different levels is often conducted.

In Section 4.2, *Chinese Pharmacopoeia*, the U.S. Pharmacopoeia (PDR for Herbal Medicine), and European Pharmacopoeia, which are commonly considered as reference standards, are briefly described. Section 4.3 discusses product specification for quality control and assurance of traditional Chinese medicine. Multilevel factorial designs that are frequently used for characterizing combinational drug products with multiple dose levels are reviewed in Section 4.4. Section 4.5 posts some practical issues that are commonly encountered during the development of traditional Chinese medicines. Some concluding remarks are given in Section 4.6.

4.2 Reference Standards

For pharmaceutical research and development, each country publishes a pharmacopoeia, which provides information on the standards of purity, description, test, dosage, precaution, storage, and strength for each drug. In this section, for illustration purpose, we briefly describe the 2010 version of Pharmacopoeia of the People's Republic of China, the USP *Chinese Pharmacopoeia*, and European Pharmacopoeia, which cover almost traditional Chinese medicines and most Western medicines and preparations.

4.2.1 *Chinese Pharmacopoeia*

The Pharmacopoeia of the People's Republic of China (PPRC), which is usually referred to as *Chinese Pharmacopoeia* (CP) by the China Food and Drug Administration (CFDA), Ministry of Health of China. The *Chinese Pharmacopoeia* 2010, which is the ninth edition of *Chinese Pharmacopoeia* since the founding of the founding of the People's Republic of China, features significant revisions and improvements as compared to the *Chinese Pharmacopoeia* 1997. The English edition of *Chinese Pharmacopoeia* 2010 compiled by the Pharmacopoeia Commission of the Ministry of Health is an official and authoritative compendium of drugs. It covers traditional Chinese medicines, most Western medicines and preparations, giving information on the standards of purity, description, test, dosage, precaution, storage, and strength for each drug. It is recognized by the World Health Organization as the official *Chinese Pharmacopoeia*.

Contents of the *Chinese Pharmacopoeia* 2010 are given in Table 4.1. The key features of the *Chinese Pharmacopoeia* 2010 are outlined below. First, it includes 4567 total monographs. Among these monographs, 1386 are for new admissions and 2228 are for revisions. Second, the *Chinese Pharmacopoeia* 2010 emphasizes (1) concepts of the wild resource protection and sustainable

Reference Standards and Product Specifications

TABLE 4.1

Contents of *Chinese Pharmacopoeia* 2010

Volume	Monographs	New Admissions	Revisions	Content
I	2165	1019	634	Chinese material medica Prepared slices of Chinese crude drugs Vegetable oils Fats and extracts Patented Chinese traditional medicines Single ingredients of Chinese crude drug preparations
II	2271	330	1500	Chemical drugs Antibiotics Biochemical preparations Radiopharmaceuticals Excipients for pharmaceutical use
III	131	37	94	Biological products

development of traditional Chinese medicines, (2) pharmaceutical safety in General Notices, Appendices, and Monographs, (3) applications of contemporary analytical technologies, and (4) the development of green standards. In the English edition, the 2005 version of *Chinese Pharmacopoeia* consists of three volumes (ISBN 7117069821) and a total of 2691 monographs (992 for traditional Chinese medicines and 1699 for modern western drugs). It is considered a compendium of almost all traditional Chinese medicines and most Western medicines and preparations. Information is given for each drug on standards of purity, description, test, dosage, precaution, storage, and strength. Volume I contains monographs of Chinese material medica and pared slice, vegetable oil/fat and its extract, Chinese traditional patent medicines, single ingredients of Chinese crude drug preparations, etc.; Volume II deals with monographs of chemical drugs, antibiotics, biochemical preparations, radiopharmaceuticals, and excipients for pharmaceutical use; Volume III contains biological products.

As compared with the 2005 *Chinese Pharmacopoeia*, the 2010 *Chinese Pharmacopoeia* has significant changes that can be outlined in the following aspects. First, on the basis of the previous edition, containing relevant species a significant increase in species containing a total of 4615 kinds of income, new varieties of 1358, an increase of 42 percent, 69 percent revision rate for the calendar version of the maximum. Second, drug test ways to increase testing, higher standards, so in the drug safety and controllability have more to upgrade. Third, standards for Chinese medicine have a breakthrough and innovation, especially in the past, Chinese herbal medicine and Chinese medicine are relatively weak pieces of new and revised standards, there were a major breakthrough. Fourth, the new Pharmacopoeia in

74 *Quantitative Methods for Traditional Chinese Medicine Development*

the Legend, variety of standards, appendix, etc. General formulations have a greater change and progress, largely with international practice. Finally, the new Pharmacopoeia of adhering to scientific, practical, standardized, and drug safety, quality control of and standards of the advanced nature of principle, seek to cover the National Essential Drugs List species and social health insurance reimbursement catalogs kinds.

Note that there are over three hundred herbs that are commonly being used today. Some of the most commonly used herbs are listed in Table 4.2.

4.2.2 PDR for Herbal Medicines

In the United States, herbal products are marketed under the provisions of the *Dietary Supplement and Health Education Act* of 1994, which prohibits their sale for the diagnosis, treatment, cure, or prevention of any disease. Enumeration of specific commercial preparations within an herbal monograph should not be construed as a claim or warranty of their efficacy for any purpose by either the manufacturer or the publisher. Furthermore, it should be understood that, just as omission of a product does not signify rejection, inclusion of a product does not imply endorsement and that the publisher is not advocating the use of any product or substance described herein.

TABLE 4.2

List of Most Commonly Used Herbs

English Name	Chinese Name
Ginseng	人参, rénshēn
Wolfberry	枸杞子
Angelica sinensis	当归, dāngguī
Astragalus	黄耆, huángqí
Atractylodes	白术, báizhú
Bupleurum	柴胡, cháihú
Cinnamon twigs	桂枝, guìzhī
Cinnamon bark	肉桂, ròuguì
Coptis	黄莲, huánglián
Ginger	姜, jiāng
Hoelen	茯苓, fúlíng
Licorice	甘草, gāncǎo
Ephedra sinica	麻黄, máhuáng
Peony	White: 白芍, báisháo Reddish: 赤芍, chìsháo
Rehmannia	地黄, dìhuáng
Rhubarb	大黄, dàhuáng
Salvia	丹参, dānshēn

Reference Standards and Product Specifications 75

The PDR for Herbal Medicines is the product of one of the most thorough and inclusive examinations of the herbal literature ever undertaken. Nevertheless, it is important to remember that it merely summarizes and synthesizes key data from the underlying research reports and of necessity includes neither every published report nor every recorded fact.

The PDR for Herbal Medicines provides with the closest available analog to FDA-approved labeling—the findings of the German Regulatory Authority's herbal watchdog agency, commonly called "Commission E." This agency has conducted an intensive assessment of the peer-reviewed literature on some 300 common botanicals, weighing the quality of the clinical evidence and identifying the uses for which the herb can reasonably be considered effective. Its conclusions represent the best expert consensus on medicinal herbs currently available. For the herbs not considered by Commission E, the PDR for Herbal Medicines provides the results of an exhaustive literature review conducted by the respected PhytoPharm U.S. Institute of Phytopharmaceuticals under the direction of noted botanist, Dr. Joerg Gruenwald. These additional monographs, now some 400 in number, provide a detailed introduction to an array of exotic botanicals that you will be hard pressed to find in any other source.

Each monograph contains title, trade name, description, actions and pharmacology, indication and usage, contraindications, precautions and adverse reactions, over dosage, dosage, and literature. The title of each specific herb is referred to by the generally accepted common name followed by the scientific name, description such as detailed botanical review of the herb including its medicinal parts (flower and fruit, leaves, stem, and root), unique characteristic, habitat, production, related plants, and additional common names and synonyms. The section of actions and pharmacology include data on the active compounds or heterogeneous mixtures found in the plant and a summary of its clinical effects. Information regarding indication and usage is listed under the categories of (1) approved by Commission E, (2) unproven uses, (3) Chinese medicine, (4) indicant medicine, and (5) homeopathic. As a few pharmacologically potent herbs should be avoided in the presence of certain medical conditions, such contraindications are summarized in the section on contraindications. The section on precautions and adverse reactions includes any restrictions on use in pregnancy or childhood and any notably side effects reported in the available literature. Whenever adverse effects of overdose have been found in the literature, they are also reported in the section on overdoses. The section on dosage describes the common modes of administration, forms and strengths of available commercial preparations, methods for preparing the natural herb, and representative dosage recommendations drawn from the literature. Although the dosage recommendation can be used only as a general guide, the potency of individual preparations and extracts is subject to substantial variation. Thus, it is suggested that the manufacturer's directions should be consulted whenever available.

76   *Quantitative Methods for Traditional Chinese Medicine Development*

For example, the scientific name of *Lotus* is *Nelumbo nucifera*. The medicinal parts are the roots, the seeds, and the aerial part of the flowering plant. The plant is indigenous to India. *Lotus* is the whole plant of *Nelumbo nucifera*. The active compounds of *Lotus* are the *alkaloids nelumbin* and *roemerine* in the leaves. The drug is an astringent. The powdered beans are often used in the treatment of digestive disorders, particularly diarrhea, while flowers are used an as astringent for bleeding. However, these usages are considered unproven. No health hazards or side effects for *Lotus* are known in conjunction with the proper administration of designated therapeutic dosages. The mode of administration for *Lotus* includes power and liquid extract for internal use.

4.2.3 European Pharmacopoeia

The 8th edition of the European Pharmacopoeia (Ph. Eur.) was published in July 2013. A new edition is updated and published every 3 years. The 8th edition of Ph. Eur. comprises two initial volumes which contain the complete set of the 7th edition texts and the texts adopted or revised at the November 2012 session of the European Pharmacopoeia Commission including 2224 monographs, 345 general chapters illustrated with diagrams or chromatograms, and 2500 descriptions of regents.

Several legal texts make the European Pharmacopoeia mandatory in Europe, including (1) Convention on the Elaboration of a European Pharmacopoeia, and amending Protocol (following accession of the European Union), and (2) European Union Directives 2001/82/EC and 2001/83/EC, as amended, and 2003/63/EC on medicines for human and veterinary use. These state the legally binding character of European Pharmacopoeia texts for marketing authorization applications. As indicated in Directive 2001/83/EC as amended, the monographs of the European Pharmacopoeia shall be applicable to all substances, preparations, and pharmaceutical forms appearing in it. In respect of other substances, each Member State may require observance of its own national pharmacopoeia. Also, in the case where starting and raw materials, active substance(s) or excipient(s) are described neither in the European Pharmacopoeia nor in the pharmacopoeia of a Member State, compliance with the monograph of a third country pharmacopoeia can be accepted. In such cases, the applicant shall submit a copy of the monograph accompanied by the validation of the analytical procedures contained in the monograph and by a translation where appropriate.

European Pharmacopoeia provides specifications in monographs for the following products: (1) active substances including antibiotics, (2) excipients, (3) biologicals, blood and plasma derivatives, vaccines and radiopharmaceutical preparations, (4) dosage forms, (5) homoeopathic preparations and homoeopathic stocks, and (6) herbal drugs, herbal drug preparations

Reference Standards and Product Specifications

TABLE 4.3

Number of Texts Included in European Pharmacopoeia

Monograph for	Number of Texts (Approximately)
APIs	1480
Excipients	370
Finished dosage forms	30
Biologicals	295
General	22
Supplementary*	3210

* 33 general texts, 258 methods of analysis, 2513 reagents, 26 materials and containers, and 1 suture.

and Traditional Chinese Medicines. The numbers of texts (approximately) included in the pharmacopoeia is summarized in Table 4.3.

Note that most monographs require at least one reference standard and the reference standard underpins the quality standard. Thus, there are about 2200 reference standards in European Pharmacopoeia.

4.2.4 Remarks

It should be noted that reference standards for specific components of a TCM such as botanical components as described in *Chinese Pharmacopoeia*, PDR for Herbal Medicines, and European Pharmacopoeia may be similar but different owing to differences in (1) locations of raw materials, (2) assay methods used, (3) experiences in different regions (e.g., Asian Pacific region and the United States), and (4) interpretation and perception of the pharmacological activity and/or therapeutic effect.

4.3 Product Specifications

As indicated by USP/NF, a drug product is said to possess good drug characteristics such as identity, strength, quality, and purity if the good drug characteristics remain within some acceptance limits (product specifications) of the good drug characteristics prior to the expiration dating period of the drug product. As an example, without loss of generality, consider manufacturing tablets of a drug product. To ensure that a drug product will meet the USP/NF (2000) standards for the identity, strength, quality, and purity of the drug product, a number of tests such as potency testing, content uniformity testing, dissolution testing, and disintegration testing are usually performed at various stages of the manufacturing process of the drug product.

78   *Quantitative Methods for Traditional Chinese Medicine Development*

In this book, we will refer to these tests as USP tests. The USP/NF provides standard testing procedure and requirements regarding sampling plan and acceptance criteria for each of these USP tests.

4.3.1 Testing Procedure

For Good Laboratory Practice (GLP), testing procedures must be clearly described with sufficient information in a way such that laboratory technicians or analysts are able to verify the compliance of the drug product up to the end of drug expiration dating period (shelf life). The analytical methods must be validated in accordance with regulatory guidelines/guidance (see, e.g., FDA 2001b). The results of analytical method validation must be documented for GLP. The testing procedure should include the description of the reference substance including its specifications and the description of the calculation formula (or an example of the calculation regardless of whether they are performed by an automatic instrument), chromatograms, and spectra furnishing the proof of the results obtained. As an example, consider dissolution testing. Dissolution testing is typically performed by placing a dosage unit in a 1000-mL transparent vessel containing a dissolution medium. A variable-speed motor rotates a cylindrical basket containing the dosage unit. The dissolution medium is analyzed to determine the percent of the drug dissolved. The dissolution test is typically performed on six units simultaneously. The dissolution medium is usually sampled at various predetermined intervals to form a dissolution profile (over time).

In practice, a testing procedure may use either an official reference substance (e.g., European Pharmacopoeia or USP/NF) or a working standard provided that the latter is standardized against the official reference substance. It should be noted that an analytical result cannot be dissociated from the method used. Thus, in practice, it is assumed that the specifications adopted for the tests and assay are established from the methods described in the Pharmacopoeia (e.g., *Chinese Pharmacopoeia*, USP/NF, and European Pharmacopoeia). Methods other than the methods described in the Pharmacopoeia may be used for control purposes providing that these methods are validated with reference to the official method and providing that these methods used enable an unequivocal decision to be made as to whether compliance with the standards of the monograph would be achieved if the official methods were used. In addition, the general methods described in the Pharmacopoeia may be used for products not described in the Pharmacopoeia or for specifications not described in individual monographs.

4.3.2 Sampling Plan and Acceptance Criteria

The USP/NF requires that a specific sampling plan for the individual USP test be employed and that specific acceptance criteria be met in order to pass

Reference Standards and Product Specifications   79

the test. In this subsection, sampling and acceptance criteria for individual USP tests are described.

4.3.2.1 Potency Testing

Let Y_i be the assay results of the potency, $i = 1, \ldots, K$. Also, let LPS and UPS denote the lower and the upper product specifications as designated in the USP/NF individual monograph. Then the requirement for potency testing is met if all of the individual assay results and the average assay results lie within (LPS, UPS), where LPS and UPS are lower and upper product specification, respectively. If the requirement is not met, additional assays may be required.

4.3.2.2 Content Uniformity Testing

For the determination of dosage uniformity by assay of individual units, the USP/NF recommends assaying 10 units individually, as directed in the assay in the individual monograph, unless specified otherwise in the test for content uniformity. Where a special procedure is specified in the test for content uniformity in the individual monograph, the results should be adjusted (see, e.g., Chow and Liu 1995). The requirements for dose uniformity are met if the amount of the active ingredient in each of the 10 dosage units conforms to the acceptance criteria given in Table 4.4. The requirements for dosage uniformity are met if the amount of active ingredient in each of the 10 dosage units lies within the range of 85–115 percent of label claim and the relative standard deviation is less than 6 percent. If one unit is outside the range of 85–115 percent of the label claim and no unit is outside the range of 75–125 percent of the label claim, or if the relative standard deviation is greater than 6 percent, or if both conditions prevail, test 20 additional units. The requirements are met if not more than one unit of the 30 units is outside the range of 85–115 percent of the label claim and no unit is outside the range 75–125 percent of the label claim and the relative standard deviation of the 30 dosage units does not exceed 7.8 percent.

TABLE 4.4

Acceptance Criteria for Content Uniformity Testing

Stage	Number Tested	Pass IF
S_1	10	1. Each of the 10 units lies within the range of 85% to 115% of the label claim. 2. The relative standard deviation is less than or equal to 6%.
S_2	20	1. No more than one unit of the 30 units ($S_1 + S_2$) is outside the range of 85% to 115% of label claim. 2. No unit is outside the range of 75% to 125% of label claim. 3. The relative standard deviation of the 30 units ($S_1 + S_2$) does not exceed 7.8%.

80 *Quantitative Methods for Traditional Chinese Medicine Development*

It should be noted that the acceptance criteria in Table 4.4 apply only if the average of the limits specified in the potency definition in the individual monograph is 100 percent or less. If the average of the limits specified in the potency definition in the individual monograph is greater than 100 percent, the requirements are the same as those given in Table 4.4 except that the words *label claim* are replaced by the words *label claim multiplied by the average of the limits specified in the potency definition in the monograph divided by 100.*

4.3.2.3 Dissolution Testing

The USP/NF provides detailed sampling plan and acceptance criteria for dissolution testing (see Table 4.5). The requirements are met if the quantities of active ingredient dissolved from the units conform to the USP/NF acceptance criteria. Let Q be the amount of dissolved active ingredient specified in the individual monograph, which is usually expressed as a percentage of label claim. The USP/NF dissolution acceptance criteria comprise a three-stage sampling plan. For the first stage (S_1), six dosage units are to be tested. The requirement for the first stage is met if each unit is not less than Q + 5%. If the product fails to pass S_1, an additional six units will be tested at the second stage (S_2). The product is considered to have passed if the average of the 12 units from S_1 and S_2 is equal to or greater than Q and if no unit is less than $Q - 15\%$. If the product fails to pass both S_1 and S_2, an additional 12 units will be tested at the third stage (S_3). If the average of all 24 units from S_1, S_2, and S_3 is equal to or greater than Q, no more than two units are less than $Q - 15\%$, and no unit is less than $Q - 25\%$, the product has passed the USP/NF dissolution test.

4.3.2.4 Disintegration Testing

The USP/NF provides a detailed sampling plan and acceptance criteria for disintegration testing (see Table 4.6). Disintegration testing is to determine

TABLE 4.5

Acceptance Criteria for Dissolution Testing

Stage	Number Tested	Pass IF
S_1	6	Each unit is not less than $Q + 5\%$
S_2	6	Average of 12 units ($S_1 + S_2$) is equal to or greater than Q, and no unit is less than $Q - 15\%$
S_3	12	Average of 24 units ($S_1 + S_2 + S_3$) is equal to or greater than Q, no more than two units are less than $Q - 15\%$, and no unit is less than $Q - 25\%$

Note: Q is the amount of dissolved active ingredient specified in the individual monograph, which is expressed as a percentage of label claim.

Reference Standards and Product Specifications

TABLE 4.6

Acceptance Criteria for Disintegration Testing

Stage	Number Tested	Pass IF
S_1	6	All of the units have disintegrated completely
S_2	12	No fewer than 16 of the total of 18 units ($S_1 + S_2$) tested disintegrate completely

compliance with the limits on disintegration as stated in the individual monograph except where the label indicates that the tablets or capsules are intended for use as troches, are to be chewed, or are designed to liberate the drug content gradually over a period of time or release the drug over two or more separate periods with a distinct interval between periods. As indicated in Table 4.6, in the first stage (S_1) of disintegration testing, six dosage units are tested. The requirements are met if all six units disintegrate completely. Complete disintegration is defined as that state in which any residual of the unit, except fragments of an insoluble coating or capsule shell that may remain on the test apparatus screen, is a soft mass with no palpably firm core. If one or two units fails to disintegrate completely, repeat the test on 12 additional units at the second stage (S_2). The requirements are met if no fewer than 16 units of the total of 18 units tested disintegrate completely.

Note that disintegration testing may be applied to uncoated tablets, plain coated tablets, enteric-coated tablets, buccal tablets, sublingual tablets, hard gelatin capsules, and soft gelatin capsules.

4.3.3 Product Specification

Product specifications are referred to as specific intervals that the sample mean and standard deviation must be contained to meet USP/NF standards for good drug characteristics such as identity, strength, quality, purity, and stability with a high probability. For example, for a pharmaceutical compound, the dissolution specifications after encapsulation may state that at 4 hours the mean percent release of 12 capsules must be between 35 and 60 percent and the standard deviation must be less than 11 percent. In this example, the specific interval (35, 60 percent) and (0, 11 percent) are the specifications on mean and standard deviation for the dissolution testing at 4 hours. For pharmaceutical development, there are two types of product specifications, namely in-house specifications and release targets, which are briefly described below.

4.3.3.1 In-House Specifications

For a given drug product, in-house specifications (acceptance limits) are often established for quality assurance/control of the drug products/substances at various stages of the manufacturing process of the drug product. In-house specifications are usually derived based on quality characteristics related to the manufacturing process of the drug product. An appropriate in-house specification for each quality characteristic during the phase of development and during the validation of the manufacturing process should be determined. At least those aspects considered to be critical should be the object of specifications routinely. In-house specifications are usually constructed based on the sample mean and standard deviation of test results. For a given sample, the idea is to construct acceptance limits for the population mean and standard deviation. If the sample mean and standard deviation fall inside the acceptance limits, there is a high probability of passing the USP tests. As an example, typical in-house specifications (acceptance limits) for potency testing are obtained as follows.

Let Y be the potency assay (percent of label claim). Assume that Y follows a normal distribution with mean μ and variance σ^2. Let s be an estimate of the standard deviation σ with v degrees of freedom. Then, there is a 5 percent chance that the mean of the next K potency assay results will be greater than or equal to $\mu + t_{0.05,v}\left(s/\sqrt{K}\right)$, where $t_{0.05,v}$ is the upper 5 percent quantile of a t distribution with v degrees of freedom. Similarly, there is a 5 percent chance that the mean of the next K potency assay results will be less than or equal to $\mu - t_{0.05,v}\left(s/\sqrt{K}\right)$. These statements can be applied to obtain a set of acceptance limits for potency testing at various stages of a manufacturing process of a drug product. Denote by L and U the lower and upper acceptance limits, respectively. L and U can be constructed by letting μ equal the lower product specification (LPS) limit in the first statement and μ equal the upper product specification (UPS) limit in the second statement. This leads to

$$L = \text{LPS} + t_{0.05,v}\left(s/\sqrt{K}\right),$$

$$U = \text{UPS} - t_{0.05,v}\left(s/\sqrt{K}\right).$$

This set of acceptance limits is then considered in-house specifications for potency testing for quality assurance and control. It should be noted, however, that the lower and upper acceptance limits are meaningful (i.e., $L < U$) only when the difference between the upper and lower product specification limits (i.e., $UPS - LPS$) is greater than $2t_{0.05,v}\left(s/\sqrt{K}\right)$. The situation for $L > U$ can occur when the variation of the potency assay result under study is large or K is too small. When L turns out to be greater than U, the assay fails the potency testing. Following a similar idea, in-house specifications for content uniformity testing, dissolution testing, and disintegration testing can be obtained (see, e.g., Chow and Liu 1995).

4.3.3.2 Release Targets

Release targets are usually referred to as in-house specifications for testing for quality characteristics such as potency testing at the time of manufacture

Reference Standards and Product Specifications

or at the time of release for use. Basically, there are two types of release targets: one is established for the final finished product at manufacture (or at release), while the other one is established for the final finished product up to the end of shelf life. In practice, the release targets of a finished product at the time of manufacture or release are often set up in such a way that the specifications proposed at the end of shelf life are guaranteed. The specifications of the finished product at manufacture may be different from those products at expiry due to potential stability loss over time. As an example, consider the same example of potency testing mentioned above, the release targets that will take stability loss up to the expiry become

$$L = \text{LPS} + t_{0.05,v}\left(s/\sqrt{K}\right) + \delta,$$

$$U = \text{UPS} - t_{0.05,v}\left(s/\sqrt{K}\right) - \delta,$$

where δ is the estimated stability loss over the drug expiration dating period (shelf life).

In certain cases, for characteristics of the product that may change during storage under the approved conditions, the quality required at the end of shelf life should be taken into account in determining appropriate specifications at the time of manufacture. For example, in the case of overages for reasons of stability, it is desirable that all specifications (characteristics and acceptance limits) of the drug product and the finished product at the time of release be presented in the form of a summary table. In this table, the limits of any likely breakdown products that may form under the approved conditions of storage should be stated.

4.3.3.3 Remarks

Note that the standard deviation or variance of a test result may consist of several variance components, depending on how the test is conducted. For example, the test may be conducted at different laboratories on different days by different analysts. In addition, the sample may be drawn from different locations of a transport or drum at different stages of a manufacturing process. An appropriate statistical model, which can account for these possible sources of variations, should be considered to obtain estimates of these variance components. In practice, estimates of these sources of variations provide valuable information regarding whether the drug product will meet the USP/NF requirements for good drug characteristics. The sources of variations include dosage unit-to-unit, batch-to-batch, laboratory-to-laboratory, day-to-day, analyst-to-analyst, and location-to-location variations. Once these sources of variations have been identified, attempts can be made to eliminate, reduce, and control these variations. The impact of these variations on the quality of the drug product can also be assessed.

4.3.4 Probability of Passing USP Tests

As discussed above, most USP tests utilize a multiple-stage sampling plan (e.g., two-stage sampling plan for dose uniformity testing and three-stage sampling plan for dissolution testing). In practice, it is of interest to evaluate the probability of passing a multiple-stage sampling test for quality assurance and control. Bergum (1990) proposed the use of a lower probability bound as a conservative approach to approximating the exact probability bound, the acceptance limits can be constructed for the sample means and variances of the test results. The acceptance limits assure that a future sample will have a high probability of passing multiple-stage sampling tests provided that the acceptance limits are met.

Following Bergum's proposal, we need to first evaluate the probability of passing a multiple-stage sampling test. Suppose there is an USP test utilizing a K-stage sampling plan. At each stage, denoted by S_i and C_{ij} the event that the ith stage is passed the event that the jth criterion for the ith stage is met, where $j = 1,\dots,m_i$ and $i = 1,\dots, K$. Also, let P_i be the probability of passing the ith stage. Then the probability of passing a multiple-stage sampling test is given by

$$P\{\text{passing a } K-\text{stage sampling test}\} = P\{S_1 \text{ or } S_2 \text{ or}\dots\text{or } S_K\}$$

$$= P(S_1) + P(\text{not } S_1)P(S_2|\text{not } S_1) + \dots$$

$$+P\{\text{not}(S_1, S_2,\dots, S_{K-1})\}P\{S_K|\text{not}(S_1, S_2,\dots, S_{K-1})\}$$

$$= P_1 + (1 - P_1)P_2 + (1 - P_1)(1 - P_2)P_3 + \dots$$

$$= P_1 + \sum_{i=1}^{K-1}\left\{\prod_{j=1}^{i}(1 - P_j)\right\}P_{i+1}$$

$$= 1 - \prod_{i=1}^{K}(1 - P_i)$$

$$\geq \max\{P_1, P_2,\dots, P_{K.}\}.$$

Furthermore, we have

$$P_i = P(S_i) = P\left\{C_{i1} \text{ and } C_{i2} \text{ and}\dots\text{and } C_{im_i}\right\}$$

$$\geq \max\left\{\sum_{j=1}^{m_i}P(C_{ij}) - (m_i - 1), 0\right\}.$$

Reference Standards and Product Specifications 85

Chow and Liu (1995) and Chow et al. (2002a) derived the lower bounds of probabilities of passing the content uniformity testing, dissolution testing, and disintegration testing. The results are summarized in Tables 4.7 through 4.9, respectively.

As indicated in Table 4.7, the lower bound (LB) for the probabilities of passing the content uniformity test can be calculated for given values of μ and σ based on the approximations by a central F distribution and a standard normal distribution. For example, with normal approximation, if μ is 98 and σ is less than 5.64, there is at least a 95 percent chance of passing the content uniformity test. For dissolution testing, as indicated by Table 4.8, the LB depends on σ^2 and the magnitude of the difference between Q and μ (i.e., $D = \mu - Q$). For example, if D is 10 percent of label claim and if σ is less than 17.4 percent of label claim, the lower bound on the probability of passing the dissolution testing test is 50 percent. It should be noted that the lower bound on the probability of passing will increase as σ decreases. For the disintegration testing, as indicated by Table 4.9, if $\mu = 15$ min and if σ is less than 14.22 min, there is at least a 50 percent chance of passing the disintegration test.

TABLE 4.7

Probability Lower Bounds of Passing
Content Uniformity Test

	σ			
	LB = 0.50		**LB = 0.95**	
μ	F	N	F	N
86	0.67	0.67	0.45	0.44
88	2.01	2.00	1.33	1.33
90	3.33	3.34	2.22	2.21
92	4.39	4.60	3.11	3.10
94	5.60	5.63	3.99	3.99
96	6.44	6.77	4.87	4.87
98	6.92	7.52	5.61	5.64
100	7.12	7.77	5.89	5.96
102	7.06	7.53	5.64	5.64
104	6.63	6.77	4.87	4.87
106	5.64	5.78	3.99	3.99
108	4.54	4.66	3.11	3.10
110	3.34	3.34	2.22	2.21
112	2.01	2.00	1.33	1.33
114	0.67	0.67	0.45	0.44

Note: F, approximation by a central F distribution; N, approximation by a standard normal distribution.

TABLE 4.8

Probability Lower Bounds of Passing Dissolution Testing

| | σ | |
$D(= \mu - Q)$	LB = 0.50	LB = 0.95
1	9.84	2.98
5	14.11	9.94
10	17.40	12.03
15	20.27	13.87
20	23.06	15.67
25	25.81	17.45
30	28.53	19.22
35	31.21	20.97
40	33.87	22.72
45	36.54	24.48
50	39.19	26.22

TABLE 4.9

Probability Lower Bounds of Passing Disintegration Test

| | σ | | | |
| | Exact Probability Bound | | Lower Probability Bound | |
μ	0.50	0.95	0.50	0.95
1	30.29	17.90	27.50	17.32
3	28.20	16.67	25.60	16.12
5	26.11	15.44	23.70	14.93
7	24.03	14.20	21.81	13.73
9	21.94	12.97	19.91	12.54
11	19.85	11.73	18.02	11.35
13	17.76	10.50	16.12	10.15
15	15.67	9.26	14.22	8.96
17	13.58	8.03	12.33	7.76
19	11.49	6.79	10.43	6.57
21	9.40	5.56	8.53	5.37
23	7.31	4.32	6.64	4.18
25	5.22	3.09	4.74	2.99
27	3.13	1.85	2.84	1.79

4.4 Product Characterization

In practice, TCM can be viewed as combination treatments because it often contains multiple components. Individual components are expected to make a contribution to the therapeutic effect on the disease under study. Combination treatments are widely used in medicine especially for cancer. The FDA regulations regarding fixed-dose, combination-dosage form prescription drugs for humans is that two or more drugs may be combined in a single-dosage form when each component makes a contribution to the claimed effects of the combination and the dosage of each component is such that the combination is safe and effective for a significant patient population requiring such concurrent therapy as defined in the labeling for the drug [21 CFR 300.50].

In clinical studies, it is expected that the combination is superior to its components in terms of effectiveness or safety. The relationship between the combination treatments and its components has been studied by Laska et al. (1997). In many diseases such as hypertension, drug treatments for the patients are administered according to a dose titration schedule. Dose-effect information is essential for drug labeling, particularly if one or both of the component drugs have dose-dependent side effects. Therefore, a multilevel factorial design trial for simultaneously studying multiple-dose combinations is often asked for during the development of combination drugs (see, e.g., Hung et al. 1990, 1994). Such a factorial design trial is also needed for studying a combination drug proposed for use as an initial therapy.

4.4.1 Fixed-Dose Combination

In practice, the following full 2×2 factorial design (Table 4.10) is often considered for evaluation of a fixed-dose combination of two drugs namely drug A and drug B, respectively (Hung 2010).

Subjects will be randomly assigned to one of the combinations: $P_A P_B$, $P_A B$, AP_B, and AB, where P_A and P_B are placebos for drug A and drug B, respectively. As can be seen from the table, the effects of drug A and drug B can be evaluated by comparing the treatment group AP_B with $P_A P_B$ and treatment group $P_A B$ with $P_A P_B$, respectively. On the other hand, the effect of drug A (B) on drug B (A) can be studied by comparing AB with $P_A B$ (AP_B). In practice, it is expected that the combination treatment (AB) is superior to drug A and

TABLE 4.10

2 × 2 Factorial Design for Combination Treatments

$P_A P_B$:	$P_A B$:
Placebo of A and Placebo of B	Placebo of A and Drug B
AP_B:	AB:
Drug A and Placebo of B	Drug A and Drug B

88   *Quantitative Methods for Traditional Chinese Medicine Development*

drug B alone. The above 2×2 factorial design is useful for verifying this hypothesis. It should be noted that the placebo-placebo combination may sometimes be voided, but usually it is preferred to include this combination. The purpose of including this combination is to check the activity of each component drug. The subjects enrolled are randomly allocated into the three or four combination cells. The allocation can be in equal or unequal proportions.

The primary statistical hypothesis of concern involves two pairwise comparisons between the combination and the two components. Both of the comparisons must succeed in order to prove the notion of contributing. This is a well-known statistical testing problem studied in the literature (see, e.g., Lehmann 1952; Berger 1982). Laska and Meisner (1989) proposed a natural joint test by taking the minimum of the individual standardized tests for the respective pairwise comparisons. In parametric testing, such as testing for mean difference, the distribution of the min test involves a primary parameter and a nuisance parameter. The primary parameter is the minimum of the values of the parameters for the two respective comparisons. The nuisance is the difference of the values of the parameters for the two comparisons. If the hypothesis pertains to a single response, then the primary parameter measures the least gain of effect by use of the combination relative to its components whereas the nuisance is the mean difference of the components.

Snapinn (1987) constructed five tests based on the min test. Each of his first four tests $(T_1–T_4)$ employs a different estimate of the nuisance parameter that is derived from the same set of the data used for testing the hypothesis of the primary parameter. As indicated by Snapinn (1987) and Hung et al. (1994), the tests could be biased in favor of the combination treatment. That is, if the true value of the nuisance parameter differs from the estimate, then the tests could lead one to falsely assert that the combination is superior to the components more often than it should be. The maximum Type I error probability for each of these tests exceeds the target α-level. Snapinn's fifth test (T_5) is the α-level min test, later presented by Laska and Meisner (1989); it requires the individual test statistics to reject the respective null hypotheses at the level of at most α. Equivalently, the individual p values for all pairwise comparisons must not exceed α. The α-level min test has existed early in the literature (see, e.g., Lehmann 1952) and its maximum Type I error probability is α. Laska and Meisner (1989) showed an optimality property of this test, the implication of which needs to be an important consideration in regulatory applications. The performance of the α-level min test as a function of the nuisance parameter has been further studied by Patel (1991), Hung (1993), Hung et al. (1994), and Wang and Hung (1997). On the other hand, Gibson and Overall (1989), Sarkar et al. (1993), and Snapinn and Sarkar (1995) also contemplated the possibility of improving the min test. It is clear that the α-level min test cannot be improved unless the true value of the nuisance parameter is known to be in a very narrow range or under a specific alternative.

Reference Standards and Product Specifications

The statistical power of the α-level min test depends on the primary parameter and the nuisance parameter discussed above. In the case of testing a mean parameter, given any fixed value of the primary parameter, the power of the α-level min test increases as a function of the absolute value of the nuisance parameter. Therefore, given any value of the primary parameter, the α-level min test has the smallest power when the nuisance parameter is null. Ideally, the sample size for a fixed-dose combination trial should be planned to ensure sufficient power for detecting an expected value of the primary parameter, assuming that the nuisance parameter is zero; i.e., the two components have an identical effect.

The problem of comparing a combination treatment with its component drugs on multiple-response variables has been studied extensively (Laska et al. 1992). The multivariate responses present more than one way of interpreting "making a contribution," depending on the claimed effects. The optimality of the α-level min test in the univariate response case also carries to the multiple-response case for showing that the combination is superior to the components on all response variables.

4.4.2 Multiple-Dose Combinations

Similarly, for multiple-dose combinations, the following multilevel factorial design is an intuitive choice for studying multiple-dose combinations of two drugs simultaneously in one trial. Thus, in a $(r + 1) \times (s + 1)$ factorial cell, A_iB_j labels the combination of the ith dose of drug A and the jth dose of drug B, and A_0 and B_0 are the placebos of drug A and drug B, respectively (see Table 4.11). The subjects enrolled are randomly allocated to the cells. As indicated by Hung et al. (1990, 1994), the above factorial design trial carries multiple objectives. For one, the study needs to provide confirmatory evidence for the assertion that the combination of the drugs is more beneficial than each component drug alone. Another objective is to obtain reliable and useful dose-effect information for writing instructions for use in drug labeling.

TABLE 4.11

Multilevel Factorial Design for Combination Treatments

A_0B_0	A_0B_1	A_0B_2	...	A_0B_s
A_1B_0	A_1B_1	A_1B_2	...	A_1B_s
A_2B_0	A_2B_1	A_2B_2	...	A_2B_s
.	.	.	...	.
.	.	.	...	.
.	.	.	...	.
A_rB_0	A_rB_1	A_rB_2	...	A_rB_s

Note: Drug A has r dose levels and drug B has s dose levels.

The definition for superiority of the combination drug over the component drugs in studying multiple-dose combination is not obvious. Hung et al. (1990) presented two distinct concepts of global superiority. In a weak sense of global superiority, the average of all the nonzero dose combinations is superior to both of the averages of the individual component doses. In a strong sense, there exist some nonzero dose combinations that are superior to the respective components in the dose region under study. The weak sense is less desirable because by showing it there is no guarantee that there is a single-dose combination superior to its components.

To demonstrate the strong sense of global superiority, the classical analysis of variance (ANOVA) using the additive model (i.e., no drug by drug interaction terms) can be a very powerful method. The additive model prescribes that the effect of each nonzero dose combination is the sum of the effects of its components. If the true effect of a dose combination is less than the sum of the component effects, the additive model will overestimate the effect of the combination. For such dose combinations, the probability of falsely asserting superiority over the components will be greater than it should be. Thus, the assumption of no drug interaction is essential to the validity of the ANOVA using the additive model. The classical global F test for testing additivity does not guarantee that nonadditivity is always detectable at each dose combination. The patterns depicted by the estimates of the drug by drug interactions for the dose combinations may be more informative for detecting the possible presence of nonadditivity at the local level.

When the validity of the ANOVA is in doubt, some alternative useful methods for testing the strong-sense global superiority are α-level AVE and MAX tests developed by Hung et al. (1993). These global tests are based on the estimate of the least gain in effect resulting from use of each combination relative to its component. The AVE test is an average of the min test statistics applied to the nonzero dose combinations under study, whereas the MAX test takes the largest min test statistic. The α-level AVE test imposes a weak control on the family-wise Type I error probability; that is, the probability of the type I error associated with the global null hypothesis that none of the dose combinations under study are superior to their respective components is maintained at α. The α-level MAX test controls at α the maximum probability of the family-wise type I error incurring in the pairwise comparisons between all nonzero dose combinations and their respective components (i.e., strong control). These tests have been extended to the incomplete factorial designs where some nonzero dose combinations are not studied and to the unbalanced designs where the cell sample sizes are not equal (see, e.g., Hung 1996, 2000).

The power functions of both the α-level AVE test and the α-level MAX test contain the nuisance parameters, each quantifying the difference of the respective component doses. The most conservative but perhaps impractical strategy of sample size planning for a multifactorial trial is one that assumes an identical effect for each dose level of both component drugs. A practical

Reference Standards and Product Specifications 91

strategy should rely on Monte Carlo simulation studies based on a number of layouts for possible expected effect sizes at all local cells.

A more informative approach is to identify a dose combination that is superior to the highest dose of Drug A and the highest dose of Drug B under study. The most natural dose combination for testing is the combination of the highest doses of Drug A and Drug B. Some other considerations may prompt testing lower dose combinations against the highest dose of each single drug alone. Strong control of type I error rate associated with testing such multiple dose combinations is generally required to assert which dose combination(s) is superior to the highest dose of either drug.

Dose-effect relationship can be studied using a biological model or an empirical statistical model, such as a quadratic polynomial model via response surface or regression analyses. The surface can provide valuable information as to whether the effect increases as a function of dose, whether the effect increases start to level off at some dose combination, or whether there may be drug by drug interactions. If the response surface model fits the dose-effect data well, then one can construct confidence surfaces to identify desirable dose combinations that have greater effects than the individual components with a desired level of confidence (Hung 1992). Other useful analysis approaches using response surface method can be found in Phillips et al. (1992).

4.4.3 Global Superiority of Combination Drug

In order to identify the optimal combination of dose levels and to investigate the potential drug-to-drug interactions, it is recommended that several or all possible combinations be explored simultaneously with multilevel factorial designs. Table 4.12 provides a cross tabulation of a full multilevel factorial design with μ_{ij} representing the average response of the combination made of dose i of component A and dose j of component B. A separate dose-response relationship of each component can be investigated by the first row for drug B or first column for drug A where the placebo is administered for

TABLE 4.12

Cross Tabulation of a Full $(a + 1) \times (b + 1)$ Factorial Design for Combination Therapy with the Mean Effects

Dose Levels for Component A	Dose Levels for Component B					Overall
	Placebo	1	2	...	b	
Placebo	μ_{00}	μ_{01}	μ_{02}	...	μ_{0b}	$\mu_{0\cdot}$
1	μ_{10}	μ_{11}	μ_{12}	...	μ_{1b}	$\mu_{1\cdot}$
2	μ_{20}	μ_{21}	μ_{22}	...	μ_{2b}	$\mu_{2\cdot}$
$\vdots$	$\vdots$	$\vdots$	$\vdots$	...	$\vdots$	$\vdots$
A	μ_{a0}	μ_{a1}	μ_{a2}	...	μ_{ab}	$\mu_{a\cdot}$
Overall	$\mu_{\cdot 0}$	$\mu_{\cdot 1}$	$\mu_{\cdot 2}$	...	$\mu_{\cdot b}$	$\mu_{\cdot\cdot}$

the other component. In order to provide a useful dose-response relationship for therapeutic applications, Hung et al. (1989) suggests that the dose ranges to be investigated must include a very low dose level and a very high dose level that are not in the effective dose range. As a result, the contribution of some doses by one component when added to the other drug may not be different from the placebo, while the contribution of the other component is quite obvious. Hence, with respect to the requirement described in Section 300.50 in Part 21 of CFR that each component makes a contribution to the claimed effects, Hung et al. (1990) defines the superiority of a combination drug over its component drugs in a global sense. Strict superiority of a combination drug is defined as the existence of at least one dose combination that is more effective than its components. Let d_{ij} be the minimum gain in efficacy obtained from combining dose i of drug A and dose j of drug B as compared to its component drugs at the same dose levels alone,

$$d_{ij} = \mu_{ij} \max(\mu_{i0}, \mu_{0j}), \ i = 1,...,a, \ j = 1,...,b. \tag{4.1}$$

The corresponding statistical hypotheses can then be formulated as

$$H_0 : d_{ij} \leq 0 \text{ for every } i = 1,...,a, \ j = 1,...,b$$

$$\text{versus } H_a : d_{ij} > 0 \text{ for some } i = 1,...,a, \ j = 1,...,b. \tag{4.2}$$

A combination drug is said to be superior to its components in the wide sense if the average of all the dose combinations is superior to both the averages of the individual monotherapy doses. Let m_A represent difference between the average responses of all (i,j) combinations over the entire range of active doses and that dose i of component A when placebo is administered for component B,

$$m_A = Ave(\mu_{ij} - \mu_{i0}).$$

Similarly,

$$m_B = Ave(\mu_{ij} - \mu_{0j}).$$

Consequently, the concept of the wide global superiority of a combination drug can be stated as

$$H_0 : m_A \leq 0 \text{ or } m_B \leq 0$$

$$\text{versus } H_a : m_A > 0 \text{ and } m_B > 0. \tag{4.3}$$

The strict global superiority of a combination drug restricts our attention to a more effective class of combinations than either component drug alone.

Reference Standards and Product Specifications 93

According to d_{ij} in the alternative hypothesis of Equation 4.2, we only need to identify one dose level that is better than mean responses $\mu_{i\cdot}$ and $\mu_{\cdot j}$ of the corresponding monotherapy of component A at dose i and of component B at dose j. However, it does not guarantee superiority of one combination over all dose levels of either monotherapy.

Consider the example given by Hung et al. (1993). Table 4.13 displays the mean reductions from the baseline in post-treatment supine diastolic blood pressure from a clinical trial that evaluated a combination drug with three dose levels for drug A and four dose levels for drug B, including the placebo (Hung et al. 1993). From Table 4.13 the mean reductions in diastolic blood pressure of all combinations are seen to be more than those at the corresponding doses of either monotherapy. As a result, the minimum gain d is positive for all combinations, which is shown in Table 4.14. From Table 4.15 suppose that the mean reduction from the baseline in diastolic blood pressure of dose 3

TABLE 4.13

Difference from Placebo in Mean Reduction in Supine Diastolic Blood Pressure (mmHg)

Dose Levels for Component A	Dose Levels for Component B			
	Placebo	1	2	3
Placebo	0	4	4	3
1	5	9	7	8
2	5	6	6	7

Source: Hung, H.M.J. et al., *Biometrics*, 49, 85–94, 1993.

TABLE 4.14

Minimum Gain of Combinations for the Data in Table 4.13

Active Dose Levels for Component A	Active Dose Levels for Component B		
	1	2	3
1	4	2	3
2	1	1	2

Source: Hung, H.M.J. et al., *Biometrics*, 49, 85–94, 1993.

TABLE 4.15

Modified Differences from Placebo in Mean Reduction in Supine Diastolic Blood Pressure (mmHg)

Dose Levels for Component A	Dose Levels for Component B			
	Placebo	1	2	3
Placebo	0	4	4	7
1	5	9	7	8
2	5	6	6	7

Source: Hung, H.M.J. et al., *Biometrics*, 49, 85–94, 1993.

for component B as monotherapy is changed from 3 to 7. Table 4.16 reveals that although the minimum gain of all combinations over their corresponding monotherapy is at least 0, only combinations (1, 1) and (1, 3) surpass the monotherapy of drug B at dose level 3. This result is desirable because the monotherapy of drug B at the highest dose may induce some severe adverse events, while the dose level of drug B in combination with a larger reduction is two levels lower than that of the monotherapy. As a result the combination of dose 1 of drug A with dose 1 of drug B provides a much safer margin and hence a larger benefit-to-risk ratio.

For assessment of wide global superiority, as outlined in the hypotheses (Equations 4.2 and 4.3), there seem to be, on the one hand, a combination that is better than its component A and, on the other, a combination that might not be the same combination but is better than its component B. Unlike strict superiority, however, this does not guarantee that there is a combination that is better than both of its components as required by the FDA regulation. Therefore, the strict global superiority meets the current regulatory requirement for approval of a combination drug product. Hung et al. (1990, 1993) propose two statistical testing procedures for hypotheses (Equations 4.2 and 4.3) under the assumption that data are normally distributed. The proposed methods reduce to the min test proposed by Laska and Meisner (1989) when only one active dose level is included in the assessment trial of a combination drug. Note that the sampling distributions of the methods proposed by Hung et al. are quite complicated and require special tables for the significance tests. Hung (1996) extends the application of these two methods to the situations (1) where the variance of the clinical endpoint is a function of its mean and (2) where an incomplete factorial design is used.

When a combination drug consists of more than two component drugs, the concept of strict global superiority for the combination drug of two components can be easily extended. Let d_{ijk} be the minimum gain in efficacy obtained by combining dose i of drug A with dose j of drug B, and dose k of drug C over its components alone at the same dose levels:

$$d_{ijk} = \mu_{ijk} - \max(\mu_{i..}, \mu_{.j.}, \mu_{..k}), \, i = 1,\ldots,a, \, j = 1,\ldots,b, \, k = 1,\ldots,c, \qquad (4.4)$$

TABLE 4.16

Minimum Gain of Combinations for the Modified Data in Table 4.15

Active Dose Levels for Component A	Active Dose Levels for Component B		
	1	2	3
1	4	2	1
2	1	1	0

Source: Hung, H.M.J. et al., *Biometrics*, 49, 85–94, 1993.

Reference Standards and Product Specifications   95

where μ_{ijk} is the mean response of the combination of dose i of drug A, dose j of drug B, and dose k of drug C, and $\mu_{i..}$, $\mu_{.j.}$, and $\mu_{..k}$ represent the mean responses of its components A, B, and C alone at the same dose levels i, j, and k, respectively, where the active agents are administered with the placebos of the other two components. The strict global superiority of a three-drug combination over its components can be formulated by the following statistical hypotheses:

$$H_0 : d_{ijk} \leq 0 \text{ for every } i = 1,\ldots,a, j = 1,\ldots,b, \text{ and } k = 1,\ldots,c$$

$$\text{versus } H_a : d_{ijk} > 0 \text{ for some } i = 1,\ldots,a, j = 1,\ldots,b, \text{ and } k = 1,\ldots,c. \quad (4.5)$$

The above hypotheses can be tested to verify the existence of strict global superiority of a combination drug. However, the extension of the methods of Hung et al. (1993) for testing the above hypotheses is not straightforward. Further research is needed.

Suppose that a combination of two component drugs is developed to treat patients with benign prostatic hyperplasia (BPH). Two primary efficacy endpoints for assessment of the combination are peak urinary flow are (mL/s) and AUA-7 symptom scores. Let c_{if} and d_{ij} be the minimum gain of combination of dose i of drug A with dose j of drug B of peak urinary flow rate and AUA-7 symptom scores, respectively. Following the suggestion by Laska and Meisner (1990), the strict global superiority for more than one clinical endpoint is defined as that where at least one combination is superior to its component drugs for at least one clinical endpoint. Hence, if a combination is better than its component drugs for at least one clinical endpoint, then the minimum gain of the combination based on both clinical endpoints must be greater than zero. The hypotheses corresponding to the strict global superiority can be formulated as follows:

$$H_0 : \min(c_{ij}, d_{ij}) \leq 0 \text{ for every } i = 1,\ldots,a, j = 1,\ldots,b$$

$$\text{versus } H_a : \min(c_{ij}, d_{ij}) > 0 \text{ for some } i = 1,\ldots,a, j = 1,\ldots,b. \quad (4.6)$$

The concept of the hypotheses (Equation 4.6) can easily be extended to an evaluation of the combination drug based on more than two endpoints. However, the definition of strict global superiority and its corresponding formulation of hypotheses and proposed statistical procedures are to verify the existence of at least one combination that is better than both of its components. Furthermore, they are hypothesis testing procedures and hence cannot describe the dose-response relationship and potential drug-to-drug interaction among components. Consequently, they fail to provide a way to search for combinations for which each component makes a contribution to the claimed effects should they exist.

4.4.4 Method of Response Surface

To overcome the drawbacks associated with the definition of the strict global superiority for a combination drug, the concept of response surface methodology (Carter et al. 1982; Carter and Wampler 1986) can provide a nice complement to the statistical testing procedures suggested by Laska and Meisner (1989) and Hung et al. (1993). For a combination trial conducted with a factorial design, if the dose levels of each component are appropriately selected, then the technique of response surface can provide valuable information regarding (1) the therapeutic dose range of the combination drug with respect to effectiveness and safety and (2) the titration process and drug-to-drug interaction. The response surface method can empirically verify a model that adequately describes the observed data. For example, we can consider the following statistical model to describe the response:

$$Y_{ijk} = f(A_i, B_j, \theta) + e_{ijk},\tag{4.7}$$

where Y_{ijk} is the clinical response of patient k who receives dose i of drug A, denoted by A_i and dose j of dose B, denoted by B_j, is a vector of unknown parameters, and e_{ijk} is the random error in observing Y_{ijk}, where $k = 1,\ldots, n_{ij}, j = 1,\ldots,b, i = 1,\ldots,a$. The component $f(A_i, B_j, \theta)$ in Equation 4.7 gives a mathematical description and an approximation to the true unknown response surface provided by the two drugs. When the primary clinical endpoints of interest are continuous variables, $f(A_i, B_j, \theta)$ is usually approximated by a polynomial. For a detailed description of response surface methodology, see Box and Draper (1987); also see Peace (1990) for applications of response surface to a phase II development of anti-anginal drugs.

If the assumed mathematical model is not too complicated, then the standard statistical estimation procedures such as least squares method or maximum likelihood method can be selected to estimate the unknown parameter θ. After substitution of the parameter in $f(A_i, B_j, \theta)$ by its estimate, an estimated response surface can be obtained that provides an empirical description of the dose-response relationship either by a three-dimensional surface or by two-dimensional contours. In addition, an optimal dose combination can be estimated to give a maximum clinical response if it exists and is unique. If the 95 percent confidence region for the optimal dose combination does not lie on both the horizontal axis representing drug A and the vertical axis representing drug B at the contours, then it is concluded that the estimated optimal combination is superior to both of its components. The technique of response surface therefore can estimate an optimal dose combination that may not be the combination of doses of both components selected for the trial given the existence of such combinations. Hung (1992) suggests a procedure to identify a positive dose-response surface for combination drugs. Hence, the response surface can also estimate a region in which the combinations are superior to their components. Estimation of a superior region is particularly appealing if safety is the major reason for the combination

Reference Standards and Product Specifications 97

drug because a combination can be chosen from the superior region with much lower doses of both components to achieve the same superiority in efficacy but with a much better safety profile. Because μ_{ij} is estimated using the information of the entire sample, if the assumed model can adequately describe the dose-response relationship of the combination, the response surface method requires fewer patients than the procedures for testing strict global superiority proposed by Hung et al. (1993).

Note that estimation of the unknown parameters, response surface, and the optimal combination dose and construction of the confidence region for the optimal combination dose are model dependent. Consequently, as indicated by Hung et al. (1990), the FDA is concerned about the application of the response surface method for the following reasons. First, the sensitivity of the methods such as lack-of-fit tests, goodness-of-fit tests, and residual plots for verification of the adequacy of the fitted models is often questionable. Second, even if there is no evidence for the inadequacy of the fitted model, the chance of selecting an inadequate model and the effect of such an error cannot be evaluated. Third, the response surface method is model dependent. Two different models that both adequately fit the given data may provide contradictory conclusions in any subsequent statistical analyses. The methods for strict global superiority and response surface methodology should play crucial but complementary roles in assessment of combination drugs. Existence of a combination superior to its components can be verified first by the model-independent statistical testing procedures proposed by Hung et al. (1993). Then the response surface technique can be applied to (1) empirically describe the dose-response relationship, (2) identify the region of superior efficacy, and (3) estimate the optimal dose combination. Also, it would be of interest to provide a scientific justification as to why the two methods yield inconsistent conclusions.

4.4.5 Remarks

Combination treatment trials present many interesting and yet difficult statistical design and inference problems. For testing a single dose combination versus its components, it is a typical intersection-union testing problem that involves the difference between the effects of the two components as the nuisance or ancillary parameter. Without a complete knowledge of the value of this parameter, the α-level min test described above is the only solution to the testing problem. From a design perspective, a good sample size plan should ensure that this test has sufficient statistical power under the worst scenario that the effects of the two component drugs are equal.

The multilevel factorial design provides an avenue for studying multiple dose combinations with multiple objectives entertained above. Depending on the study objective, sample size planning requires careful attention. If the objective is to assert that at least one dose combination is superior to its respective components, then the sample sizes need to be carefully allocated to all dose combination cells under testing. If, however, the objective is to identify which dose combination(s) is superior to the highest dose of each drug, then the tested dose combinations need to be loaded with the major portion of the total sample size. Multiple comparison adjustments need to be incorporated in sample size planning. Consequently, the dose-response exploration that will involve other dose combinations will be based on much smaller sample sizes.

4.5 Practical Issues

For most TCMs, it is not uncommon to have 5–10 individual components. Some TCMs may consist of more than 10 individual components. These components could be active components or inactive components. In practice, pharmacological activities of some of these components may be known and available in Pharmacopeia such as *Chinese Pharmacopoeia*, USP/NF, and European Pharmacopeia. One of the major concerns, however, is that pharmacological activities for some components may be unknown. There may exist unknown relationships among the active and/or inactive components. Besides, it is not clear whether there exist possible component-to-component interactions among these components.

In addition, the relative proportions (ratios) among the individual components that will lead to the optimal therapeutic effects are also unknown. If the relative proportions of the individual components are known for a given subject or some subjects, it is a concern whether this relative proportion is applicable to other subjects as the TCM is meant to be individualized treatment with flexible dose and/or treatment duration for minimizing intrasubject variability and consequently maximizing (optimizing) the therapeutic effect. In practice, it is very difficult, if it is not impossible, to address the above questions even if a large scale of multilevel factorial design is employed.

4.6 Concluding Remarks

In pharmaceutical research and development, the establishment of product specifications is important for meeting reference standards for (1) manufacturing process validation and (2) quality assurance and control of the final product before it is released for use. The USP/NF provides reference standards for various drug products and substances in terms of some good drug characteristics (e.g., dosage content uniformity, dissolution and disintegration for tablet manufacturing). The USP/NF also provides detailed

Reference Standards and Product Specifications

information regarding sampling plan, acceptance criteria, and testing procedures for various tests to assist the sponsors to meet the reference standards. In practice, it is of interest to set up product specifications based on the test results in such a way that if we pass a specific test, there will be a high probability of passing the test for future products manufactured by the same manufacturing process.

For drug products with single active ingredients, reference standards for various drug products and substances are available in Pharmacopeia (e.g., European Pharmacopeia and US Pharmacopeia). Statistical methods for establishment of product specifications (e.g., in-house specification for in-process materials and/or release targets for final finished products) based on sampling plan, acceptance criteria, and testing procedure as described in the Pharmacopeia are well established. For drug products with multiple components such as TCMs, on the other hand, the multiple components are usually unknown and/or not well understood. Besides, the pharmacological activities of these individual components could vary widely and their relative ratios (or proportions) for achieving optimal therapeutic effect are usually unknown. In this case, not only are reference standards for individual components not available, product specifications for individual components and/or the product are often difficult, if not impossible to obtain. Thus, it is suggested that analytical methods for quantitation of the pharmacological activity of individual components be developed for establishing reference standards and consequently specifications for individual components. The established reference standards and specifications can then be applied for quality assurance and quality control during the manufacturing process and final finished product after manufacture.

For a given TCM with multiple components, in practice, it is desired to obtain acceptance limits for these components, which guarantee that future samples will pass the USP tests for good drug characteristics such as potency, strength, quality, and purity with a high probability. Such acceptance limits are usually constructed based on the sample means and standard deviations of the test results of these components. For a given USP test (e.g., potency testing), the idea is to construct a joint confidence region for the population means and standard deviations of these components. The probability of passing the USP test for each population mean and standard deviation in the confidence region can then be evaluated. The confidence region is obtained as the set of all possible sample means and standard deviations such that the probability of passing the USP test is greater than a pre-specified probability for all points in the confidence region. The confidence region is usually referred to as the acceptance region.

5

QOL-Like Quantitative Instrument for Evaluation of TCM

5.1 Introduction

In clinical research, a quantitative instrument (or questionnaire) is often used to provide objective measurement of safety and efficacy of a test treatment under investigation across various therapeutic areas. In practice, although there exist many instruments such as Hamilton-D (Hamilton scale for depression) and Hamilton-A (Hamilton scale for anxiety) for central nervous system (CNS) and quality of life (QOL) assessment in cancer trials, the investigators frequently face the need to develop new ones. A typical example is the development of an objective instrument for evaluation of clinical benefits including safety, efficacy, and/or quality of life of traditional Chinese herbal medicines. This need arises because proper development/validation or modification of instruments can achieve specific purposes relative to specific target patient populations. While the existing instruments may include one that has been developed for the target patient population and the desired purpose, new research questions often require new instruments or modification of existing instruments for measurement. Validation of the developed instrument is important to ensure a proper sampling and a valid measurement of the content of the subjective state, behavior, or disease to be measured. In this chapter, without loss of generality and for illustrative purposes, we will focus on validation of a developed instrument for assessment of QOL in cancer trials. The performance characteristics for validation of QOL instruments can be applied to other instruments for other purposes such as the evaluation of safety and efficacy of TCMs across therapeutic areas.

In cancer clinical trials, it has been a concern that the treatment of disease or survival may not be as important as the improvement of QOL, especially for patients with chronic and/or life-threatening diseases. Enhancement of life beyond absence of illness to the enjoyment of life is considered more important than the extension of life. QOL not only can provide information as to how patients feel about drug therapies but also appeals to the physician's desire for the best clinical practice. It can be used as a predictor of

101

compliance of the patient. In addition, it may be used to distinguish between therapies that appear to be equally efficacious and equally safe at the stage of marketing strategy planning. The information can be potentially used in advertising for the promotion of the drug therapy. However, unlike the analytic instrument, no known standards exist that can be used as a reference. In addition, the QOL instrument is a very subjective tool, which is expected to have a large variation. It is then a concern as to whether the adopted QOL instrument can accurately and reliably quantify patients' QOL. To ensure the accuracy and reliability of QOL assessment in clinical trials, the adopted QOL instrument is necessarily validated in terms of some performance characteristics. In practice, a QOL instrument is usually validated based on some classic validation parameters such as validity, reliability, test-retest reproducibility, responsiveness, and sensitivity. However, it is not clear whether the classic validation can actually verify the instrument. In other words, can the classic validation address whether the questions are the right ones for assessment of QOL?

In Section 5.2, we briefly review background and statistical methods for QOL assessment. In Section 5.3, we provide statistical evaluation for the validation of a QOL instrument in terms of performance characteristics of validity, reliability, and test-retest reproducibility. Responsiveness and sensitivity are discussed in Section 5.4. The validation of utility analysis and calibration is discussed in Section 5.5. The use of QOL-like instrument for evaluation of TCMs is discussed in Section 5.6. A controversial issue concerning parallel assessments of TCM is discussed in Section 5.7. A brief discussion concerning the use of an instrument for evaluation of TCMs is given in the last section.

5.2 QOL Assessment

In general, there exists no universal definition for QOL. It may vary from one patient population to another and from one therapeutic area to another. For example, Williams (1987) defined QOL as a collective term that encompasses multiple components of a person's social and medical status. However, Smith (1992) interpreted QOL as the way a person feels and how he or she functions in day-to-day activities. The concept of QOL can be traced back to the mid-1920s. Peabody (1927) pointed out that the clinical picture of a patient is an impressionistic painting of the patient surrounded by his home, work, friends, joys, sorrows, hopes, and fears. In 1947, the World Health Organization (WHO) stated that health is a state of complete physical, medical, and social well-being and not merely the absence of disease or infirmity. In 1948, Karnofsky published his performance status index to assess the usefulness of chemotherapy for cancer patients. The New York Heart Association proposed a refined version of its functional classification to assess the effects

QOL-Like Quantitative Instrument for Evaluation of TCM

of cardiovascular symptoms on performance of physical activities in 1964. In the past several decades, QOL has attracted much attention. Since 1970, several research groups have been actively working on the assessment of QOL in clinical trials. For example, Kaplan et al. (1976) developed the *Index of Well-Being* to provide a comprehensive measure of QOL. Torrance (1976) and Torrance and Feeny (1989) introduced the concept of utility theory to measure the health state preferences of individuals and quality-adjusted life-year to summarize both quality of life and quantity of life. Bergner et al. (1981) developed the Sickness Impact Profile to study perceived health and sickness-related QOL. Ware (1987) proposed a set of widely used scales for the Rand Health Insurance Experiment and Williams (1987) studied the effects of QOL on hypertensive patients.

In clinical trials, QOL is usually assessed by means of a global physician's assessment or a QOL instrument that consists of a number of questions. The global physician's assessment, such as an analog scale ranging from 0 to 10, is easy to apply by simply asking the question "How is your QOL?" However, it cannot capture the whole spectrum of QOL. In addition, if the drug therapy does improve QOL, no information as to which domain of QOL is provided. The global physician's assessment generally produces large variability and low reproducibility. For a QOL instrument, the questionnaire may be assessed by patients, their spouses/significant others, reviewers (e.g., nurses or social workers), and/or physician through direct observation or face-to-face or teleconference interview. It can be self-administered or supervised self-administered. On the basis of the collected data, the health-related QOL can be quantified. Generally, health-related QOL may be described by a number of major domains (or dimensions). The most commonly considered QOL domains include physical functioning and morbidity, emotional or psychological status and well-being, disease-specific symptoms and somatic discomfort, and cognitive function. Other domains, such as intimacy and sexual functioning, economic status and personal productivity, employment, and laboratory test values, are less often used.

In the QOL instrument, for each patient, scores associated with each question are usually referred to as items. In practice, there may be a larger number of items and it is not practical to analyze the data by item. Thus, items are usually grouped to form subscales, which are often used to evaluate different components of QOL. However, analysis of individual subscales often produces inconsistent results across subscales; consequently, no overall conclusion can be made. As an alternative, these subscales may be combined to form the so-called composite scores, which can be used to assess major domains of QOL.

As a result, QOL may be assessed by analyzing items, subscales, composite scores, and/or total score. Unlike multivariate analysis (e.g., Morrison 1976), Tandon (1990) applied global statistics to combine the results of univariate analysis of each subscale. His approach is useful; yet, it does not reveal the underlying correlation structure of subscales. As an alternative approach, Olschewski and Schumacher (1990) proposed the use of aggregated measures to reduce the dimension of the measurements. Their method uses the standardized scoring coefficients from factor analysis as data-oriented weights for combining subscales that neglects small coefficients. The disadvantage of their method is that the selected coefficients are neither unique nor have optimal properties. To overcome these problems, Ki and Chow (1995) suggest the use of factor analysis in conjunction with the analysis of principal components for combining subscales. The proposed method provides statistical justification for the use of composite scores.

5.3 Performance Characteristics

In practice, commonly considered performance characteristics for validation of an instrument include, but are not limited to, accuracy (or validity), precision (or reliability), and reproducibility (see, e.g., USP/NF 2000, 2012; NCCLS 2001), which are briefly described below.

5.3.1 Validity

Validity of a QOL instrument is defined as the extent to which the QOL instrument measures what it is designed to measure. In other words, it is a measure of bias of the instrument. The bias of an instrument can reflect the accuracy of the instrument.

In clinical trials, as indicated earlier, the QOL of a patient is usually quantified based on responses to a number of questions related to several components or dimensions of QOL. It is a concern that the questions may not be the right questions to assess the components or domains of QOL of interest. To address this concern, consider a specific component (or domain) of QOL that consists of K items (or subscales), i.e., X_i, $i = 1,\ldots, K$. Also, let Y be the QOL component (or domain) of interest that is unobservable. Suppose that Y follows a normal distribution with mean θ and variance τ^2 and can be quantified by X_i, $i = 1,\ldots, K$. In other words, there exists a function f such that

$$f(X) = f(X_1, X_2,\ldots, X_K) = Y,$$

where $X = (X_1, X_2,\ldots, X_K)'$. Suppose X follows a distribution with mean $\mu = (\mu_1,\ldots, \mu_K)$ and variance Σ. Thus, θ can be estimated by

$$\hat{\theta} = \hat{f}(X_1, X_2,\ldots, X_K),$$

and the bias is given by

$$Bias(\hat{\theta}) = E(\hat{\theta} - \theta) = E(\hat{f}(X_1, X_2,\ldots, X_K)) - \theta.$$

QOL-Like Quantitative Instrument for Evaluation of TCM

In practice, for convenience, the unknown function f is usually assumed to be the mean of X_i, i.e.,

$$f(X) = f(X_1, X_2, \ldots, X_K) = \frac{1}{K} \sum_{i=1}^{K} X_i = Y.$$

Thus, it is desired to have the mean of X_i, $i = 1, \ldots, K$ closes to 0 and $\bar{\mu} = \frac{1}{K} \sum_{i=1}^{K} \mu_i = 0$. As a result, we may claim that the instrument is validated in terms of its validity if

$$\left| \mu_i - \bar{\mu} \right| < \delta \ \forall i = 1, \ldots, K.$$

To verify this, we may consider a simultaneous confidence interval for $\mu_i - \bar{\mu}$, $i = 1, \ldots, K$. Let $\mu_i - \bar{\mu} = a_i' \mu$, where $a_i' = \left(-\frac{1}{K} 1_{i-1}, 1 - \frac{1}{K}, -\frac{1}{K} 1_{K-i} \right)$. Suppose the QOL questionnaire is administered to N patients. Let

$$\hat{\mu} = \frac{1}{N} \sum_{j=1}^{N} X_j = \bar{X}.$$

Then, the $(1 - \alpha) \times 100\%$ simultaneous confidence intervals for $\mu_i - \bar{\mu}$, $i = 1, \ldots, K$ are given by

$$a_i' \hat{\mu} - \sqrt{\frac{1}{N} a_i' S a_i} \, T(\alpha, K, N - K) \le a_i' \mu \le a_i' \hat{\mu} + \sqrt{\frac{1}{N} a_i' S a_i} \, T(\alpha, K, N - K),$$

$$i = 1, \ldots, K,$$

where

$$S = \frac{1}{N-1} \sum_{j=1}^{N} (X_j - \bar{X})(X_j - \bar{X})',$$

$$T^2(\alpha, K, N - K) = \frac{(N-1)K}{N-K} F(\alpha, K, N - K),$$

and

$$P(T^2(K, N - K) \le T^2(\alpha, K, N - K)) = 1 - \alpha.$$

We may also consider Bonferroni adjustment of an overall α level as follows:

$$a_i'\hat{\mu} - \sqrt{\frac{1}{N}a_i'Sa_i}\,T\left(\frac{\alpha}{2K}, N-1\right) \le a_i'\mu \le a_i'\hat{\mu} + \sqrt{\frac{1}{N}a_i'Sa_i}\,T\left(\frac{\alpha}{2K}, N-1\right).$$

We then compare the confidence interval with $(-\delta, \delta)$ and reject the null hypothesis that

$$H_0 : |\mu_i - \bar{\mu}| < \delta \; \forall i = 1, \ldots, K$$

if any confidence interval falls completely outside $(-\delta, \delta)$.

Note that it is also important to establish concurrent validity in practice. Concurrent validity is established for a new instrument by demonstrating a good correlation with an already existing tool that is widely accepted as measuring the same construct(s). For example, a clinical evaluation by a physician might be considered the *gold standard* diagnosis. Or a well-recognized and accepted diagnostic criterion that is widely used by practitioners in the area may exist. In the case that the existing tool is continuous, a Pearson or Spearman's correlation coefficient can be computed. In the case of a dichotomous diagnostic tool, the area under the Receiver Operating Characteristics curve (ROC) can be used to establish a good relationship. If no such *gold standard* exists, one option is to compare the new instrument to existing instruments that measure similar or related constructs. This is referred to as convergent validity (discussed below). For example, all instruments in the same general area of general well-being should show some degree of relationship. Furthermore, all instruments or domains designed to measure general well-being should show a somewhat closer relationship to one another than they do to other domains, even if they have been developed on varying populations.

5.3.2 Reliability

The reliability of a QOL instrument reflects the other part of measurements and refers to the freedom from random error. The reliability of an instrument measures the variability of the instrument, which directly relates to the precision of the instrument. Therefore, the items are considered reliable if the variance of Y is small. To verify the reliability of estimating θ by Y, we consider the following hypothesis:

$$H_0 : Var(Y) < \Delta \text{ for some fixed } \Delta.$$

The variance of Y is given below

$$Var(Y) = Var\left(\frac{1}{K}\sum_{i=1}^{K}X_i\right) = \frac{1}{K^2}1'\Sigma1.$$

QOL-Like Quantitative Instrument for Evaluation of TCM

The sample distribution of

$$\sum_{j=1}^{N}(Y_j - \bar{Y})/Var(Y)$$

Has a chi-square distribution with $N - 1$ degrees of freedom. Thus, a $(1 - \alpha) \times 100\%$ one-sided confidence interval for $Var(Y)$ as follows:

$$Var(Y) \geq \frac{\sum_{j=1}^{N}(Y_j - \bar{Y})^2}{\chi^2(\alpha, N-1)} = \xi(Y).$$

If $\xi(Y) > \Delta$, then we reject the null hypothesis and conclude that the items are not reliable in estimating θ. As indicated earlier, patients' response to a QOL instrument may vary from one patient population to another and from one therapy to another. Therefore, it is recommended that the variability of QOL scores be studied before and after medication intervention.

Since the items $X_1, X_2, \ldots, X_K$ are relevant to a QOL component, they are expected to be correlated. In classical validation, a group of items with high intercorrelation between items are considered to be internally consistent. The Cronbach's α defined below is often used to measure the intercorrelations between items:

$$\alpha_C = \frac{K}{K-1}\left(1 - \frac{\sum_{i=1}^{K}\sigma_i^2}{\sum_{i=1}^{K}\sigma_i^2 + 2\sum\sum_{i<l}\sigma_{il}}\right),$$

where $\sigma_i^2 = Var(X_i)$ and $\sigma_{il} = Cov(X_i, X_l)$. When the covariance between items is high compared to the variance of each item, α_C is large. To ensure that the items are measuring the same component of QOL, the items under the component should be positively correlated, i.e., $\alpha_C \geq 50\%$. However, if the intercorrelations between items are too high, i.e., α_C is close to 1, it suggests that some of the items are redundant. Note that the variance of Y given below

$$Var(Y) = \left(\frac{1}{K-(K-1)\alpha_C}\right)\frac{1}{K}\sum_{i=1}^{K}Var(X_i)$$

Increases with α_C for fixed K and K and $Var(X_i)$, $i = 1,\ldots,K$. By including redundant items we cannot improve the precision of the result. It is desired to have independent items reflect the QOL component at different perspective.

Quantitative Methods for Traditional Chinese Medicine Development

However, in that case, it is hard to validate whether the items are measuring the same targeted component of QOL. Therefore, we suggest using items with moderate α_C i.e., α_C is somewhere between 50 and 80 percent.

5.3.3 Reproducibility

Reproducibility is defined as the extent to which repeat administrations of the same QOL measure yield the same result, assuming no underlying changes have occurred. The assessment of reproducibility involve expected and/or unexpected variabilities that might occur in the assessment of QOL. It includes inter-time (between time) point and inter-rater (between rater) reproducibility.

For the assessment of reproducibility, the technique of test-retest is often employed. The same QOL instrument is administered to patients who have reached stable conditions at two different time points. These two time points are generally separated by a sufficient length of time that is long enough to wear off the memory of the previous evaluation but not long enough to allow any change in environment. The Pearson's product moment correlation coefficient, ρ, of the two repeated results is then studied. In practice, a test-retest correlation of 80 percent or higher is considered acceptable. To verify this, the sample correlation between test-retest, denoted by r, is calculated from a sample of N patients. The following hypotheses are then tested.

$$H_0 : \rho \geq \rho_0 \text{ versus } H_a : \rho < \rho_0.$$

When N is large,

$$Z(r) = \frac{1}{2} \ln\left(\frac{1+r}{1-r}\right)$$

is approximately normally distributed with mean $Z(\rho)$ and variance $1/(N-3)$. The null hypothesis is rejected if

$$\sqrt{N-3}(Z(r) - Z(\rho_0)) < z(1-\alpha),$$

where $z(1-\alpha)$ is the αth quantile of the standard normal distribution. Note that a shift in mean of the score at test-retest may be detected by using a simple paired t-test. The inter-rater reproducibility can be verified by the same method.

5.4 Responsiveness and Sensitivity

The responsiveness of a QOL instrument is usually referred to as the ability of the instrument to detect a difference of clinical significance within a

QOL-Like Quantitative Instrument for Evaluation of TCM 109

treatment. The sensitivity is a measure of the ability of the instrument to detect a clinically significant difference between treatments. A validated instrument should be able to detect a difference if there is indeed a difference and should not wrongly detect a difference if there is no difference. Chow and Ki (1994) proposed precision and power indices to assess the responsiveness and sensitivity of a QOL instrument when comparing the effect of drugs on QOL between treatments. The precision index measures the probability of not detecting a false difference and the power index reflects the probability of detecting a meaningful difference. The precision and power indices for measuring responsiveness and sensitivity under a time series model proposed by Chow and Ki (1994) are described below.

5.4.1 Statistical Model

For a given QOL index, let X_{ijt} be the response of the ith subject to the jth question (item) at time t, where $i = 1,...,N$, $j = 1,...,J$, and $t = 1,...,T$. Consider the average score over J questions:

$$y_{it} = \bar{X}_{i \cdot t} = \frac{1}{J}\sum_{j=1}^{J} X_{ijt}.$$

Since the average scores $y_{i1},...,y_{iT}$ are correlated, the following autoregressive time series model is an appropriate statistical model for y_{it}.

$$y_{it} = \mu + \psi(y_{i,t-1} - \mu) + e_{it}, \ i = 1,..., N, \ t = 1,...,T, \tag{5.1}$$

where μ is the overall mean, $|\psi| < 1$ is the autoregressive parameter, and e_{it} are independent identically distributed random errors with mean 0 and variance σ_e^2. It can be verified that $E(e_{it}, e_{jt'}) = 0$ for all i, j and $t \neq t'$, and $E(e_{it}, y_{it'}) = 0$ for all $t' < t$. The autoregressive parameter ψ can be used to assess the correlation of consecutive responses y_{it} and $y_{i,t+1}$. From the above model, it can be shown that the autocorrelation of response with k lag times is ψ^k, which is negligible when k is large. Based on the observed average scores on the ith subject, i.e., $y_{i1}, y_{i2},...,y_{iT}$, we can estimate the overall mean μ and the autoregressive parameter ψ. The ordinary least squares estimators of μ and ψ can be approximated by

$$\hat{\mu}_i = \bar{y}_{i \cdot},$$

$$\hat{\psi}_i = \frac{\sum_{t=2}^{T}(y_{it} - \bar{y}_{i \cdot})(y_{i,t-1} - \bar{y}_{i \cdot})}{\sum_{t=2}^{T}(y_{it} - \bar{y}_{i \cdot})^2} r_{it'}$$

which are the sample mean and sample autocorrelation of consecutive observations. Under model (Equation 5.1), it can be verified that the variance of $\hat{\mu}_i$ is

$$Var(\bar{y}_{i\cdot}) = \frac{\gamma_{i0}}{T}\left[1 + 2\sum_{k=1}^{T-1}\frac{T-k}{T}\psi^k\right],$$

where $\gamma_{i0} = Var(y_{it})$. The standard error of $\hat{\mu}_i$ is then given by

$$s(\bar{y}_{i\cdot}) = \left[\frac{c_{i0}}{T}\left(1 + 2\sum_{k=1}^{T-1}\frac{T-k}{T}r_{i1}^k\right)\right]^{1/2},$$

in which

$$c_{i0} = \sum_{i=1}^{T}\frac{(y_{it} - \bar{y}_{i\cdot})^2}{T-1}.$$

Suppose that the N subjects are from the same population with same variability and autocorrelation. The QOL measurements of these subjects can be used to estimate the mean average scores μ. An intuitive estimator of μ is the sample mean

$$\hat{\mu} = \bar{y}_{\cdot\cdot} = \frac{1}{N}\sum_{i=1}^{N}\bar{y}_{i\cdot}.$$

Under model (Equation 5.1), the variance and standard error of $\hat{\mu}$ are given by, respectively,

$$Var(\bar{y}_{\cdot\cdot}) = \frac{1}{N^2}\sum_{i=1}^{N}Var(\bar{y}_{i\cdot}),$$

and

$$s(\bar{y}_{\cdot\cdot}) = \frac{1}{N}\left\{\sum_{i=1}^{N}[s(\bar{y}_{i\cdot})]^2\right\}^{1/2}$$

$$= \frac{1}{N}\left\{\frac{c_0}{T}\sum_{i=1}^{N}\left[1 + 2\sum_{k=1}^{T-1}\frac{T-k}{T}r_1^k\right]\right\}^{1/2} \tag{5.2}$$

$$= \left\{\frac{c_0}{NT}\left[1 + 2\sum_{k=1}^{T-1}\frac{T-k}{T}r_1^k\right]\right\}^{1/2},$$

QOL-Like Quantitative Instrument for Evaluation of TCM

where

$$c_0 = \frac{1}{N(T-1)} \sum_{i=1}^{N} \left[\sum_{t=1}^{T} (y_{it} - \bar{y}_{i.})^2 \right],$$

$$r_1 = \frac{1}{N} \sum_{i=1}^{N} r_{i1}.$$

As a result, an approximate $(1 - \alpha) \times 100\%$ confidence interval for μ can then be constructed as follows:

$$\bar{y}_{..} \pm z_{1-1/2\alpha} s(\bar{y}_{..}), \tag{5.3}$$

where $z_{1-1/2\alpha}$ is the $100(1 - \alpha/2)$th percentile of a standard normal distribution and $s(\bar{y}_{..})$ is given in Equation 5.2. As a matter of fact, the assumption that all the QOL measurements over time are independent is a special case of model (Equation 5.1) with $\psi = 0$. In practice, it is suggested that model (Equation 5.1) be used to account for the possible positive correlation between measurements over test time period. Under model (Equation 5.1), it can be seen that the confidence interval given in Equation 5.3 with $r_1 > 0$ is wider than that when $\psi = 0$.

Note that, for the statistical validation of an instrument, at a fixed confidence level, the width of the confidence interval in Equation 5.3 is inversely proportional to the prevision of the estimator $\bar{y}_{..}$ and may be used as an indicator of the validity of the instrument. For example, if the width of a confidence interval is too wide, the instrument may not be sensitive due to low power for detecting a positive difference or an equivalence. In what follows, the precision and power indices of QOL instruments will be evaluated under model (Equation 5.1).

5.4.2 Precision Index

Suppose that a homogeneous group is divided into two independent groups A and B that are known to have the same QOL. A *good* QOL instrument should have a small chance of *wrongly* detecting a difference. Let $y_i = (y_{i1}, y_{i2}, \ldots, y_{it}, \ldots, y_{iT})'$ be the average scores observed on the ith subject in group A at different time points over a fixed time period. Similarly, denote the average scores for the jth subject in group B over time period by $w_j = (w_{j1}, w_{j2}, \ldots, w_{jt}, \ldots, w_{jT})'$. The objective is to compare mean average scores between groups to see whether the instrument reflects the expected result statistically. On the basis of y_i, $i = 1, \ldots, N$ and w_j, $j = 1, \ldots, M$, the difference in mean average scores between groups A and B can be assessed by testing the following hypotheses that $H_0 : \mu_y = \mu_w$ versus $H_a : \mu_y \neq \mu_w$, where μ_y and μ_w are the mean average scores for groups A and B, respectively. Under the null hypothesis, the following test statistic

$$Z = \frac{\bar{y}_{..} - \bar{w}_{..}}{[s^2(\bar{y}_{..}) + s^2(\bar{w}_{..})]^{1/2}}$$

is approximately distributed as a standard normal distribution when N and M are both large. Therefore, we would reject the null hypothesis if $|Z| > z_{1-\alpha/2}$.

Note that the above test is a uniform most powerful test. The level of significance of the test is α. The confidence interval for $\mu_y - \mu_w$ and the rejection region are given, respectively, by

$$(L, U) = \bar{y}_{..} - \bar{w}_{..} \pm d_\alpha \text{ and } \left| \bar{y}_{..} - \bar{w}_{..} \right| > d_\alpha,$$

where

$$d_\alpha = z_{1-\alpha/2} [s^2(\bar{y}_{..}) + s^2(\bar{w}..)]^{1/2}.$$

In general, an interval estimator of $\mu_y - \mu_w$ is given by

$$(\bar{y}_{..} - \bar{w}_{..}) \pm d, \tag{5.4}$$

which is used for detecting a difference in means. A difference is detected if zero lies outside the interval, i.e.,

$$\left| \bar{y}_{..} - \bar{w}_{..} \right| > d.$$

The precision index, denoted by P_d, of an instrument is defined as the probability of the interval (Equation 5.4) not detecting a difference when there is no difference between groups, i.e.,

$$\begin{aligned} P_d &= P\left\{ \left| \bar{y}_{..} - \bar{w}_{..} \right| \leq d \,|\, \mu_y = \mu_w \right\} \\ &= P\left\{ |Z| \leq d \left[\sigma^2(\bar{y}_{..}) + \sigma^2(\bar{w}_{..}) \right]^{-1/2} \right\}, \end{aligned} \tag{5.5}$$

where

$$Z = \frac{(\bar{y}_{..} - \bar{w}_{..}) - (\mu_y - \mu_w)}{[\sigma^2(\bar{y}_{..}) + \sigma^2(\bar{w}_{..})]^{1/2}}$$

QOL-Like Quantitative Instrument for Evaluation of TCM

is the standardized random variable that is approximately distributed as a standard normal when N and M are large. It can be seen that the precision index of an instrument is $1 - \alpha$ at $d = d_\alpha$. Note that P_d is the confidence level of the interval estimator given in Equation 5.4, which increases as d increases. When d is too big, although the interval has a very high probability to capture the true difference, it may not have sufficient power for detecting a positive difference.

5.4.3 Power Index

On the other hand, if the QOL instrument is administered to two groups of subjects who are known to have different QOL, then the QOL instrument should be able to correctly detect such a difference with a high probability. The power index of an instrument for detecting a meaningful difference, denoted by $\delta_d(\varepsilon)$, is defined as the probability of detecting a meaningful difference ε. That is,

$$\delta_d(\varepsilon) = P\left\{\left|\bar{y}_{..} - \bar{w}_{..}\right| > d \,\middle|\, \left|\mu_y - \mu_w\right| = \varepsilon\right\}$$

$$= P\left\{Z > (d-\varepsilon)[\sigma^2(\bar{y}_{..}) + \sigma^2(\bar{w}_{..})]^{-1/2}\right\} \tag{5.6}$$

$$+ P\left\{Z < -(d+\varepsilon)[\sigma^2(\bar{y}_{..}) + \sigma^2(\bar{w}_{..})]^{-1/2}\right\}.$$

For $d = d_\alpha$, $\delta_d(\varepsilon)$ is the power, which can be calculated as follows.

$$\delta_d(\varepsilon) = P\left\{\left|\bar{y}_{..} - \bar{w}_{..}\right| > z_{1-\alpha/2}[s^2(\bar{y}_{..}) + s^2(\bar{w}_{..})]^{1/2} \,\middle|\, \left|\mu_y - \mu_w\right| = \varepsilon\right\}$$

$$\doteq P\left\{Z < -z_{1-\alpha/2} - \frac{\varepsilon}{[s^2(\bar{y}_{..}) + s^2(\bar{w}_{..})]^{1/2}}\right\}$$

$$+ P\left\{Z > z_{1-\alpha/2} - \frac{\varepsilon}{[s^2(\bar{y}_{..}) + s^2(\bar{w}_{..})]^{1/2}}\right\}.$$

Note that for a fixed ε, $\delta_d(\varepsilon)$ decreases as d increases. We consider an instrument to be responsive in detecting a difference if both P_d and $\delta_d(\varepsilon)$ are above some reasonable limits for a given ε.

In practice, two groups are considered to have equivalent QOL if their mean QOL measurements only differ by less than a meaningful difference η. In this case, it is of interest to detect an equivalence rather than a difference. Denote the acceptable limits for the difference between two group means by $(-\Delta, \Delta)$. When the confidence interval of $\mu_y - \mu_w$ given in Equation 5.4 is within the acceptable limits, we conclude that the two groups have equivalent effect on QOL. We will refer to the probability of detecting an equivalence as the power index of an instrument for detecting an equivalence when the true group means differ by less than a meaningful difference η. The power index is then defined as

$$\phi_\Delta(\eta) = \inf_{|\mu_y-\mu_w|} P\{(L,U) \subset (-\Delta,\Delta) \mid |\mu_y - \mu_w| < \eta\}$$

$$= P\{(L,U) \subset (-\Delta,\Delta) \mid \mu_y - \mu_w = \eta\},$$

(5.7)

where (L, U) is a confidence interval of $\mu_y - \mu_w$ as given in Equation 5.4. Note that $\phi_\Delta(\eta)$ can be obtained as follows:

$$\phi_\Delta(\eta) = P\{(L,U) \subset (-\Delta,\Delta) \mid \mu_y - \mu_w = \eta\}$$

$$= P\left\{(\bar{y}_{..} - \bar{w}_{..} - d, \bar{y}_{..} - \bar{w}_{..} + d) \subset (-\Delta,\Delta) \mid \mu_y - \mu_w = \eta\right\}$$

$$= P\left\{\frac{(\bar{y}_{..} - \bar{w}_{..}) - \eta}{\left[\sigma^2(\bar{y}_{..}) + \sigma^2(\bar{w}_{..})\right]^{1/2}} > \frac{-(\Delta - d) - \eta}{\left[\sigma^2(\bar{y}_{..}) + \sigma^2(\bar{w}_{..})\right]^{1/2}} \text{ and } \right.$$

$$\left. \frac{(\bar{y}_{..} - \bar{w}_{..}) - \eta}{\left[\sigma^2(\bar{y}_{..}) + \sigma^2(\bar{w}_{..})\right]^{1/2}} < \frac{(\Delta - d) - \eta}{\left[\sigma^2(\bar{y}_{..}) + \sigma^2(\bar{w}_{..})\right]^{1/2}}\right\}$$

$$= P\left\{\frac{-(\Delta - d) - \eta}{\left[\sigma^2(\bar{y}_{..}) + \sigma^2(\bar{w}_{..})\right]^{1/2}} < Z < \frac{(\Delta - d) - \eta}{\left[\sigma^2(\bar{y}_{..}) + \sigma^2(\bar{w}_{..})\right]^{1/2}}\right\},$$

(5.8)

which can be approximated by

$$\phi_\Delta(\eta) \doteq \Phi\left[\frac{(\Delta - d) - \eta}{\left[\sigma^2(\bar{y}_{..}) + \sigma^2(\bar{w}_{..})\right]^{1/2}}\right] - \Phi\left[\frac{-(\Delta - d) - \eta}{\left[\sigma^2(\bar{y}_{..}) + \sigma^2(\bar{w}_{..})\right]^{1/2}}\right],$$

where Φ is the cumulative distribution function of a standard normal distribution.

5.4.4 Sample Size Determination

Because QOL response may vary widely from patient to patient, a large sample size is usually required to attain reasonable precision and power. Under model (Equation 5.1) and the setting as described above, some useful formulae for determination of sample size can be derived based on normal approximation. The formulae can also be applied to many clinical research studies with time-correlated outcome measurements, e.g., 24-hour monitoring of blood pressure, heart rates, hormone levels, and body temperature.

QOL-Like Quantitative Instrument for Evaluation of TCM 115

For a fixed precision index (e.g., $1 - \alpha$), to ensure a reasonable high power index δ for detecting a meaningful difference ε, the sample size per treatment group should not be less than

$$N_\delta = \frac{c[z_{1-\alpha/2} + z_\delta]^2}{\varepsilon^2} \text{ for } \delta > 0.5, \tag{5.9}$$

where

$$c = \frac{\gamma_y}{T} \left[1 + 2 \sum_{k=1}^{T-1} \frac{T-k}{T} \psi_y^k \right] + \frac{\gamma_w}{T} \left[1 + 2 \sum_{k=1}^{T-1} \frac{T-k}{T} \psi_w^k \right].$$

For a fixed precision index (e.g., $1 - \alpha$), if the acceptable limit for detecting an equivalence between two treatment means is $(-\Delta, \Delta)$, to ensure a reasonable high power ϕ for detecting an equivalence when the true difference in treatment means is less than a small constant η, the sample size for each treatment group should be at least

$$N_\phi = \frac{c}{(\Delta - \eta)^2} [z_{1/2+1/2\phi} + z_{1-\alpha/2}]^2. \tag{5.10}$$

If both treatment groups are assumed to have some variability and autocorrelation coefficient, the constant c in Equations 5.9 and 5.10 can be simplified as

$$c = \frac{2\gamma}{T} \left[1 + 2 \sum_{k=1}^{T-1} \frac{T-k}{T} \psi^k \right].$$

When $N = \max(N_\phi, N_\delta)$, it ensures that the QOL instrument will have precision index $1 - \alpha$ and power of no less than δ and ϕ in detecting a difference and an equivalence, respectively. It should be noted that the required sample size is proportional to the variability of the average scores considered. The higher the variability, the larger the sample size that would be required.

As an example, suppose that there are two independent groups A and B. A QOL index containing 11 questions is administered to subjects at weeks 4, 8, 12, and 16. The mean scores are analyzed to assess group difference. Denote the mean of QOL score of the subjects in group A and B by Y_{it} and W_{jt}, respectively, where $i, j = 1,\ldots, N$, and $t = 1, 2, 3, 4$. We assume that Y_{it} and W_{jt} have distributions that follow the time series model described in model (Equation 5.1) with common variance $\gamma = 0.5$ sq. unit and have moderate autocorrelation between scores at consecutive time points, say $\psi = 0.5$. For a fixed

95 percent precision index, by Equation 5.9, 87 subjects per group will provide a 90 percent power for detection of a difference of 0.25 unit in means. If the chosen acceptable limits are $(-0.35, 0.35)$, by Equation 5.10, 108 subjects per group will have a power of 90 percent that the 95 percent confidence interval of difference in group means will correctly detect an equivalence with $\eta = 0.1$ unit. If the sample size is chosen to be 108 per group, it ensures that the power indices for detecting a difference of 0.25 unit or an equivalence are not less than 90 percent.

5.5 Utility Analysis and Calibration

5.5.1 Utility Analysis

Gains in quantity of life can be measured in terms of life years gained, while gains in quality of life should be measured by an instrument that incorporates a broad spectrum of health status, including physical/mobility function, psychological function, cognitive function, social function, and so forth. Feeny and Torrance (1989) proposed a utility approach to measure the health-related QOL. Utility is a single summary score, which ranges from zero (for dead) to one (for perfect health). Torrance and Feeny (1989) used QOL utility as quantity-adjustment weights for quality adjusted life years, which are highly used in cost-effectiveness analysis.

The utility of hypothetical or actual health states may be evaluated by an individual. Utility is the preference of an individual for a health state. The preference of health state can be measured by some standard technique, such as rating scale, standard gamble, and time tradeoff. However, the utility measurements are not very precise. The within-subject variability is around 0.13 and the intersubject variability is approximately 0.3 for the general public and 0.2 for patients experiencing the health state (Feeny and Torrance 1989). An individual either is experiencing the disease state or understands the hypothetical description of the disease state. A rating scale consists of a line with the least preferred state (e.g., death) on one end and the most preferred state (perfect health) on the other end. An individual will rate the disease state on the line between these two extreme states. Usually, the utility value obtained by this technique has high variability. A utility value of a disease state can be assigned by the standard gamble technique. An individual is given the choice of remaining at the disease state for an additional t years or the alternative, which consists of perfect health for an additional t years with probability p and immediate death with probability $(1 - p)$. The probability p is varied until the individual is indifferent between the two alternatives. Then the preference/utility of that disease state is p. The preference value of a disease state can also be assigned by using a time tradeoff technique. An individual is offered two alternatives: (1) at the disease state with life expectancy of t years or (2) in perfect health for x years. Then x is varied until the individual is indifferent between the two alternatives. Then, the preference value of the disease state is x/t. The time tradeoff technique is easier for an individual to understand; however, the preference value is the true utility provided that the individual's utility function for additional healthy years is linear in time. If the utility function for additional healthy years is concave, the preference value by time tradeoff method will underestimate the true utility value of the disease state. For more details regarding the performance of the above utility measuring techniques, readers should refer to Torrance (1987).

The utility values should be validated for test and retest reproducibility before they are used to measure any change in health state. For interpretation of improvement in utility, Torrance and Feeny (1989) related the utility values of some marker states. If there are utility values for some marker states, A, B, and C at 0.8, 0.7, and 0.4, respectively, an average improvement of 0.1 in utility of outcome health state from a trial may be described as equivalent to improving from outcome B to A average over all patients in the trial.

Although aggregation of utilities across individuals is commonly used in analysis of data, it should be done with caution. The utility function may not be the same across subjects. The anchor states, perfect health and death, should be well defined for the same understanding across all subjects. To evaluate the effect of a therapy, the life years gained should be adjusted by the quality of life. The quality-adjusted life years is the area under the profile of quality of life utility over time. The quality-adjusted life years gained is usually used in evaluation of the effectiveness of therapy.

5.5.2 Calibration

Besides the validation of a QOL instrument, another issue of particular interest is the interpretation of an identified significant change in QOL score. For this purpose, Testa et al. (1993) considered the calibration of change in QOL against change in life events. A linear calibration curve was used to predict the relationship between the change in QOL index and change in life event index. Only negative life events were considered. The study was not designed for calibration purposes and the changes in life events were collected as auxiliary information. The effect of change of life event was confounded with the effect of medication. If we want to use calibration to interpret the impact of change in QOL score, further research in the design and analysis method is necessary. Because the impact of life events is subjective and varies from person to person, it is difficult to assign numerical scores/indices to life events. The relationship between QOL score and life event may not be linear. More complicated calibration functions or transformations may be required. We expect that the QOL score has a positive correlation with life event score; however, the correlation may not be strong enough to give a precise calibration curve.

118   *Quantitative Methods for Traditional Chinese Medicine Development*

Besides the calibration of the QOL score with the life event score, changes in the QOL score may be related to changes in disease status.

5.6 QOL-Like Instrument for Evaluation of TCM

Kondoh et al. (2005) indicated that a QOL-like instrument is a useful instrument for measurement of the efficacy of herbal medicine. As a first step of the clinical study for the efficacy of herbal drugs, Kondoh et al. (2005) evaluated the feasibility of modified dermatology life quality index (DLQI) based questionnaires (QOL sheet). The QOL sheet consisted of 10 questions, each referring to the DLQI (Finlay and Khan 1994). The DLQI designed for routine clinical use has 10 questions concerning the QOL and provides a total score. It is applicable to patients with any skin disease (Finlay and Khan 1994). The original DLQI has check box answers only. Because the original DLQI is in English, Kondoh et al. (2005) used its translated Japanese version with Japanese patients. The reliability of the Japanese DLQI was subsequently validated. However, Kondoh et al. (2005) made slightly modifications to the original QOL-like instrument to evaluate the efficacy of the herbal medicine (Table 5.1). In the modified QOL questionnaire, the patients were also asked to assess the visual analog scale (VAS). Higher scores of DLQI reflect greater impairment. In comparing VAS and DLQI, higher VAS scores indicate greater impairment in the modified QOL questionnaire. The modified QOL questionnaire was supplemented with three original questions that concerned therapy using herbal medicines. The AQ were used for a combined evaluation with other scores.

By using the modified QOL questionnaire, Kondoh et al. (2005) compared the scores of before, 2 and/or 4 weeks after receiving herbal medication. Kondoh et al. (2005) also evaluated the symptoms of patients clinically at 2 and/or 4 weeks after the herbal medication. The scores of the questions 1 to 10 that were made as DLQI in Japanese were graded according to the original scoring rule as described by Finlay and Khan (1994). The VAS scores were also assessed by patients.

As indicated by Kondoh et al. (2005), herbal medicines have been used widely by physicians in Japan. In dermatology, some reports showed the effectiveness of the herbal medicines for skin diseases (see, e.g., Ikawa and Imayama 1983; Kimura et al. 1985; Yabe 1985; Satoh et al. 1995; Abeni et al. 2002; Inagi 2003; Suzugamo et al. 2004). Some dermatologists who are less familiar with traditional Chinese herbal medicines, however, often hesitate at their use because the herbal medicines can be somewhat ambiguous in a comprehensive assessment of clinical efficacy. For this reason, Kondoh et al. (2005) studied the applicability of the QOL-related scoring methods to assessing the efficacy of the herbal medicines. In their study, Kondoh et al. (2005)

TABLE 5.1
QOL-like Questionnaire for Assessment of Efficacy of Chinese Herbal Medicine

Patients	1	2	3	4	7	8	9	10	11
Age	73	75	86	79	77	18	76	69	82
Sex*1	M	M	M	F	F	M	F	M	M
Disease*2	2	1	4	2	2	1	2	3	1
Prescription*3	6	6	6	86	6	6	6	86	6
Period*4	0, 5	4, 5	2, 4	0, 4	2, 2, n	0, 2	0, 2, 2, n	0, 2	2, 0, 2
DLQ1	16, 5, 13, 9, 6	13, 9	10	10, n	6, 2	11, 2	23, 2	6, 5	1, 0
VAS	53.1, 7.9, 10.3, 14.2	13.1, 31.1, 24.7	26.4	29.4, n	4.9, n	45.6, 4	64.6, n	15.3, 8.7	8.7, 5
Clinical impression*5	1, 0	−1	0, 1	0, 1	1, 1	2	1	1	1

(Continued)

TABLE 5.1 (CONTINUED)

QOL-like Questionnaire for Assessment of Efficacy of Chinese Herbal Medicine

Patients		12			13			14			15			16		17		18		19	
Age		69			70			45			60			52		65		42		74	
Sex*1		M			M			M			M			F		M		F		M	
Disease*2		2			1			1			1			1		1		3		1	
Prescription*3		6			86			6			6			6		6		86		6	
Period*4	0	2	4	0	2	4	0	2	4	0	2	4	0	2	4	0	2	0	2	0	2	4
DLQ1	13	6	2	7	8	8	2	1	0	1	2	2	1	0	0	6	7	17	13	4	5	6
VAS	70.9	64.3	53.4	22.5	24.2	20.2	2.6	0.1	0	2.2	5	4	0.4	0	0	14.6	6.1	59.6	53.5	12.2	12.2	19.5
Clinical impression*5		1			0	0		1	1		−1	−1		1	1		0		1		0	−1

Note: *1: M: male F: female; *2: 1: seborrheic dermatitis, 2: asteatotic eczema, 3: pruritus, 4: others; *3: 6: *jumi-haidoku-tou*, 86: *touki-inshi*; *4: 0: before, 2: 2 weeks after, 4: 4 weeks after; *5: 2: the effect was high, 1: improving, 0: same, −1: worsening; n: no data.

proposed the use of QLQI for patients with any skin diseases. The results indicate that herbal medicines are clinically effective for the chronic skin diseases (Table 5.2). Statistically, the changes in the DLQI and VAS scores agreed with the clinically proven effectiveness of the herbal medicines ($P < 0.05$). No significant difference was found between the clinical impressions and the DLQI with the AQ or the VAS with the AQ ($P > 0.05$). Thus, the results indicate that the modified QOL questionnaire is found useful for evaluation of the efficacy of the herbal medicine. The QOL sheet appears particularly useful in evaluating the efficacy of the herbal medicines for some skin diseases such as puritis without skin lesions and the patients with uncertain changes of the clinical symptoms (e.g., patient No. 2, 3, 13, and 17).

Note that the number of cases determined "effective" by the changes in the DLQI or VAS scores was 11 and 10, respectively. On the other hand, the number of cases classified as effective by the score changes in the DLQI with the AQ or the VAS with the AQ was 9 and 9, respectively. When evaluated by the DLQI with the AQ or VAS with the AQ, the number of effective cases was fewer than that obtained by the DLQI or VAS alone. Because these additional questions were related to the negative elements of herbal medicines, the scoring with the AQ can necessarily be higher, leading to poorer effectiveness than that revealed by the clinical symptoms, DLQI or VAS. It may be necessary to reconsider the contents of the additional questions. In conclusion, we showed that the QOL sheet is useful to evaluate the efficacy of herbal medicines. However, it may be necessary to reconsider the contents of our original questions. Further studies with larger samples are required to fully establish both the applicability and reliability of the QOL-based evaluation of the herbal medications in patients with skin diseases.

5.6.1 Remarks

For development of an instrument for evaluation of herbal medicines, one may consider developing questions for different purposes in order to improve the accuracy and precision of the instrument for assessment of the herbal medicines. For example, one may consider developing questionnaires at the following different levels:

Level 1 questions – identifying the type of diseases;
Level 2 questions – determining the affected organ;
Level 3 questions – describing the signs and symptoms.

On the basis of the results of the above different levels of questions, individualized treatment (dose) is possible. As a result, the treatment effect of the herbal medicine can then be evaluated by comparing the data collected via the instrument before and after the herbal medicine.

TABLE 5.2
Assessment of QLQI, VAS, and AQ for Patients with Skin Diseases

Patients	1			2			3			4			7			8			9			10			11	
Periods*4	0	2	4	0	2	4	0	2	4	0	2	4	0	2	4	0	2	4	0	2	4	0	2	4	0	2
AQ11	0	6.3	5.3	0.9	0	1.8	0	1	0	0.8	n	0	0	n	5	0	0	0	3.7	7	0	0	0	0	0	6.8
AQ12	0	0	0	1	2	1	0	1	0	0	n	0	0	n	0	0	0	0	1	0	0	0	0	1	0	0
AQ13	0	0	0	9	2.1	0.3	0	0	0	0	n	0.2	0	n	0	0	0	0	0	0.2	0	0	1	0	0	0
total	0	6.3	5.3	1.9	4.1	3.1	0	2	0	0.8	n	0.2	0	n	5	0	0	0	4.7	7.2	0	0	0	1	0	6.8
DLQ1+AQ	16	11.3	10.3	6.9	10.1	16.1	9	12	9	10.8	n	0.2	2	n	7	11	2	27.7	9.2	6	6	1	6.8
VAS+AQ	53.1	14.2	15.6	16.1	17.2	34.2	24.7	28.4	n	30.2	n	0.2	6.9	n	n	45.6	4	69.3	n	15.3	8.7	5	6.8

(Continued)

TABLE 5.2 (CONTINUED)

Assessment of QLQI, VAS, and AQ for Patients with Skin Diseases

Patients	12			13			14			15			16			17		18		19		
periods*4	0	2	4	0	2	4	0	2	4	0	2	4	0	2	4	0	2	0	2	0	2	4
AQ11	0	0.4	0.7	0	0	0	0	0	0	0	0	0	0	0.3	0	0	0.8	0	6	0	0.5	0.5
AQ12	0	0	0	0	0	0	1	1	0	0	0	0	0	0	0	0	0	0	1	0	0	0
AQ13	0	0	0	0	0.1	0.1	0	0.1	0.2	0	0	0	0	0.2	0.2	0	0.1	0	0	0	0	0
total	0	0.4	0.7	0	0.1	0.1	1	1.1	0.2	0	0	0	0	0.5	0.2	0	0.9	0	7	0	0.5	0.5
DLQ1+AQ	13	6.4	2.7	7	8.1	8.1	3	2.1	0.2	1	2	2	1	0.5	0.2	6	7.9	17	20	4	5.5	6.5
VAS+AQ	70.9	64.7	54.1	22.5	24.3	20.3	3.6	0.2	0.2	2.2	5	4	0.4	0.5	0.2	14.6	7	59.6	60.5	12.2	12.7	20

Note: *4: 0: before, 2:2 weeks after, 4:4 weeks after; n: no data.

124   *Quantitative Methods for Traditional Chinese Medicine Development*

In practice, it is always a concern that the QOL-like instrument for evaluation of safety and efficacy of TCMs may exhibit large within-rater and between-rater variabilities, which have a negative impact on the assessment of TCMs. As a result, it is suggested that the within-rater and between-rate variabilities should be avoided, eliminated, or controled whenever possible for an accurate and reliable assessment of the TCMs under investigation.

5.7 Parallel Assessments

In practice, QOL-like instrument for evaluation of TCMs may be assessed in parallel by a Chinese doctor and a Western clinician. The variability of the rating is expected to vary between the Chinese doctor and the Western clinician. Although the scores can be analyzed separately based on individual ratings, they may lead to different conclusions. In this case, determining which rating should be used to assess the treatment effect has become a controversial issue. On one hand, it is suggested that the Chinese doctors' ratings should be considered as the primary analysis because they are more familiar with the TCM under investigation. On the other hand, it is suggested that Western clinicians' assessment should be considered because their assessments are considered more objective and evidence-based.

In practice, a typical approach is to analyze each rating separately. This approach, however, may cause the loss of some important information from the responses provided by the different perspectives. Besides, the assessment based on each rating alone may lead to a totally different conclusion. To fully use the information contained in the two ratings, as an alternative, it is suggested that a composite index that combines both parallel ratings be considered. In this case, "Should the individual ratings carry the same weights as the parallel ratings?" has become an interesting question. If the Chinese doctor's rating is considered to be more reliable than others, it should carry more weight in the assessment of TCM under investigation; otherwise, it should carry less weight in the analysis. Along this line, Ki and Chow (1994) considered the following weighted score function:

$$Z = aX + bY,$$

where X and Y denote the ratings of a Chinese doctor and a Western clinician, respectively, and a and b are the corresponding weights assigned to X and Y. Note that if $a = 1$ and $b = 0$, then the score function reduces to the Chinese doctor's rating. On the other hand, when $a = 0$ and $b = 1$, the score function represents the Western clinician's rating. When $a = b = 1/2$, the score function is the average of the two ratings; that is, the Chinese doctor's rating and the Western clinician's rating are considered equally important.

QOL-Like Quantitative Instrument for Evaluation of TCM

If one believes that one rating is more reliable than the other rating, then the more reliable rating should carry more weight for the assessment of the TCM under investigation. The choice of a and b in the above score function determines the relative importance of the ratings in the evaluation of the TCM under investigation. Ki and Chow (1994) proposed using the technique of principal components to determine a and b based on the observed data. The idea is to derive a one-dimensional function of both ratings, which can retain as much information as possible as compared to the two-dimensional vector $W = (X, Y)'$. Assume that W follows a bivariate joint distribution with mean $\mu = (\mu_X, \mu_Y)'$ and covariance matrix

$$\Sigma = \begin{pmatrix} \sigma_X^2 & \rho\sigma_X\sigma_Y \\ \rho\sigma_X\sigma_Y & \sigma_Y^2 \end{pmatrix},$$

where σ_X and σ_Y are the standard deviation of X and Y, respectively, and ρ is the linear correlation coefficient between X and Y. Then, the mean and covariance matrix of W can be estimated based on observed ratings $W_i = (X_i, Y_i)'$, $i = 1,\dots, N$, as follows:

$$\hat{\mu} = \bar{W} = (\bar{X}, \bar{Y}),$$

where

$$\bar{X} = \frac{1}{N}\sum_{i=1}^{N} X_i \text{ and } \bar{Y} = \frac{1}{N}\sum_{i=1}^{N} Y_i,$$

and

$$\hat{\Sigma} = S = \frac{1}{N-1}\sum_{i=1}^{N}(W_i - \bar{W})(W_i - \bar{W})' = \begin{pmatrix} S_X^2 & rS_X S_Y \\ rS_X S_Y & S_Y^2 \end{pmatrix}.$$

The above sample covariance matrix contains not only the information about the variations of the Chinese doctor and the Western clinician ratings but also the correlation between the two ratings. For the determination of a and b, one approach is to employ the technique of principal components based on both ratings. The first principal component of the observed data $\{W_i, i = 1,\dots, N\}$ possesses the maximum sample variance, that is,

$$A'SA = a^2 S_X^2 + b^2 S_Y^2 + 2abr S_X S_Y$$

among all coefficient vectors satisfying

$$A'A = a^2 + b^2 = 1.$$

It can be shown that the numbers in the characteristic vector A associated with the largest characteristic root of S are the coefficients of the first principal component. The characteristic roots of S can be obtained from the characteristic equation

$$|S - \lambda I| = 0.$$

This leads to

$$\begin{vmatrix} S_X^2 - \lambda & rS_X S_Y \\ rS_X S_Y & S_Y^2 - \lambda \end{vmatrix} = 0.$$

Therefore,

$$\lambda = \frac{1}{2}\left(S_X^2 + S_Y^2\right) \pm \frac{1}{2}\Delta_{XY},$$

where

$$\Delta_{XY} = \sqrt{\left(S_X^2 + S_Y^2\right)^2 - 4S_X^2 S_Y^2 (1 - r^2)}.$$

The largest root is then given by

$$\lambda_1 = \frac{1}{2}\left(S_X^2 + S_Y^2\right) + \frac{1}{2}\Delta_{XY}.$$

The first principal component can be obtained by solving the following equations:

$$\left(S_X^2 - \lambda_1\right)a + brS_X S_Y = 0,$$

$$a^2 + b^2 = 1.$$

This leads to

$$a = \left(1 + \frac{\left(\lambda_1 - S_X^2\right)^2}{r^2 S_X^2 S_Y^2}\right)^{-1/2}$$

and

$$b = \frac{\left(\lambda_1 - S_X^2\right)a}{rS_X S_Y}.$$

The sample covariance of the first principal component $y = A'W$ is the largest characteristic root $\lambda_1 = A'SA$ and the percentage of variation expressed by this component is

$$\frac{\lambda_1}{tr(S)},$$

where $tr(S)$ is the trace of S, which is given by

$$tr(S) = S_X^2 + S_Y^2.$$

Note that if the sample covariance matrix S is singular, then there is only one nonzero characteristic root. The first principal component explains all the variation in the observations. The percentage of sample variation presented by the first principal component reflects how much information from the observations is retained by the first principal component and the usefulness of the component in representing the observations in a one-dimensional setting. If a large proportion of the variation of the observations can be accounted for by a single principal component, then most of the variation generated by the observations in a two-dimensional space can be expressed along a one-dimensional vector. This appeals to dimensional reduction and the coefficients (a, b) indicate the direction and relative importance of each rating toward TCM assessment.

As an example, suppose that the sample covariance matrix of X and Y is

$$S = \begin{pmatrix} 1 & r \\ r & 1 \end{pmatrix},$$

where $r > 0$. The largest characteristic root of S is $1 + r$ and its corresponding characteristic vector is $A = \left(\sqrt{2}/2, \sqrt{2}/2\right)$. The score function is then given by

$$Z = \frac{\sqrt{2}}{2}X + \frac{\sqrt{2}}{2}Y,$$

which gives equal weight to both ratings. The percentage of variation retained by Z is $100 \times (1 + r)/2$. The amount of variation expressed by Z for different values of the linear correlation coefficient r is summarized in Table 5.3. When

TABLE 5.3

Percentage of Variation Expressed by Z for Various r

r	Variation Expressed by Z
0.9	95%
0.7	85%
0.5	75%
0.0	50%

the two ratings X and Y are highly correlated, the score function retains a very high percentage of variation. When the correlation is moderate, say 0.7, the score function can still retain 85 percent of the variation of the data. As can be seen from Table 5.3, the score function proposed in this section is simple and easy to use. It reduces a two-dimensional problem to a univariate problem. It uses the information from both ratings and gives a better power for statistical tests.

Suppose the instrument is assessed before drug therapy (at baseline) and at the end of the therapy (endpoint) by the Chinese doctor and the Western clinician. The hypothesis of interest is one of no drug effect. Denote the endpoint change from baseline in the Chinese doctor's rating by X and that of the Western clinician's rating by Y. When X and Y are analyzed separately, the probabilities of all possible conclusions are summarized in Table 5.4. As can be seen from Table 5.4, the probability of observing inconsistent conclusion is given by $P = P_{AR} + P_{RA}$. For a particular case, when X and Y are bivariate normal with linear correlation coefficient ρ, the probabilities of observing inconsistent conclusions can be calculated and are presented in Table 5.5. Analysis of treatment effect can be done on the score function Z to avoid the potential problem of inconsistent results that may occur when the ratings are analyzed separately.

TABLE 5.4

Probabilities of All Possible Conclusions

	Accepted H_0	Reject H_0
X	P_{RA}	P_{RR}
Y	P_{AA}	P_{AR}

TABLE 5.5

Probability of Inconsistent Conclusions

ρ	$P = P_{AR} + P_{RA}$
−0.9	0.0407
−0.8	0.0561
−0.7	0.0669
−0.6	0.0751
−0.5	0.0815
−0.4	0.0865
−0.3	0.0902
−0.2	0.0929
−0.1	0.0945
−0.0	0.0950
0.1	0.0945
0.2	0.0929
0.3	0.0902
0.4	0.0865
0.5	0.0815
0.6	0.0751
0.7	0.0669
0.8	0.0561
0.9	0.0407

Note: X and Y are bivariate normal with correlation ρ.

5.8 Concluding Remarks

The modernization of TCMs is to convert the experience-based TCMs into evidence-based TCMs by scientifically documenting the experience of clinical practice of TCMs which include diagnosis of the disease under study, individualized treatment of the diagnosed disease, and evaluation of the prescribed TCM. In practice, it has been criticized that the diagnosis of a given disease using the four Chinese diagnostic techniques, individualized treatment of the diagnosed disease, and the evaluation of the prescribed TCMs are subjective rather than objective. Besides, large within-rater (e.g., the Chinese doctor or Western clinician) and between-rater (i.e., between Chinese doctors or between Western clinicians) variabilities are expected. As a result, the collected data may be biased and not reliable. Consequently, the treatment effect cannot be assessed accurately and reliably.

As discussed earlier, the QOL-like instrument is a useful tool for evaluation of herbal medicines if one can identify, eliminate/avoid, or control the within-rater and between-rater variabilities. For this purpose, a pilot study is necessarily conducted to train the raters who participate in the study using the developed instrument.

Kondoh et al. (2005) suggested the use of a modified dermatology life quality index (DLQI) for evaluation of herbal medicines. The resultant DLQI instrument has been shown to be a useful tool for evaluating the efficacy of herbal medicines in patients with skin diseases. However, it is suggested that the contents of the original questions be reconsidered in order to reduce within-rater and between-rater variabilities for improving accuracy and reliability of the estimated treatment effect. Further studies with larger samples are required to fully establish both the applicability and reliability of the DLQI for evaluation of the herbal medications in patients with skin diseases.

6

Factor Analysis and Principal Component Analysis

6.1 Introduction

As indicated earlier, most Western medicines contain single active ingredients for treating patients with the specific disease (e.g., cancer) under study. Statistical methods for clinical evaluation of the active ingredient in terms of some well-defined study endpoints (e.g., response rate, time to disease progression, and median survival time) are well established. Unlike Western medicines, most traditional Chinese medicines (TCMs) often consist of multiple components (active and inactive). Thus, standard methods for clinical evaluation of Western medicines cannot be applied directly to evaluate the safety and efficacy of TCMs. In practice, TCMs can be viewed as combinational drug products with known or unknown ratio of combination of the multiple components. In practice, it is difficult to evaluate the safety and efficacy of traditional Chinese medicine due the following reasons that (1) there is a large number of components (e.g., say up to 12–15), (2) some individual components cannot be characterized, (3) it is not clear which components are active and which components are inactive, (4) the relationships among these components are unknown, and (5) the ratio of the combination is often unknown.

For drug products with multiple components, intuitively, under certain assumptions, one may consider a multivariate analysis for evaluation of the safety and efficacy of TCMs. However, the analysis results may be biased and hence misleading due to the obstacles described above. In practice, because the pharmacological activities of individual components are often unknown, it is suggested dividing the components into two groups: one is the group of primary active components and the other one is the group of secondary (or less) active components. For this purpose, factor analysis and principal component analysis for dividing all of the variables into two groups of variables (primary and secondary) are helpful.

Factor analysis is a statistical approach that is often used to analyze large number of interrelated variables and to categorize these variables using their

131

common aspects. The approach involves finding a way of representing correlated variables together to form a new smaller set of derived variables with minimum loss of information. In other words, factor analysis is a method used to describe variability among observed, correlated variables in terms of a potentially lower number of unobserved variables, which are referred to as factors. In practice, if it is possible, factor analysis is to identify three or four factors that can reflect the variations of the large number of interrelated variables. Factor analysis is a correlational technique to determine meaningful clusters of shared variance, which finds relationships or natural connections where minimally correlated with other variables, and then groups the variables accordingly. Thus, factor analysis is sometimes referred to as a collection of statistical methods for reducing correlational data into a smaller number of dimensions or factors.

There are two main types of factor analysis, namely, principal component analysis and common factor analysis. Principal component analysis provides a unique solution so that the original data can be reconstructed from the results. Thus, this method not only provides a solution but also works the other way around, i.e., provides data from the solution. The solution generated includes as many factors as there are variables. Common factor analysis—this technique uses an estimate of common difference or variance among the original variables to generate the solution. Owing to this, the number of factors will always be less than the number of original factors. So, factor analysis actually refers to common factor analysis. Factor analysis is related to principal component analysis (PCA), but the two are not identical. Latent variable models, including factor analysis, use regression modeling techniques to test hypotheses producing error terms, while PCA is a descriptive statistical technique. There has been significant controversy in the field over the equivalence or otherwise of the two techniques (see exploratory factor analysis versus principal components analysis).

In Section 6.2, factor analysis is briefly outlined, while principal component analysis is introduced in Section 6.3. An example is given in Section 6.4 to illustrate the use of factor analysis and principal component analysis for evaluation of drug products with multiple components. Section 6.5 provides some concluding remarks.

6.2 Factor Analysis

Factor analysis is a commonly employed statistical method in multivariate analysis. The goal of factor analysis is data reduction of multiple measurements into a smaller number of factors that are not directly observable (latent outcomes). In practice, the factors are derived by decomposing the covariance or correlation matrix of the observed data. The development of factor

Factor Analysis and Principal Component Analysis 133

analysis can be traced back to early 1900 when researchers sought to measure intelligence (Spearman 1904). Factor analysis has become very popular especially in the social sciences and health research such as quality assessment (see, e.g., Bartholomew 1981; Gould 1981; Everitt 1984; Sammel and Ryan 1996, 2002; Laden et al. 2000; Henley et al. 2004).

There are two approaches to the implementation of factor analysis namely exploratory and confirmatory. The goal of the exploratory approach is to identify the latent structure that is data driven, while confirmatory factor analysis begins with a proposed structure or model and then evaluates the structure or model by performing goodness-of-fit to the observed data. For introductory purposes, we will focus on the exploratory approach for factor analysis.

6.2.1 Statistical Model

The purpose of factor analysis is to partition the covariance matrix of the data into two components, one is common to all the variables and the other one is to each variable. Let $X = (x_1, \ldots, x_p)'$ be a p-variate random vector with mean $\mu = (\mu_1, \ldots, \mu_1)'$ and covariance matrix $\Sigma = [\sigma_{ij}]_{p \times p}$. The vector X is assumed to be linearly dependent on a set of m random, unobserved common factors $f = (f_1, \ldots, f_m)$. Also, let $\varepsilon = (\varepsilon_1, \ldots, \varepsilon_p)$ be residual or specific factors. Assume that $E(f) = 0$, $Cov(f) = I$, $E(\varepsilon) = 0$, $Cov(\varepsilon) = \Psi = diag(\Psi_1, \ldots, \Psi_p)$, and $Cov(f, \varepsilon) = 0$. Thus, we have

$$X - \mu = Lf + \varepsilon,$$

where $L = [l_{ij}]_{p \times m}$ is a matrix of loadings or regression weights. Thus, the covariance matrix is given by

$$\Sigma = LL' + \Psi,$$

where

$$\sigma_{ii}^2 = \sum_{i=1}^{m} l_{ij}^2 + \Psi_i = h_i^2 + \Psi_i.$$

Note that h_i^2 is known as the ith communality that explains the variance associated with the ith variable, while Ψ_i is called the unique or specific variance. The above model can be generalized to the case where the common factors are intercorrelated by assuming that $Cov(f) = \Phi$ rather than $Cov(f) = I$ (in this case, the factors are orthogonal to one another).

6.2.2 Parameter Estimation

Let $x_1, \ldots, x_n$ be a sample of size n observations of random vector X. The factors and loadings can be derived from the sample variance/covariance matrix S,

134 *Quantitative Methods for Traditional Chinese Medicine Development*

which is an estimate of the true variance/covariance matrix Σ. Because the solution may not be unique, initial solutions are often obtained by imposing further constraints. The most commonly used methods for obtaining the initial solution are the methods of principal component, principal factor, and maximum likelihood. The solution is usually rotated for an easy interpretation of the data. The most commonly considered method for rotation is probably the varimax rotation proposed by Kaiser (1958, 1959), which selects the orthogonal matrix T that maximizes the sum of variances of the squared loadings of each factor.

As indicated by Sammel et al. (2010), other useful orthogonal rotations including the quarimax and equamax rotations can also be used. As indicated earlier, in many cases, $Cov(f) = \Phi \neq I$. In other words, the factors are not orthogonal to one another. In this case, we may consider rotating the oblique factors again to achieve the orthogonality using the method of promax rotation proposed by Hendrickson and White (1964) as follows. Let

$$QQ = [q_{ij}]_{p \times m}$$

be structured such that

$$q_{ij} = \left| l_{ij}^{r-1} \right| l_{ij},$$

where $r > 1$ is the power of the rotation. In this case, oblique factors have been demonstrated to replicate better than orthogonal solutions (see, e.g., Coste et al. 1995).

6.2.3 Number of Factors

As indicated earlier, TCMs often consists of a large number of components or variables. The goal of factor analysis is to reduce the number of variables. Thus, one of the key questions is how many factors to include in the model, as different m's will lead to different solutions and interpretations. Parameter estimation is conditional on a pre-specified number of factors. Statistically, when the population is normally distributed, a likelihood ratio test can be used to test the adequacy of the choice of the number of factors (Bartlett 1954). However, this test may lead to selecting an m such that the final factor(s) is significant with no additional value or insight into the data.

For selection of the number of factors, although several methods such as using (1) factors with unrotated eigenvalues greater than one, (2) factors that account for approximately 70 to 80 percent of the original variation in the data, and (3) factors with *large* values on a scree plot of the sample eigenvalues of $S - \Psi$ are available, there is no one method giving the correct answer. Thus, in practice, trying a few values of m is recommended, with the final choice being driven by the subject matter and the interpretability of the solution.

6.2.4 An Example

For illustration purposes, consider the example concerning data collected from the Interstitial Cystitis Database (ICDB) study where the measured variables are mixed types of normal, binary, and ordinal (Sammel et al. 2010). As indicated by Simon et al. (1997), interstitial cystitis (IC) is a chronic syndrome characterized by urinary frequency, urgency, and/or pain in the absence of any identifiable cause. The ICDB cohort study was to follow the natural history of IC in treated patients. One of the goals of the study was to investigate the association of IC symptoms with pathologic bladder features. An instrument with 39 items was designed to capture a wide range of potential processes affecting the development of IC-related symptoms (Tomaszewski et al. 2001).

Sammel et al. (2010) selected a subset of 24 items that had a low percentage of missing data and at least some variability among responses to analyze the correlation among biopsy features for identifying some of the biologic processes contributing to IC and the key features affected by these processes. The data set contains one continuous variable, 16 binary variables, and 7 ordinal variables constitute these items. Of the 211 subjects who underwent bladder biopsy, 203 had complete data for the selected items and were included in these analyses. Two factor analyses were performed. The first assumes that all of the variables are normally distributed, while the second accounts for the fact that the distributions are of different types. Estimation of model parameters was done using the method of ordinary unweighted least squares. The method of scree plots was used to determine the number of factors. In both analyses, a three-factor model was suggested because the slope of the plot was steepest through the third factor (see Figures 6.1 and 6.2).

Factor loadings and groupings of the variables based on their factor loadings are given in Table 6.1 (under normality assumption) and Table 6.2

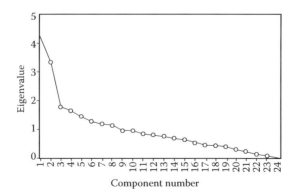

FIGURE 6.1
Scree plot of eigenvalues (assuming all observed variables are normally distributed). (From Sammel, M.D. et al., Factor analysis. In *Encyclopedia of Biopharmaceutical Statistics*, 3rd Edition, Ed. Chow, S.C., Taylor & Francis, New York, 2010.)

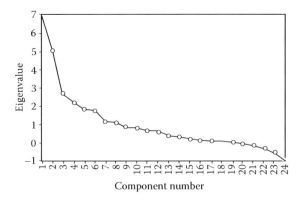

FIGURE 6.2
Scree plot of eigenvalues (assuming mixed outcome types of continuous, binary, and ordered categorical). (From Sammel, M.D. et al., Factor analysis. In *Encyclopedia of Biopharmaceutical Statistics*, 3rd Edition, Ed. Chow, S.C., Taylor & Francis, New York, 2010.)

(under distribution assumptions of different data types). The largest factor loading in absolute value for each variable has been marked in boldface, indicating the factor to which that variable is most strongly related. As can be seen in Tables 6.1 and 6.2, factor 2 is clearly defined in both analyses and is related to items 9a, 9b, 11, 22, and 25, which record the amount of urothelium lost and the capacity for urothelial regeneration. The remaining items are related most strongly to factors 1 and 3, although the grouping of the variables differs somewhat between the two analyses. These factors represent the role of mastocytosis and cellular inflammation in the development of IC. Factor loadings obtained under normality assumption are smaller than those obtained under distribution assumptions of different data types, while the correlations among the factors are larger (see Table 6.3). This leads to less certainty about variable groupings and less clearly defined factors.

Most standard statistical software packages such as SAS, S-PLUS, and SPSS have functions or procedures for performing factor analysis. All packages have the most popular methods for initial estimation and rotations. Each package also has a variety of other techniques available. Estimation of the unobservable factors is often a goal and can be produced by these software packages (see, e.g., Johnson and Wichern 1992).

6.3 Principal Component Analysis

Principal component analysis is a multivariate technique that analyzes a data table in which observations are described by several intercorrelated

Factor Analysis and Principal Component Analysis

TABLE 6.1

Factor Loadings under the Assumption that All Observed Variables Are Normally Distributed

Variable (Codes)	Factor 1	Factor 2	Factor 3
5: Mast cell counts	0.15	−0.07	**0.24**
9a: Urothelium completely denuded	0.10	**0.98**	0.11
9b: Urothelial discontinuities	−0.10	**−0.93**	−0.11
10: Granulation tissue lamina propria	**0.76**	0.07	−0.07
11: Percent of mucosa denuded of urothelium	0.22	**0.68**	−0.07
12: Submucosal hemorrhage	−0.09	0.16	**0.92**
13a: Submucosal hemorrhage aggregated	−0.07	0.01	**0.70**
13d: Submucosal hemorrhage diffuse	−0.09	0.07	**0.60**
14: Percentage of submucosa with granulation tissue	**0.86**	0.15	−0.01
16b: Eosinophilia in lamina propria	**0.15**	0.06	0.14
17: Mononuclear endothelitis	**0.55**	0.07	−0.21
18: Transmural mononuclear vasculitis	**0.47**	−0.13	−0.21
20: Mucosal edema	**0.12**	−0.09	**0.12**
22: Reactive urothelial change	0.18	**−0.35**	−0.03
23: Urothelial hyperplasia	**−0.10**	−0.08	0.04
25: Urothelial hematopoietic cells	0.10	**−0.32**	0.24
26: Lamina propria hematopoietic cells	**0.56**	−0.08	0.27
27a: Lamina propria infiltrate aggregated	**0.64**	0.08	−0.02
27d: Lamina propria infiltrate diffuse	0.23	−0.17	**0.28**
30: Lamina propria collage dense	−0.06	0.03	**0.11**
32: Percentage of lamina propria with nerves	**0.41**	−0.02	0.15
34: Percentage of lamina propria with S100 positive mononuclear cells	**0.12**	−0.07	0.00
36: Percentage of lamina propria with vessels	0.25	0.06	**0.26**
37: Vessels in lamina propria clustered	0.13	−0.06	**0.26**

Source: Sammel, M.D. et al., Factor analysis. In *Encyclopedia of Biopharmaceutical Statistics*, 3rd Edition, Ed. Chow, S.C., Taylor & Francis, New York, 2010.

quantitative dependent variables. Principal component analysis is related to factor analysis described in the previous section, but the two are not identical. As indicated by Abdi and Williams (2010), the goals of principal component analysis are multifold. First, it is to extract the most important information from the data table. Second, it is to compress the size of the data set by keeping only this important information. Third, it is to simplify the description of the data set. Finally, it is to analyze the structure of the observations and the variables.

TABLE 6.2

Factor Loadings under the Assumption of Mixed Outcome Types (Continuous, Binary, and Ordered Categorical)

Variable Code	Factor 1	Factor 2	Factor 3
5: Mast cell counts (continuous)	**0.28**	−0.16	−0.03
9a: Urothelium completely denuded (0,1)	0.33	**1.04**	−0.10
9b: Urothelial discontinuities (0,1)	−0.30	**−0.90**	0.12
10: Granulation tissue lamina propria (0,1)	**0.84**	0.30	0.05
11: Percent of mucosa denuded of urothelium (0–4)	0.38	**0.88**	0.07
12: Submucosal hemorrhage (0–3)	**0.47**	−0.29	0.17
13a: Submucosal hemorrhage aggregated (0,1)	**0.42**	−0.34	0.26
13d: Submucosal hemorrhage diffuse (0,1)	**0.38**	−0.28	0.17
14: Percentage of submucosa with granulation tissue (0–3)	**1.04**	0.39	0.20
16b: Eosinophilia in lamina propria (0,1)	**0.55**	−0.01	−0.41
17: Mononuclear endothelitis (0,1)	**0.77**	0.44	−0.58
18: Transmural mononuclear vasculitis (0,1)	0.62	0.11	**−0.74**
20: Mucosal edema (0,1)	0.48	−0.04	**0.75**
22: Reactive urothelial change (0,1)	0.14	**−0.47**	−0.08
23: Urothelial hyperplasia (0,1)	−0.09	−0.18	**−0.37**
25: Urothelial hematopoietic cells (0–3)	0.13	**−0.83**	−0.12
26: Lamina propria hematopoietic cells (0–3)	**0.76**	−0.23	−0.32
27a: Lamina propria infiltrate aggregated (0,1)	**0.77**	0.20	−0.22
27d: Lamina propria infiltrate diffuse (0,1)	0.39	**−0.44**	0.01
30: Lamina propria collage dense (0,1)	0.04	0.03	**0.43**
32: Percentage of lamina propria with nerves (0–3)	**0.57**	−0.03	−0.09
34: Percentage of lamina propria with S100 positive mononuclear cells (0,1)	0.27	−0.15	**−0.65**
36: Percentage of lamina propria with vessels (0–2)	**0.56**	0.05	0.05
37: Vessels in lamina propria clustered (0,1)	**0.33**	−0.19	0.03

Source: Sammel, M.D. et al., Factor analysis. In *Encyclopedia of Biopharmaceutical Statistics*, 3rd Edition, Ed. Chow, S.C., Taylor & Francis, New York, 2010.

TABLE 6.3

Correlations among the Factors for Analyses 1 and 2

	Analysis 1		Analysis 2	
	Factor 1	**Factor 2**	**Factor 1**	**Factor 2**
Factor 2	0.021		−0.211	
Factor 3	0.383	−0.331	−0.030	−0.142

Source: Sammel, M.D. et al., Factor analysis. In *Encyclopedia of Biopharmaceutical Statistics*, 3rd Edition, Ed. Chow, S.C., Taylor & Francis, New York, 2010.

Factor Analysis and Principal Component Analysis 139

6.3.1 Singular Value Decomposition

Let $X = [x_{ij}]_{I \times J}$ be the data table to be analyzed, where x_{ij} is the ith observation from the jth variable, where $i = 1,\ldots,I$ and $j = 1,\ldots,J$. Also, let L be the rank of the matrix X. Then, we have $L \leq \min (I, J)$. In practice, the data table X is usually pre-processed such that the columns of X will be centered and the mean of each column is equal to 0 (i.e., $X'1 = 0$, where 0 is a J by 1 vector of zeros and 1 is an I by 1 vector of ones). Furthermore, if each element of X is divided by $\sqrt{I}$ (or $\sqrt{I-1}$), then $X'X$ become the covariance matrix. In this case, the analysis is usually referred to as a covariance principal component analysis. If each variable is standardized, the analysis is called a correlation principal component analysis because the matrix $X'X$ has become a correlation matrix.

As indicated by Takane (2002) and Abdi (2007a,b), the matrix X has the singular value decomposition (SVD), which is a generalization of the eigendecomposition. The SVD decomposes a rectangular matrix into three simple matrices: two orthogonal matrices and one diagonal matrix. In other words, if A is a rectangular matrix, its SVD gives

$$A = P\Delta Q',$$

where P is the (normalized) eigenvectors of the matrix AA' (i.e., $P'P = I$), Q is the (normalized) eigenvectors of the matrix $A'A$ (i.e., $Q'Q = I$), and Δ is the diagonal matrix of the singular values, $\Delta = \Lambda^{1/2}$ with Λ being the diagonal matrix of the eigenvalues of matrix AA' and of the matrix $A'A$ (as they are the same). Note that the columns of P are called the left singular vectors of A, while the columns of Q are called the right singular vectors of A. The SVD is a straightforward consequence of the eigendecomposition of positive semidefinite matrices (see also Abdi and Williams 2010). Thus, we have

$$X = P\Delta Q',$$

where P is the $I \times L$ matrix of left singular vectors, Q is the $J \times L$ matrix of right singular vectors, and Δ is the diagonal matrix of singular values. Note that Δ^2 is equal to Λ which is the diagonal matrix of the (nonzero) eigenvalues of $X'X$ and XX'.

6.3.2 Principal Components

In general, principal component analysis computes new variables called principal components, which are obtained as linear combinations of the original variables. The first principal component is required to have the largest possible variance (i.e., this component will explain the largest part of the inertia of the data table). The second component is computed under the constraint of being orthogonal to the first component and to have the largest possible inertia. The other components can be similarly computed. The values of these new variables for the observations are called factor scores, and these factor scores can be interpreted geometrically as the projections of the observations onto the principal components. In principal component analysis, the components are obtained from the SVD of the data table X. Specifically, with $X = P\Delta Q'$, the $I \times L$ matrix of factor scores, denoted by F, can be obtained as

$$F = P\Delta.$$

The matrix Q gives the coefficients of the linear combinations used to compute the factor scores. This matrix can also be interpreted as a projection matrix because multiplying X by Q gives the values of the projections of the observations on the principal components. This can be shown as

$$F = P\Delta = P\Delta Q'Q = XQ.$$

The above expression shows that matrix Q is a projection matrix that transforms the original data matrix into factor scores. This matrix can be used to compute factor scores for observations that were not included in the principal component analysis. Note that the matrix X can also be interpreted as the product of the factor score matrix by the loading matrix as

$$X = FQ'$$

with $F'F = \Delta^2$ and $Q'Q = I$.

6.3.3 Interpretation of Principal Components

The importance of a component is reflected by its inertia or by the proportion of the total inertia explained by this factor. In principal component analysis, the eigenvalue associated with a component is equal to the sum of the squared factor scores for this component. Therefore, the importance of an observation for a component can be obtained by the ratio of the squared factor score of this observation to the eigenvalue associated with that component. This ratio is called the contribution of the observation to the component.

Denote the contribution of observation i to component l by $C_{i,l}$, which can be obtained as

$$C_{i,l} = \frac{f_{i,l}^2}{\sum_i f_{i,l}^2} = \frac{f_{i,l}^2}{\lambda_l},$$

Factor Analysis and Principal Component Analysis 141

where λ_l is the eigenvalue of the lth component. For a given component, the value of a contribution is between 0 and 1 and the sum of the contributions of all observations is equal to 1. The larger the value of the contribution, the more the observation contributes to the component. In practice, it is helpful in interpreting the contribution of a given component by comparing its contribution with the average contribution (i.e., $1/I$). The observations with high contributions and different signs can then be opposed to help interpret the component because these observations represent the two endpoints of this component. The factor scores of the supplementary observations are not used to compute the eigenvalues, and therefore their contributions are generally not computed.

Note that the squared cosine shows the importance of a cosine indicates the contribution of a component to the squared distance of the observation to the origin. It corresponds to the square of the cosine of the angle from the right triangle made with the origin, the observation, and its projection on the component and is computed as (see, e.g., Abdi and Williams 2010):

$$Cos_{i,l}^2 = \frac{f_{i,l}^2}{\sum_l f_{i,l}^2} = \frac{f_{i,l}^2}{d_{i,g}^2},$$

where $d_{i,g}^2$ is the squared distance of a given observation to the origin. The squared distance, $d_{i,g}^2$ can be computed as the sum of the squared values of all the factor scores of this observation. Components with a large value of $Cos_{i,l}^2$ contribute a relatively large portion to the total distance, and therefore these components are important for that observation. The value of $Cos_{i,l}^2$ can help find the components that are important to interpret both active and supplementary observations.

In principal component analysis, the correlation (i.e., loading) between a component and a variable estimates the information they share. The sum of the squared coefficients of correlation between a variable and all the components is equal to 1. Consequently, the squared loadings are easier to interpret than the loadings (because the squared loadings give the proportion of the variance of the variables explained by the components). Note that, in general, different meanings of loadings lead to equivalent interpretations of the components. This happens because the different types of loadings differ mostly by their type of normalization. In practice, the variables are often plotted as points in the component space using their loadings as coordinates. This representation differs from the plot of the observations: The observations are represented by their projections, but the variables are represented by their correlations. Note that the sum of the squared loadings for a variable is equal to 1. As a result, when the data are perfectly represented by only two components, the sum of the squared loadings is equal to 1.

6.4 Application of QOL in Hypertensive Patients

6.4.1 Background

QOL is typically assessed by a QOL instrument, which consists of a number of questions (or items). To collect information on various aspects of QOL, a QOL instrument with a large number of questions is found necessary and helpful. For a simple analysis and easy interpretation, these questions or items are often grouped to form subscales, composite scores, or overall QOL. The items (or subscales) in each subscale (or composite score) are correlated. As a result, the structure of responses to a QOL instrument is multidimensional, complex and correlated. In addition, the following questions are of particular concern when subscales and/or composite scores are to be analyzed for the assessment of QOL. First, how many subscales or composite scores should be formed? Second, which items (subscales) should be grouped in each subscale (composite score)? Third, what are the appropriate weights for obtaining subscales (composite scores)? These questions are important because the components and/or domains of QOL may vary from drug therapy to drug therapy. For example, for the assessment of the effect of antihypertensive treatment on QOL, it may be of interest to quantify the patient's QOL in terms of the following QOL components: physical state, emotional state, performance of social roles, intellectual function, and life satisfaction (Testa 1987; Hollenberg et al. 1991). For treatment of breast cancer, four aspects of QOL, namely, mobility, side effects, pain, and psychological stress are usually considered (Zwinderman 1990). Olschewski and Schumacher (1990) proposed to use the standardized scoring coefficients from factor analysis as a criterion for selecting subscales for grouping of composite scores. The idea is to drop those subscales with small coefficients. This method of grouping is attractive because it is a selection procedure based on data-oriented weights. However, this methods suffers the drawbacks that (1) the factorization of the correlation matrix is not unique, (2) the standardization scoring coefficients used in combining subscales vary across different rotations of the factor system, (3) each composite score is a linear combination of all the subscales (unless some subscales with small coefficients are dropped), and (4) the resulting composite score does not have optimal properties. To overcome these drawbacks, Ki and Chow (1995) proposed an objective method for grouping subscales. The idea is to apply principal component analysis and factor analysis to determine (1) an appropriate number of composite scores, (2) the subscales to be grouped in each composite score, and (3) optimal weights for forming a composite score with each group.

6.4.2 Development of QOL Instrument

To illustrate the method of grouping described above, consider the study published by Testa et al. (1993). A QOL instrument was administered to

Factor Analysis and Principal Component Analysis

TABLE 6.4

QOL Subscales

Subscale	QOL Component	No. of Items
1	GHS: General health status	3
2	VIT: Vitality	4
3	SLP: Sleep	4
4	EMO: Emotional ties	2
5	GPA: General positive affect	12
6	LIF: Life satisfaction	1
7	ANX: Anxiety	11
8	BEC: Behavioral/emotional control	3
9	DEP: Depression	10
10	SEX: Sexual functioning	5
11	WRX: Work well-being	11

TABLE 6.5

QOL Composite Scores

Composite Score	QOL Dimension	Subscales
I (PSD)	Psychological distress	7, 8, 9
II (GPH)	General perceived health	1, 2, 3
III (PWB)	Psychological well-being	4, 5, 6

341 hypertensive patients before drug therapy. The instrument consists of 11 subscales as given in Table 6.4. Table 6.5 lists the three composite scores, which are established by psychologists and health experts, used by Testa et al. (1993). The sample covariance matrix and the correlation matrix of these 11 subscales are given in Tables 6.6 and 6.7, respectively. It is desirable to combine some subscales for simple analysis and easy interpretation. An overall QOL score combining the information of all subscales may be used to give a general summary of the results.

6.4.2.1 Principal Component Analysis

A principal component analysis was performed on the data. The coefficient of the principal components and the percentage of variation explained by each principal component are given in Table 6.8. It can be seen from Table 6.8 that three components could retain 80 percent of the total variation of the data. Most variation of the data could be captured by a three-dimensional space without much loss of information. If a one-dimensional summary score were used, the first principal component would give optimal weights for combining the subscales. The weights were close to the usual uniform

TABLE 6.6

Covariance Matrix of the 11 QOL Subscales

Subscale	GHS	VIT	SLP	EMO	GPA	LIF	ANX	BEC	DEP	SEX	WRX
GHS	7133										
VIT	3790	6272									
SLP	3338	5205	8667								
EMO	2744	3736	3503	13,333							
GPA	2801	4299	4169	6340	6566						
LIF	2201	2843	2415	3976	3672	5025					
ANX	2865	3615	3972	3828	4360	2418	5698				
BEC	1877	2397	2544	3334	3140	1931	3032	2608			
DEP	2767	3558	3551	4512	4370	2755	4198	2931	5031		
SEX	1364	2063	1231	1208	1148	1046	675	664	1190	23,379	
WRX	2727	3777	3469	2949	3530	2592	2751	2006	2949	966	3875

Factor Analysis and Principal Component Analysis

TABLE 6.7

Correlation Matrix of the 11 QOL Subscales

Subscale	GHS	VIT	SLP	EMO	GPA	LIF	ANX	BEC	DEP	SEX	WRX
GHS	1.00*										
VIT	0.57*	1.00*									
SLP	0.42	0.71*	1.00*								
EMO	0.28	0.41	0.33	1.00*							
GPA	0.41	0.67*	0.55*	0.68*	1.00*						
LIF	0.37	0.51*	0.37	0.49	0.64*	1.00*					
ANX	0.45	0.60*	0.57*	0.44	0.71*	0.45	1.00*				
BEC	0.44	0.59*	0.54*	0.57*	0.76*	0.53*	0.79*	1.00*			
DEP	0.46	0.63*	0.54*	0.55*	0.76*	0.55*	0.78*	0.81*	1.00*		
SEX	0.11	0.17	0.09	0.07	0.09	0.10	0.06	0.09	0.11	1.00*	
WRX	0.52*	0.77*	0.60*	0.41	0.70*	0.59*	0.59*	0.63*	0.67*	0.10	1.00*

* Significance at 5% level.

TABLE 6.8

Principal Component Analysis on the Covariance Matrix of 11 Subscales

	Total Variance = 87,587		
Principal Component	Characteristic Root	Proportion of Variance Explained	Cumulative Proportion
1st	38558.2	0.440227	0.44023
2nd	22565.1	0.257630	0.69786
3rd	9064.0	0.103486	0.80134
4th	3954.2	0.052414	0.85376
...	...	...	...
11th	573.1	0.006544	1.00000
	1st	**2nd**	**3rd**
GHS	0.259955	−0.036307	0.312788
VIT	0.329832	−0.034736	0.277338
SLP	0.337983	−0.078279	0.416114
EMO	0.420902	−0.132316	−0.770326
GPA	0.361128	−0.100137	−0.109206
LIF	0.243912	−0.053006	−0.073678
ANX	0.298467	−0.094213	0.119421
BEC	0.211205	−0.058717	−0.006907
DEP	0.302104	−0.071833	0.016791
SEX	0.235259	0.969770	−0.043750
WRX	0.249063	−0.055368	0.157592

weights. Thus, for simplicity, a simple average of the subscales might be used to summarize the information.

6.4.2.2 Factor Analysis

Because principal component analysis suggested that the variation of the data could be appropriately explained by a three-dimensional space, a factor analysis model with three common factors is an appropriate statistical model for explaining the correlation matrix given in Table 6.7. All subscales are highly correlated with one another except for sexual functioning. The initial factor pattern and the partial correlation matrix controlling for the three common factors are summarized in Tables 6.9 and 6.10, respectively. The partial correlations between the subscales controlling for the factors were very small, which indicated that three common factors could reasonably explain the correlations among the subscales. The initial factor loading patterns given in Table 6.9, however, were hard to interpret. All subscales except Sexual functioning (SEX) had heavy positive loadings on factor 1, and a mix of positive and negative loading for factors 2 and 3. The loadings of all three common factors for SEX were very small. This is because the correlation

Factor Analysis and Principal Component Analysis 147

TABLE 6.9

Initial Factor Pattern

	Factor Pattern Loading		
	Factor 1	**Factor 2**	**Factor 3**
GPA	0.88*	−0.20	0.14
DEP	0.86*	−0.15	−0.14
BEC	0.85*	−0.21	−0.17
VIT	0.81*	0.36	0.06
WRK	0.81*	0.22	0.12
ANX	0.81*	−0.09	−0.31
SLP	0.68*	0.28	−0.09
LIF	0.65*	−0.09	0.26
EMO	0.62*	−0.32	0.21
GHS	0.57*	0.24	0.00
SEX	0.13	0.09	0.07

* Significance at 5%.

between SEX and other subscales was low. Therefore, a rotation was necessary to produce a more easily understood factor pattern. The resulting factor pattern of a varimax rotation is given in Table 6.11. Note that varimax rotation is an orthogonal rotation of the factor axes to maximize the variance of the squared loadings of a factor (column) on all the variables (rows) in a factor matrix, which has the effect of differentiating the original variables by extracted factor. Each factor will tend to have either large or small loadings of any particular variable. The rotated factor patterns given in Table 6.11 suggested that subscales Anxiety (ANX), Behavior/emotional control (BEC), and Depression (DEP) could be grouped together as a composite score, which is referred to as Psychological Distress (PSD); the subscales Vitality (VIT), Work well-being (WRK), Sleep (SLP), and General health status (GHS) are grouped to form the composite of General Perceived Health (GPH), and the subscales Emotional ties (EMO), General positive affect (GPA), and Life satisfaction (LIF) could be grouped together as a composite score as Psychological Well-Being (PWB). Each subscale is grouped under the factor with which it has highest correlation. The subscale SEX, however, could be left as a single scale because it was not highly related to any factor.

6.4.3 Analysis Results

Principal component analysis was then performed on each group of subscales to determine the optimal weights for forming a composite score which can retain as much information as possible. The results of principal component analyses are summarized in Table 6.11. The weights for combining

TABLE 6.10

Partial Correlations between Subscales Controlling for the Three Factors

Subscale	GHS	VIT	SLP	EMO	GPA	LIF	ANX	BEC	DEP	SEX	WRX
GHS	1.00*										
VIT	0.06	1.00*									
SLP	−0.05	0.18	1.00*								
EMO	0.02	0.03	0.03	1.00*							
GPA	−0.13	0.08	0.07	0.15	1.00*						
LIF	0.03	−0.04	−0.07	0.00	0.04	1.00*					
ANX	0.03	−0.01	0.03	−0.07	0.11	−0.02	1.00*				
BEC	0.01	−0.07	0.00	0.04	−0.04	0.01	0.11	1.00*			
DEP	0.03	−0.03	−0.07	0.00	−0.06	0.02	0.10	0.09	1.00*		
SEX	0.02	0.07	−0.03	0.00	−0.03	0.00	−0.03	0.02	0.05	1.00*	
WRX	0.01	0.07	−0.03	−0.12	0.06	0.12	−0.06	0.03	0.07	−0.06	1.00*

* Significance at 5% level.

Factor Analysis and Principal Component Analysis 149

TABLE 6.11

Results of Varimax Rotation on the Factor Loadings

	Orthogonal Transformation Matrix R		
	1	2	3
1	0.61335	0.56975	0.54697
2	−0.16670	0.77032	−0.61548
3	−0.77202	0.28632	0.56746
	Rotated Factor Pattern Loadings		
	Factor 1	**Factor 2**	**Factor 3**
ANX	0.76 A	0.30	0.32
BEC	0.69 A	0.28	0.50
DEP	0.67 A	0.33	0.48
VIT	0.39	0.76 B	0.26
WRX	0.37	0.67 B	0.38
SLP	0.44	0.58 B	0.16
GHS	0.31	0.50 B	0.17
SEX	0.01	0.16	0.06
GPA	0.47	0.39	0.68 C
EMO	0.27	0.16	0.66 C
LIF	0.22	0.38	0.56 C

Note: A = psychological distress (PSD); B = general perceived health (GPH); C = psychological well-being (PWB).

subscales in the first principal component were standardized such that the sum of weights equals unity, and the composite scores were

PSD = 0.39 (ANX) + 0.25 (BEC) + 0.36 (DEP)

GPH = 0.27 (VIT) + 0.19 (WRK) + 0.30 (SLP) + 0.23 (GHS)

PWB = 0.48 (EMO) + 0.31 (GPA) + 0.21 (LIF).

These three composite scores explained about 76 percent of the total variation of the 10 subscales (excluding SEX). The results based on the analysis of these composite scores provide an easy interpretation compared to that from the analysis of the original subscales. These composite scores are similar to those used by Testa et al. (1993). The above analysis provided an objective justification of the use of composite scores, which were developed by psychologists, in the study population.

6.5 Concluding Remarks

Common factor analysis and principal component analysis have a common goal of reducing a set of p observed variables to a set of m new variables

($m < p$). The reduction of observed variables has two purposes. First, the pattern matrix can be interpreted to describe the relationship between the original variables and the new variables. Second, scores for the m new variables can be used to replace the original observed scores and these scores are intended for subsequent analysis. Because common factor analysis and principal component analysis are two broad classes of procedures that share a common goal and many important mathematical characteristics, it is obvious which analysis should be used in practice. Velicer and Jackson (1990) studied some algebraic similarities and differences at the sample level between the two methods. Specifically, the issue regarding the number of components (factors) should be retained is discussed. As indicated by Velicer and Jackson (1990), if factor analysis is the procedure of choice, at least one of the following situations is assumed to exist: (1) the number of factors is known *a priori*, (2) the asymptotic chi-square statistic will accurately determine how many factors to retain, or (3) the problem is trivial and of no interest. For determination of the number of factors, the most widely employed criterion is the so-called Kaiser's criterion, i.e., eigenvalue greater than unity rule (Kaiser 1960), which has been criticized for retaining too many factors. Typically, the number of factors retained equals one third of the number of original variables as determined by the Kaiser rule. Dziuban and Harris (1973) indicated that the number of factors may be related to the conflict over the similarity-dissimilarity of common factor analysis and principal component analysis solutions.

Common factor analysis and/or principal component analysis are useful methods for multivariate analysis such as quality of life assessment in cancer trials and/or the evaluation of safety and efficacy of drug products with multiple components. Although factor analysis and principal component analysis may be useful in assessment of safety and efficacy of TCMs, there are still concerns that may limit the application of the factor analysis and principal component analysis. For example, the pharmacological activities of some of the components are unknown and cannot be characterized or fully understood. The relationships (or possible component-to-component or drug-to-drug interaction) among the components are also not known. If we consider TCMs as combinational drug products, the relative ratios among the components are often unknown. In many cases, a small change or variation of a specific component could lead to a drastic change in clinical outcomes.

7

Statistical Validation of Chinese Diagnostic Procedures

7.1 Introduction

In recent years, the search for new medicines for treating life-threatening diseases such as cancer has become the center of attention in pharmaceutical research and development. As a result, many pharmaceutical companies have begun to focus on the modernization of traditional Chinese medicines (TCM). Modernization of a TCM is based on scientific evaluations of the efficacy and safety of the TCM in terms of well-established clinical endpoints for a Western indication through clinical trials on humans. However, it should be recognized that there are fundamental differences in the scientific evaluation of the efficacy and safety of a TCM as compared to a typical Western medicine (WM) even though they are for the same indication (Chow et al. 2006; Tse et al. 2006). For example, most WMs contain a single active ingredient, while most TCMs consist of a mixture of components or constituents, which may or may not be active pharmacologically. In addition, the traditional Chinese diagnostic procedure (CDP) for a TCM is quite different from that of a WM. Typically, the CDP consists of four major categories, namely, inspection, auscultation and olfaction, interrogation, and pulse taking and palpation. Basically, each category can, in fact, be thought of as an instrument (or questionnaire), consisting of a number of questions to collect different information regarding the patient's activity/ function, disease status, and/or disease severity. For instance, the Chinese diagnosis for stroke is called *Tsu Chung*. The CDP for stroke consists of wind syndrome (six categories), fire-heat syndrome (nine categories), sputum syndrome (seven categories), stasis syndrome (five categories), deficiency syndrome (eight categories), and overabundant syndrome (nine categories). On the other hand, WM uses the NIH Stroke Scale (NIHSS) developed by the US National Institute of Neurologic Disorder and Stroke (NINDS) from the original scale devised at the University of Cincinnati to measure the neurological impact of stroke (Lyden et al. 1999).

151

152   *Quantitative Methods for Traditional Chinese Medicine Development*

An experienced Chinese doctor usually prescribes a TCM for the patient based on the combined information obtained from the four major categories and his/her best judgment. As a result, the relative proportions of the components could vary even within an individual patient. In practice, the use of a CDP has raised the following questions. First, it is of interest to determine how accurate and reliable this subjective diagnostic procedure is for the evaluation of patients with certain diseases. Second, it is also of interest to determine how a change of an observed unit in the CDP can be translated to a change in a well-established clinical endpoint for Western indication.

In this chapter, we will examine these two questions by studying the calibration and validation of the CDP for evaluation of a TCM with respect to a well-established clinical endpoint for evaluation of a Western medicine. In Section 7.2, the CDP will be briefly introduced. A proposed study design for the clinical trial is described in Section 7.3. Under the study design, the calibration of the CDP with respect to a well-established clinical endpoint is examined in Section 7.4. In Section 7.5, the CDP is then validated against the well-established clinical endpoint under the established calibration model. A numerical example is given in Section 7.6 to illustrate the proposed methods. Some concluding remarks are given in Section 7.7.

7.2 Chinese Diagnostic Procedure

TCM is an over a few thousand years old holistic medical system encircling the entire scope of human experience. It combines the use of Chinese herbal medicines, acupuncture, massage, and therapeutic exercise, e.g., *Qi Gong* (the practice of internal *air*) and *Tai Chi* for both treatment and prevention of disease. With its unique theories of etiology, diagnostic systems, and abundant historical literature, TCM itself consists of Chinese culture and philosophy, clinical practice experiences, and materials including usage experiences of many medical herbs.

TCM drug treatment typically comprises complicated prescriptions of a combination of a few components. And the combination is derived based on the CDP. The diagnostic procedure for TCM consists of four major techniques, namely, inspection, auscultation and olfaction, interrogation, and pulse taking and palpation. All these diagnostic techniques aim mainly at providing an objective basis for differentiation of syndromes by collecting symptoms and signs from the patient. Inspection involves observing the patient's general appearance (strong or week, fat or thin), mind, complexion (skin color), five sense organs (eye, ear, nose, lip, and tongue), secretions, and excretions. Auscultation involves listening to the voice, expression, respiration, vomit, and cough. Olfaction involves smelling the breath and body odor. Interrogation involves asking questions about specific symptoms and

Statistical Validation of Chinese Diagnostic Procedures 153

the general condition including history of the present disease, past history, personal life history, and family history. Pulse taking and palpation can help to judge the location and nature of a disease according to the changes of the pulse. The smallest detail can have a strong impact on the treatment scheme as well as on the prognosis. While the pulse diagnosis and examination of the tongue receive much attention due to their frequent mention, the other aspects of diagnosis cannot be ignored.

After these four diagnostic techniques have been performed, the TCM doctor has to configure a syndrome diagnosis, describing the fundamental substances of the body and how they function in the body based on the eight principles, five element theory, five *Zang* and six *Fu*, and information regarding channels and collaterals. Eight principles consist of *Yin* and *Yang* (i.e., negative and positive), cold and hot, external and internal, and *Shi* and *Xu* (i.e., weak and strong). Eight principles can help the TCM doctors to differentiate syndrome patterns. For instance, *Yin* people will develop disease in a negative, passive, and cool way (e.g., diarrhea and back pain), while *Yang* people will develop disease in an aggressive, active, progressive, and warm way (e.g., dry eyes, tinnitus, and night sweats). The five elements (earth, metal, water, wood, and fire) correspond to particular organs in the human body. Each element operates in harmony with the others.

Five *Zang* (or *Yin* organs) include heart (including the pericardium), lung, spleen, liver, and kidney, while six *Fu* (or *Yang* organs) include gall bladder, stomach, large intestine, small intestine, urinary bladder, and three cavities (i.e., chest, epiastrium, and hypogastrium). *Zang* organs can manufacture and store fundamental substances. These substances are then transformed and transported by *Fu* organs. TCM treatments involve a thorough understanding of the clinical manifestations of *Zang Fu* organ imbalance and knowledge of appropriate acupuncture points and herbal therapy to rebalance the organs. The channels and collaterals are the representation of the organs of the body. They are responsible for conducting the flow of energy and blood through the entire body.

In addition to providing diagnostic information, these elements of TCM can also help to describe the etiology of disease including six exogenous factors (i.e., wind, cold, summer, dampness, dryness, and fire), seven emotional factors (i.e., anger, joy, worry, grief, anxiety, fear, and fright), and other pathogenic factors. Once all this information is collected and processed into a logical and workable diagnosis, the traditional Chinese medical doctor can determine the treatment approach.

For example, wind, fire, phlegm, and stasis are four main pathological factors of stroke recognized by the TCM theory. These factors can weaken the internal organs including the kidney and the spleen and thus cause deficiencies of chi, blood, and yin. Deficiencies of chi, blood, or yin will result in stroke-related symptoms such as liver yang rising, stasis of chi or blood, phlegm combining with fire, liver wind, or wind in the energy pathways. In practice, Chinese medicine can identify two general types of stroke: the most severe type attacks the internal organs as well as the energy pathways; the milder type only attacks the energy pathways. For patients with the severe type, acupuncture and Chinese herbal formulas are used to loosen spasm, suppress wind, open the orifices, resolve phlegm, and lower blood pressure. In treating the milder type of stroke, acupuncture is primarily used to open the energy pathways and promote chi and blood flow (Liu and Gong 2015).

7.3 Proposed Study Design

When planning a clinical trial, it is suggested that the study objectives should be clearly stated in the study protocol. Once the study objectives are confirmed, a valid study design can be chosen and the primary clinical endpoints can be determined accordingly. On the basis of the primary clinical endpoint, sample size required for achieving a desired power can then be calculated. For evaluation of treatment effect of a TCM, however, the commonly used clinical endpoint is usually not applicable owing to the nature of the CDP as described in Section 7.2. The CDP is, in fact, an instrument (or questionnaire), consisting of a number of questions to capture the information regarding patient's activity, function, disease status, and disease severity. As required by most regulatory agencies, such a subjective instrument must be validated before it can be used for assessment of treatment effect in clinical trials. However, without a reference marker, not only can the CDP not be validated, but we also do not know whether the TCM has achieved any clinically significant effect at the end of the clinical trial. Therefore, before the CDP for evaluation of a TCM can be validated with respect to a well-established clinical endpoint for evaluation of a WM, a calibration between the scale obtained from the CDP and the well-established clinical endpoint is necessary. Similar to the calibration of an analytical method, we may consider the calibration models as suggested by the US FDA (see, e.g., Chow and Liu 1995; Tse and Chow 1995). On the basis of the calibration model, a difference detected by the CDP can be translated to the well-established clinical endpoint. In addition, the CDP can also be validated against the well-established clinical endpoint.

In practice, the diagnostic procedure of a TCM could vary from one Chinese doctor to another. Although it may reduce within-patient variability, it could increase the between-rater variability, which could significantly bias the evaluation of the efficacy and safety of the TCM under study. To address this issue, a standardized diagnostic procedure is usually developed prior to conducting a clinical trial. The standardized diagnostic procedure usually contains the four categories, which, in turn, consist of a number of questions agreed by the community of the Chinese doctors. These questions are designed to quantitatively capture the information regarding patient activity/function, disease status, and disease severity. For validation of such an instrument, similar to the validation of a typical quality of life instrument, we will consider the following validation performance characteristics: validity (or accuracy), reliability (or precision), and ruggedness (or rater-to-rater's variability) (see, e.g., Chow and Ki 1994, 1996).

To address these issues described above, Hsiao et al. (2009) proposed a study design, which allows calibration and validation of a CDP with respect to a well-established clinical endpoint for WM (as a reference marker). Subjects will be screened based on criteria for Western indication. Qualified subjects will be diagnosed by the Chinese diagnostic procedure to establish baseline. Qualified subjects will then be randomized to receive either the test TCM or an active control (a well-established Western medicine). Participating physicians including Chinese doctors and Western clinicians will also be randomly assigned to either the TCM arm or the arm of WM. As a result, this study design will result in three groups:

Group 1: Subjects who receive WM but are evaluated by both a Chinese doctor and a Western clinician.

Group 2: Subjects who receive TCM and are evaluated by Chinese doctor A.

Group 3: Subjects who receive TCM and are evaluated by Chinese doctor B.

The schema of our proposed study design is shown in Figure 7.1. Group 1 can be used to calibrate the Chinese diagnostic procedure against the well-established clinical endpoint, while groups 2 and 3 can be used to validate the Chinese diagnostic procedure based on the established standard curve for calibration.

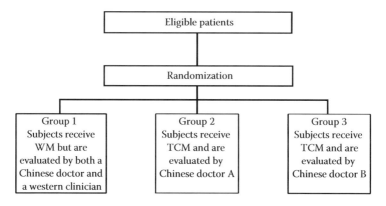

FIGURE 7.1
Schema of the proposed study design.

7.4 Calibration of Chinese Diagnostic Procedure

Let N be the number of patients collected in group 1. For the data in group 1, let x_j be the measurement of the well-established clinical endpoint of the jth patient for WM. For simplicity, we assume that the measurement of well-established clinical endpoint for WM is continuous. Suppose that the TCM diagnostic procedure consists of K items. Let z_{ij} denote the TCM diagnostic score of jth patient from the ith item, $i = 1, ..., K, j = 1, ..., N$. Let y_j represent the score of the jth patient summarized from the K TCM diagnostic items. For simplicity, we assume that

$$y_j = \sum_{i=1}^{K} z_{ij}.$$

Here we use the baseline measurements for calibration because the relationship between y and x might be confounded with the effect of medication. On the basis of these measurements of WM clinical endpoint (standards) and their corresponding TCM scores, an estimated calibration curve can be obtained by fitting an appropriate statistical model between these standards and their corresponding TCM scores. The estimated calibration curve is also known as the standard curve. Similar to calibration of an analytical method (cf. Chow and Liu 1995), we will consider the following four candidate models:

Model 1: $y_j = \alpha + \beta x_j + e_j$,
Model 2: $y_j = \beta x_j + e_j$,
Model 3: $y_j = \alpha x_j^{\beta} e_j$,
Model 4: $y_j = \alpha e^{\beta x_j} e_j$,

where α, β, β_1, and β_2 are unknown parameters and e's are independent random errors with $E(e_j) = 0$ and finite $Var(e_j)$ in models 1, and 2, and $E(\log(e_j)) = 0$ and finite $Var(\log(e_j))$ in models 3 and 4.

Model 1 is a simple linear regression model, which is probably the most commonly used statistical model for establishment of standard curves for calibration. When the standard curve passes through the origin, model 1 reduces to model 2. When there is a nonlinear relationship between y and x, models 3 and 4 are useful. Note that both models 3 and 4 are equivalent to simple linear regression model after logarithm transformation. The standard curve under each model can be obtained by estimating the corresponding parameters through the least squares method for a given data set observed from group 1. Then, the selected standard curve is used to evaluate the unknown WM clinical endpoint x_0 for a given TCM score y_0. The

Statistical Validation of Chinese Diagnostic Procedures 157

unknown WM clinical endpoint is determined by solving x based on the standard curve, which assumes the parameter estimates are the true values of the parameters. This, however, would introduce bias and variability to the WM result due to the backward transformation. We can thus develop a procedure to identify the best model for the estimation of x_0. The details are outlined below:

Step 1: The *adequacy* of the model can be assessed by the *lack-of-fit* test and the significance of the parameters (Draper and Smith 1980). Eliminate those models that fail the lack-of-fit test or the *significance* test.

Step 2: For each remaining model, calculate the corresponding R^2 value. Denote $R^2_{\max}$ to be the maximum of the R^2 values among the remaining models. For each model, define $r = R^2/R^2_{\max}$. Eliminate those models with r value less than r_0, where r_0 is a predetermined critical value. In general, we recommend r_0 to be 0.8.

Step 3: For the remaining models, identify the *best* model by comparing the mean squared error (MSE) of the estimate of x_0. The one with the smallest MSE is considered to be the *best* model. A more detailed discussion is given by Tse and Chow (1995).

7.5 Validation of Chinese Diagnostic Procedure

As indicated earlier, the standardized TCM diagnostic instrument usually contains the four categories or domains, which, in turn, consist of a number of questions agreed by the community of the Chinese doctors. For validation of such an instrument, we will consider the following validation performance characteristics (parameters): validity (or accuracy), reliability (or precision), and ruggedness (rater-to-rater variability). In several respects our development parallels that of Chow and Ki (1994, 1996), and thus we omit some of the details.

7.5.1 Validity

The validity of a TCM instrument is referred to as the extent to which the TCM instrument measures what it is designed to measure. That is, it is a measure of bias of the TCM instrument. The bias can reflect the accuracy of the TCM instrument. As mentioned earlier, a TCM instrument usually consists of a number of questions agreed by the community of Chinese doctors. It is a great concern that the questions may not be the right questions to capture the information regarding patient activity/function, disease status, and disease severity. We will use group 2 to validate the CDP based on the previously established standard curve for calibration. Let X be the unobservable measurement of the well-established clinical endpoint for WM that can be quantified by the TCM items, Z_i, $i = 1, \ldots, K$, based on the estimated standard curve in Section 7.4. Because both models 3 and 4 in Section 7.4 can be transformed into a linear model using a log transformation, for convention, we simply choose a linear model to illustrate the proposed methods for validation of the CDP. That is, we assume that

$$X = (Y - \alpha)/\beta,$$

where $Y = \sum_{i=1}^{K} Z_i$. That is, model 1 in Section 7.4 was used for calibration. Suppose that X is distributed as a normal distribution with mean θ and variance τ^2. Let $Z = (Z_1, \ldots, Z_K)'$. Again, suppose Z follows a distribution with mean $\mu = (\mu_1, \ldots, \mu_K)'$ and variance Σ. To assess the validity, it is desired to see whether the mean of Z_i, $i = 1, \ldots, K$ is close to $(\alpha + \beta\theta)/K$. Let $\bar{\mu} = \frac{1}{K}\sum_{i=1}^{K}\mu_i$. Then $\theta = (\bar{\mu} - \alpha)/\beta$. Consequently, we can claim that the instrument is validated in terms of its validity if

$$|\mu_i - \bar{\mu}| < \delta, \forall i = 1, \ldots, K, \tag{7.1}$$

for some small pre-specified δ. In fact, we can write

$$\mu_i - \bar{\mu} = a_i'\mu, \ i = 1, \ldots, K,$$

where

$$a_i = \begin{pmatrix} -\frac{1}{K}1_{i-1} \\ 1-\frac{1}{K} \\ -\frac{1}{K}1_{K-i} \end{pmatrix}, 1_i = \begin{pmatrix} 1 \\ \vdots \\ 1 \end{pmatrix}_{(i-1)\times 1}, \text{ and } 1_{K-i} = \begin{pmatrix} 1 \\ \vdots \\ 1 \end{pmatrix}_{(K-i)\times 1}.$$

Assume that the TCM instrument is administered to N patients from group 2. Let $\hat{\mu} = \frac{1}{N}\sum_{j=1}^{N} Z_j = \bar{Z}$. To verify Equation 7.1, it is desired to test the null hypothesis

$$H_0 : |\mu_i - \bar{\mu}| \geq \delta \text{ for at least one } i. \tag{7.2}$$

Statistical Validation of Chinese Diagnostic Procedures

In this case, we can apply the approach of two one-sided tests. For each fixed i, a size α test based on the two one-sided tests approach rejects the hypothesis that $|a_i'\mu| > \delta$ if and only if (η_{i-}, η_{i+}) is within $(-\delta, \delta)$, where

$$\eta_{i\pm} = a_i'\hat{\mu} \pm t_{1-\alpha; N-1}\sqrt{\frac{1}{N}a_i'Sa_i},$$

where $t_{1-\alpha; N-1}$ is the $(1 - \alpha)$th quantile of the t-distribution with $N - 1$ degrees of freedom. Then, using the approach of intersection union, a size α test rejects the null hypothesis (Equation 7.2) and concludes that the TCM instruments is validated if and only if (η_{i-}, η_{i+}) is within $(-\delta, \delta)$ for all i.

7.5.2 Reliability

The calibrated, well-established clinical endpoints derived from the estimated standard curve are considered reliable if the variance of X is small. In this regard, we can test the hypothesis

$$H_0: \tau^2 \geq \Delta \text{ versus } H_a: \tau^2 < \Delta, \tag{7.3}$$

for some fixed Δ to verify the reliability of estimating θ by X. We will use group 2 to verify the reliability based on the previously established standard curve for calibration. On the basis of the estimated standard curve, we can derive that

$$\tau^2 = \frac{1}{\beta^2} \text{Var}\left(\sum_{i=1}^{K} Z_i\right)$$

$$= \frac{1}{\beta^2} 1'\Sigma 1.$$

It should be noted that the sample distribution of

$$\sum_{j=1}^{N}(X_j - \bar{X})^2/\tau^2$$

has a chi-square distribution with $N - 1$ degrees of freedom. According to Lehmann (1986), we may reject the null hypothesis of Equation 7.3 at the α level of significance if

$$Q = \frac{\sum_{j=1}^{N}(X_j - \bar{X})^2}{\Delta} < \chi^2(1-\alpha, N-1),$$

160   *Quantitative Methods for Traditional Chinese Medicine Development*

where $\chi^2(1 - \alpha, N - 1)$ is the $(1 - \alpha)$th upper quantiles of a central chi-square distribution with $N - 1$ degrees of freedom.

7.5.3 Ruggedness

In addition to validity and reliability, an acceptable TCM diagnostic instrument should produce similar results on different raters. In other words, it is desirable to quantify the variation owing to rater and the proportion of rater-to-rater variation to the total variation. We will use the one-way random model to evaluate instrument ruggedness (Chow and Liu 1995). A model describing a one-way random model is

$$x_{ij} = \nu + A_i + e_{ij}, i = 1 \text{ (group 2)}, 2 \text{ (group 3)}; j = 1, \ldots, N,$$

where x_{ij} is the calibrated well-established clinical endpoint of the jth patient obtained from the ith rater derived from the estimated standard curve, ν is the overall mean, A_i denotes the effect of the ith rater and is assumed to be distributed i.i.d. $N\left(0, \sigma_A^2\right)$, and e_{ij} denotes the random error of jth patient's scale derived from the ith rater, which is assumed to be distributed i.i.d. $N(0, \sigma^2)$. It is also assumed that A_i and e_{ij} are independent variables (Searle et al. 1992). Two sums of squares are the sum of squares within, SSE, and the sums of squares between, SSA. That is,

$$\text{SSE} = \sum_{i=1}^{2} \sum_{j=1}^{N} \left(x_{ij} - \bar{x}_{i\cdot}\right)^2,$$

and

$$\text{SSA} = N \sum_{i=1}^{2} \left(\bar{x}_{i\cdot} - \bar{x}_{\cdot\cdot}\right)^2,$$

where $\bar{x}_{i\cdot} = \dfrac{1}{N} \sum_{j=1}^{N} x_{ij}$ and $\bar{x}_{\cdot\cdot} = \dfrac{1}{2N} \sum_{i=1}^{2} \sum_{j=1}^{N} x_{ij} = \dfrac{1}{2} \sum_{i=1}^{2} \bar{x}_{i\cdot}$. Let MSA and MSE denote mean squares for factor A and mean square error. Then

$$\text{MSA} = \text{SSA}$$

and

$$\text{MSE} = \text{SSE}/[2(N - 1)].$$

Statistical Validation of Chinese Diagnostic Procedures 161

As a result, the analysis of variance estimators of σ^2 and σ_A^2 can be obtained as follows:

$$\hat{\sigma}^2 = \text{MSE}$$

and

$$\hat{\sigma}_A^2 = \frac{\text{MSA} - \text{MSE}}{N}.$$

To show that the rater-to-rater variability is within an acceptable limit ω, we can test the hypothesis

$$H_0: \sigma_A^2 \geq \omega \text{ versus } H_1: \sigma_A^2 < \omega. \tag{7.4}$$

Because there exists no exact $(1 - \alpha) \times 100\%$ confidence interval for σ_A^2, we can then derive the Williams-Tukey interval (Williams 1962), (L_A, U_A), with a confidence level between $(1 - 2\alpha) \times 100\%$ and $(1 - \alpha) \times 100\%$ for σ_A^2. Here

$$L_A = \frac{\text{SSA}(1 - F_U/F_A)}{N\chi_{UA}^2},$$

$$U_A = \frac{\text{SSA}(1 - F_L/F_A)}{N\chi_{LA}^2},$$

where $F_L = F[1 - 0.5\alpha, 1, 2(N - 1)]$ and $F_U = F[0.5\alpha, 1, 2(N - 1)]$ represent the $(1 - 0.5\alpha)$th and (0.5α)th upper quantiles of a central F distribution with 1 and $2(N - 1)$ degrees of freedom, $\chi_{LA}^2 = \chi^2(1 - 0.5\alpha, 1)$ and $\chi_{UA}^2 = \chi^2(0.5\alpha, 1)$ are the $(1 - 0.5\alpha)$th and (0.5α)th upper quantiles of a central chi-square distribution with 1 degree of freedom, and $F_A = \text{MSA}/\text{MSE}$. The null hypothesis (Equation 7.4) is rejected at the α level of significance if $U_A < \omega$.

7.6 A Numerical Example

We use a modified data set taken from Chang Gung Memorial Hospital in Taiwan to illustrate the methods discussed in this section. The example is a randomized trial to study the effect of acupuncture for treating stroke patients. Patients with an acute ischemic stroke between 4 and 10 days were allocated into three groups. The diagnostic criteria of acute ischemic stroke were based on the typical presentations of acute onset of focal neurological deficits, and excluded other possible organic brain lesions by brain computed tomography (CT) and/or magnetic resonance imaging (MRI). In this study, 30 stroke patients received aspirin 100 mg per day and were evaluated by a Chinese doctor and a Western clinician (group 1), 30 stroke patients received acupuncture and were evaluated by Chinese doctor A (group 2), and 30 stroke patients received acupuncture and were evaluated by Chinese doctor B (group 3). The combination of scalp and body acupoints that fit the Chinese traditional theory was applied in patients from groups 2 and 3. The 12 acupoints include: (1) Qianding-GV21, (2) Baihui-GV20 (scalp acupuncture line, Dingzhongxian-MS5), (3) upper 1/5 of the Dingnie, Qianxiexian-MS6, (4) middle 2/5 of the Dingnie, Qianxiexian-MS6 (scalp acupuncture line), (5) Jianyu-LI15, (6) Quchi-LI11, (7) Waiguan-TE5, (8) Hegu-LI4 (upper limb), (9) Xuehui-SP10, (10) Zusanli-S36, (11) Sanyinjiao-SP6, and (12) Taichong-LR3 (lower limb). The TOKKI-III type stimulator (NihonRiko Medical Corporation, Nagasaki, Japan) was used on the scalp needles. On the paretic side, eight body needles were inserted. The special needle sensation called *obtaining-qi* was evoked at all body acupoints for patients and stimulated by the manual means of *moving qi* in the real acupuncture group. Then, the needles would be kept *in situ* for 30 min. The measurement that the Western clinician used was the NIHSS, whereas the TCM diagnostic instruments considered in this study were wind and fire-heat syndromes. That is, patients in group 2 have both NIHSS and TCM scores, while patients in group 2 and group 3 have only TCM scores. Outcome assessments were recorded at randomization, 14 days, one month, 3 months, and 6 months after treatment.

Table 7.1 summarizes the rating scales of the wind and fire-heat syndromes. The wind syndrome is a rating scale in six categories: onset conditions (0–8), limbs conditions (0–7), tongue body (0–7), eyeballs conditions (0–3), string-like pulse (0–3), and head conditions (0–2). Patients with a total score of over 7 were considered having wind syndrome. On the other hand, the fire-heat syndrome consists of nine categories: tongue conditions (0–6), tongue fur (0–5), stool (0–4), spirit (0–4), facial and breath conditions (0–3), fever (0–3), pulse (0–2), mouth (0–2), and urine (0–1). Again, patients with a total score of >7 forecasts fire-heat syndrome. In both syndromes, the larger the scale is, the more severe the syndrome is.

In this example, we summarize the TCM instruments based on the wind and fire-heat syndromes. That is, $K = 2$. Let y represent the sum of the scores of wind and fire-heat syndromes and x represent the NIH stroke score. Note that we use the baseline measurements for calibration because the relationship between y and x might be confounded with the effect of medication. From group 1, we fit the four models discussed in Section 7.4. We also calculate the R^2 value and conduct a test on the lack of fit of each of four proposed model. Table 7.2 summarizes the results. The summary statistics in Table 7.2 show that the R^2 values

Statistical Validation of Chinese Diagnostic Procedures 163

TABLE 7.1

Wind and Fire-Heat Syndromes

Wind Syndrome			Fire-Heat Syndrome		
Category	Syndrome	Score	Category	Syndrome	Score
Onset conditions	Peaking in 48 hours	2	Tongue conditions	Red tongue	5
	Peaking in 24 hours	4		Crimson tongue	6
	Changeable condition	6	Tongue fur	Yellow thin tongue fur	2
	Peaking at onset	8		Yellow thick tongue fur	3
Limbs conditions	Clenched hands	3		Dry tongue fur	4
	Clenched jaw	3		Gray-black and dry tongue fur	5
	Jerking of limbs	5	Stool	Dry stool and difficult evacuation	2
	Hypertonia of the limbs	7		Dry stool and absence of evacuation for three days	3
	Rigid and neck	7		Dry stool and absence of evacuation for 5 days or more	4
Tongue body	Tremulous tongue body	5	Spirit	Heart vexation and irascibility	2
	Deviated and tremulous tongue body	7		Agitation	3
Eyeballs conditions	Moving eyeballs	3		Clouded spirit and delirious speech	4
	Eyeballs fixed in one position and not moving	3	Facial and breath conditions	Loud voice	2
String-like pulse	String-like pulse	3		Rough breathing	2
Head conditions	Dizzy head	1		Hasty breathing	3
	Headache with pulling sensation	1		Bad breath	3
	Dizzy head and vision	2		Dry red lips	2

(Continued)

164 *Quantitative Methods for Traditional Chinese Medicine Development*

TABLE 7.1 (CONTINUED)

Wind and Fire-Heat Syndromes

Wind Syndrome			Fire-Heat Syndrome		
Category	Syndrome	Score	Category	Syndrome	Score
				Red facial completion	3
				Red eyes	3
			Fever	Fever	3
			Pulse	Rapid, large, and forceful pulse	2
				String-like and rapid	2
				Slippery and rapid	2
			Mouth	Bitter taste in the mouth	1
				Dry pharynx	1
				Thirst with desire for cold drinks	2
			Urine	Reddish (tea-colored) urine	1

TABLE 7.2

Fitted Results and Lack-of-Fit Tests Based on Models 1, 2, 3, and 4 for Data in Group 1

	Model			
	1	2	3	4
Estimates	α: 7.3578	β: 2.7097	α: 7.5814	α: 9.7172
	(<0.001)	(<0.001)	(<0.001)	(<0.001)
	β: 1.8608		β: 0.5251	β: 0.0961
	(<0.001)		(<0.001)	(<0.001)
R^2	0.9862	0.7082	0.9466	0.9567
Lack-of-fit test				
F ratio	0.9461	43.3773	1.6450	2.1959
p value	0.5297	<0.0001	0.1743	0.0714

Statistical Validation of Chinese Diagnostic Procedures

TABLE 7.3

Bias and MSE of the Estimate of the WM Clinical Endpoint x_0 That Gives TCM Score y_0 Based on Models 1, 2, 3, and 4

y_0		Model			
		1	2	3	4
10	$\hat{x}_0$	1.4	3.7	1.7	0.3
	Bias	−0.0050	0.0093	0.1248	−0.0197
	MSE	0.0171	0.0218	1.1260	0.0738
12	$\hat{x}_0$	2.5	4.4	2.4	2.2
	Bias	−0.0039	0.0111	0.2494	−0.0136
	MSE	0.0129	0.0302	3.6173	0.0453
16	$\hat{x}_0$	4.6	5.9	4.1	5.2
	Bias	−0.0017	0.0149	0.7211	−0.0039
	MSE	0.0079	0.0513	21.9758	0.0239
21	$\hat{x}_0$	7.3	7.7	7.0	8.0
	Bias	0.0009	0.0195	1.9058	0.0052
	MSE	0.0081	0.0853	117.0957	0.0303
27	$\hat{x}_0$	10.6	10.0	11.2	10.6
	Bias	0.0041	0.0251	4.5740	0.0137
	MSE	0.0179	0.1375	538.2488	0.0593
34	$\hat{x}_0$	14.3	12.5	17.4	13.0
	Bias	0.0079	0.0316	10.0503	0.0214
	MSE	0.0424	0.2139	2151.7481	0.1053

of the four models are around 95 percent or higher except for model 2. The parameter estimates are also statistically significant. However, model 2 fails the lack-of-fit test and would be eliminated for further consideration. In Table 7.3, we present the bias and MSE of the estimate of the WM clinical endpoint x_0 that gives TCM score y_0 based on models 1, 2, 3, and 4. Although model 2 should be eliminated as stated previously, we also list the corresponding results for comparison purposes. Several values of y are considered. On the basis of the MSEs of the estimates of x_0, Model 1 gives overall *good* estimate of x_0.

The estimated standard curve based on the model 1 is given as

$$y = 7.358 + 1.861x.$$

To provide a better understanding, the estimated regression line as well as the original data is presented in Figure 7.2. As shown in Figure 7.2, the correlation between the NIH stroke score and the TCM is very strong so that a precise calibration curve can be derived. However, the relationship between the TCM score and the well-established WM clinical endpoint may vary from disease to disease. In some cases, the correlation may not be strong enough to establish the standard curve. On the other hand, if larger variability occurs, the ordinary least squares estimators may not be efficient.

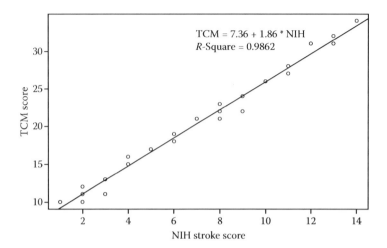

FIGURE 7.2
Scatterplot of sum of Wind syndrome score and Fire-Heat syndrome score versus NIH stroke score for the data in group 1 and the estimated standard curve.

Alternatively, a weighted least squares method can be considered to incorporate the heterogeneity of the variability.

We use group 2 to validate the CDP based on the previously established standard curve. In other words, we will claim that the instruments of wind and fire-heat syndromes are validated if

$$|\mu_i - \bar{\mu}| < \delta, \forall i = 1, 2,$$

for some small pre-specified δ. It can be seen from group 2 that

$$\hat{\mu}_1 = 8.633 \text{ and } \hat{\mu}_2 = 4.300.$$

From Section 7.5, (η_{1-}, η_{1+}) and (η_{2-}, η_{2+}) are respectively given by $(1.507, 2.826)$ and $(-2.826, -1.507)$. In this case, we can reject the null hypothesis (Equation 7.2) if $\delta = 3$.

Group 2 is also used to evaluate the reliability of the items for the TCM instrument. That is, the wind and fire-heat syndromes for the TCM instrument are considered reliable if the variance of X derived from the previously established standard curve is small. Assume that $\Delta = 15$. From group 2,

$$Q \geq \frac{\sum_{j=1}^{30}(X_j - \bar{X})^2}{\Delta}$$

$$= 27.13/15 = 1.81,$$

Statistical Validation of Chinese Diagnostic Procedures 167

TABLE 7.4

Analysis of Variance Table for Data in Groups 2 and 3

Source of Variation	DF	Sum of Squares	Mean Square	F Value	p Value
Rater	1	10.111	10.111	120.02	<0.0001
Error	58	4.886	0.084		
Total	59	14.997			

which is less than $\chi^2(0.95, 29) = 17.71$, thus we can reject the null hypothesis (Equation 7.3) at the 5 percent level of significance and conclude that the TCM instrument is validated in terms of its precision. Selection of Δ should reflect the considerable information existed in previous studies. It also varies from disease and disease.

Groups 2 and 3 are used to quantify the variation due to raters. The response variable was logarithmically transformed to normalize their distributions. The ANOVA table is given in Table 7.4. From Table 7.4, SSA = 10.11 and SSE = 4.886. Hence, estimates for σ_A^2 and σ^2 are given by $\hat{\sigma}_A^2 = 0.334$ and $\hat{\sigma}^2 = 0.084$, respectively. Because $F = 120.02$ with a p value less than 0.0001, we can reject the null hypothesis $H_0: \sigma_A^2 = 0$ at the 5 percent level of significance. The Williams-Tukey interval with a confidence level between $(1 - 2\alpha) \times 100\%$ and $(1 - \alpha) \times 100\%$ for σ_A^2 is given by (0.064, 343.184). This suggests that there is larger rater-to-rater variation. Larger variation due to raters implies either the CDP instrument is defective or the TCM doctors might have different TCM practices or experience. For the former case, the CDP instrument needs to be refined. For the latter case, the rater should revisit the established Chinese diagnostic criteria in order to ensure that consistency is maintained.

7.7 Concluding Remarks

The validation of a standard quantitative instrument in a TCM clinical trial is critical to provide an accurate and reliable assessment of the safety and effectiveness of the TCM under investigation. The calibration of the quantitative instrument with respect to a well-established clinical endpoint provides the clinicians a better understanding whether the observed significant difference from the quantitative instrument is clinically meaningful. On the basis of a well-calibrated and validated quantitative instrument, the sample size required for achieving a desired power for detecting a clinically meaningful difference can then be accurately estimated.

In clinical development of some TCMs, validated quantitative instruments for the diseases under study may not be available. In this case, it is suggested a small-scale validation pilot study be conducted to validate the quantitative instrument to be used in the intended clinical trials for a valid assessment of the safety and efficacy of the TCM under investigation. If such a small-scale pilot study is not feasible, a concurrent validation using a similar study design as described previously may be useful. In many case, a retrospective validation may also be considered.

There are several points we wish to make. In this study, the four commonly used statistical models for the calibration of the CDP with respect to a well-established clinical endpoint are introduced. The relationship between the CDP (y) and the well-established WM clinical endpoint (x) may vary from disease to disease. For some diseases, the relationship between y and x can be described by a linear regression model. In some cases, a nonlinear model may be more appropriate for describing the relationship between y and x. Therefore, to use calibration to interpret the relationship between the CDP and WM, intensive research in the design and analysis method might be necessary. The relationship between the TCM score and the WM endpoint may not be one of the four candidate models. In this case, more complicated calibration functions or transformations may be required. We may expect that the TCM score has positive correlation with the WM endpoint. However, the correlation may not be strong enough to give a precise calibration curve.

In this study, we assume that the scores of the TCM items are distributed as a multivariate normal distribution. Provided there are enough data, the central limit theorem states that the data are roughly normally distributed regardless of the original distributions of the TCM items. Severe nonnormality might encourage the use of transformations or other complicated methods. Note that the design of this study may have limitations in assessing the inter-rater reliability. For the assessment of inter-rater reliability, the technique of test-retest can be employed. The same patient is evaluated by two different TCM doctors. The Pearson's product moment correlation coefficient of the two repeated results is then studied. In practice, a test-retest correlation of 80 percent or higher is considered acceptable. At the design stage, we can also involve TCM doctor B from group 3 to evaluate the patients in group 2. Then group 2 can be used to assess the inter-rater reliability.

In practice, both NIHSS and CDP are rating scales based on the subjective judgment of qualified neurologists and TCM doctors respectively. That is, both Western clinical endpoints and CDP are subject to measurement errors. Although measurement error may probably be the most important variation that is difficult to detect and/or control, it can be reduced by specifying standard procedures for measuring NIHSS and CDP in the protocol. In this case, standardization of the procedure for rating NIHSS and CDP in the protocol by the clinicians and TCM doctors within the same center as well as by investigators at different centers is considered crucial in order to reduce measurement error and produce reliable, consistent, and reproducible results. Another issue we wish to address is the systemic error at the medical decision points for CDP. For example, a patient with ischemic stroke is defined to have improvement if his/her NIH Stroke Score reduces greater than 4 points from the baseline. It would be of interest to know the corresponding decision points for CDP and their associate systemic errors. This may require further research on statistical approaches for systemic error models.

8

Statistical Test for Consistency

8.1 Introduction

Unlike most Western medicines (WM), which typically contain a single active ingredient, TCM usually contain a number of components. However, the pharmacological activities, interactions, and relative proportions of these components are usually unknown. In practice, TCM is usually prescribed subjectively by an experienced Chinese doctor. As a result, the actual dose received by each individual varies depending on the signs and symptoms as perceived by the Chinese doctor. Although the purpose of this medical practice is to reduce the within-subject (or intrasubject) variability, it could also introduce non-negligible variability such as variations from component to component and from one Chinese doctor to another. Consequently, the reproducibility or consistency of clinical results is questionable. Thus, how to ensure the reproducibility or consistency of the observed clinical results has become a concern to regulatory agencies in the review and approval process (e.g., DOH 2004a,b; FDA 2004). In addition, it is also a great concern to the sponsor in the post-approval manufacturing process for assuring consistency of raw materials, in-process materials, and final products.

To address the question of reproducibility or consistency, it is suggested to implement a valid statistical quality control process on the raw materials, in-process materials, and final product (Chow and Liu 1995). In practice, raw materials are often from different resources and the final product may be manufactured by different sites. As a result, variabilities from different resources such as site to site, within site component-to-component are inevitable. Thus, testing for consistency in raw materials, in-process materials, and/or final product has become an important step in the quality control process in TCM research and development.

Tse et al. (2006) proposed a statistical quality control (QC) method for assessing consistency of raw materials and/or final product. The idea is to construct a 95 percent confidence interval for a proposed consistency index under a sampling plan. If the constructed 95 percent confidence lower limit is greater than a pre-specified QC lower limit, we then claim that the raw materials or final product has passed the QC and hence can be released for

171

172 *Quantitative Methods for Traditional Chinese Medicine Development*

further processing or use. Otherwise, the raw materials and/or final product should be rejected. For a given component (the most active component if possible), a sampling plan is developed to ensure that there is a desired probability for establishing consistency between sites when truly there is no difference in raw materials or final products between sites.

In Section 8.2, the concept of consistency between raw materials or final products between sites or laboratories is introduced. Statistical methods for estimating the proposed consistency index are also studied in this section. In Section 8.3, sampling plans for statistical QC of raw materials and/or final products are developed under various specifications and/or user parameters. Hypotheses testing results are also developed for the consistency index. An example concerning statistical QC of raw materials from two sites is given in Section 8.4. A brief discussion regarding a possible extension of the results to multiple active components is discussed in the last section.

8.2 Consistency Index

Let U and W be the characteristics of the most active component among the multiple components of a TCM from two different sites, where $X = \log U$ and $Y = \log W$ follows normal distributions with means μ_X, μ_Y and variances V_X, V_Y, respectively. Similar to the idea of using $P(X < Y)$ to assess reliability in statistical quality control (Enis and Geisser 1971; Church and Harris 1970), we propose the following probability as an index to assess the consistency of raw materials and/or final product from two different sites

$$p = P\left(1 - \delta < \frac{U}{W} < \frac{1}{1 - \delta}\right), \tag{8.1}$$

where $0 < \delta < 1$ and is defined as a limit that allows for consistency. We will refer p as the consistency index. Thus p tends to 1 as δ tends to 1. For a given δ, if p is close to 1, materials U and W are considered to be identical. It should be noted that a small δ implies the requirement of high degree of consistency between material U and material W. In practice, it may be difficult to meet this narrow specification for consistency. Under the normality assumption of $X = \log U$ and $Y = \log W$, Equation 8.1 can be rewritten as

$$p = P[\log(1 - \delta) < \log U - \log W < -\log(1 - \delta)]$$

$$= \Phi\left(\frac{-\log(1 - \delta) - (\mu_X - \mu_Y)}{\sqrt{V_X + V_Y}}\right) - \Phi\left(\frac{\log(1 - \delta) - (\mu_X - \mu_Y)}{\sqrt{V_X + V_Y}}\right).$$

Statistical Test for Consistency

where $\Phi(z_0) = P(Z < z_0)$ with Z being a standard normal random variable. Therefore, the consistency index p is a function of the parameters $\theta = (\mu_X, \mu_Y, V_X, V_Y)$, i.e., $p = h(\theta)$. Suppose that observations $X_i = \log U_i$, $i = 1, \ldots, n_X$ and $Y_i = \log W_i$, $i = 1, \ldots, n_Y$ are collected in an assay study. Then, using the invariance principle, the maximum likelihood estimator (MLE) of p can be obtained as

$$\hat{p} = \Phi\left(\frac{-\log(1-\delta)-(\bar{X}-\bar{Y})}{\sqrt{\hat{V}_X + \hat{V}_Y}}\right) - \Phi\left(\frac{\log(1-\delta)-(\bar{X}-\bar{Y})}{\sqrt{\hat{V}_X + \hat{V}_Y}}\right), \tag{8.2}$$

where $\bar{X} = \dfrac{1}{n_X}\sum_{i=1}^{n_X} X_i$, $\bar{Y} = \dfrac{1}{n_Y}\sum_{i=1}^{n_Y} Y_i$, $\hat{V}_X = \dfrac{1}{n_X}\sum_{i=1}^{n_X}(X_i - \bar{X})^2$, and $\hat{V}_Y = \dfrac{1}{n_Y}\sum_{i=1}^{n_Y}(Y_i - \bar{Y})^2$. In other words, $\hat{p} = h(\hat{\theta}) = h(\bar{X}, \bar{Y}, \hat{V}_X, \hat{V}_Y)$. Furthermore, it can be easily verified that the following asymptotic result holds.

Theorem 8.1

$\hat{p}$ as given in Equation 8.2 is asymptotically normal with mean $E(\hat{p})$ and variance $\mathrm{var}(\hat{p})$. In other words,

$$\frac{\hat{p} - E(\hat{p})}{\sqrt{\mathrm{var}(\hat{p})}} \to N(0, 1) \tag{8.3}$$

where $E(\hat{p}) = p + B(p) + o\left(\dfrac{1}{n}\right)$ and $\mathrm{var}(\hat{p}) = C(p) + o\left(\dfrac{1}{n}\right)$. ∎

Proof

On the basis of the definitions of $\bar{X}$ and $\hat{V}_X$, it is easy to show that $E(\bar{X}) = \mu_X$, $E(\hat{V}_X) = \dfrac{n_X - 1}{n_X} V_X$, $\mathrm{var}(\bar{X}) = \dfrac{V_X}{n_X}$, and $\mathrm{var}(\hat{V}_X) = \dfrac{2(n_X - 1)}{n_X^2} V_X^2$. Similarly, $E(\bar{Y}) = \mu_Y$, $E(\hat{V}_Y) = \dfrac{n_Y - 1}{n_Y} V_Y$, $\mathrm{var}(\bar{Y}) = \dfrac{V_Y}{n_Y}$, and $\mathrm{var}(\hat{V}_Y) = \dfrac{2(n_Y - 1)}{n_Y^2} V_Y^2$.

Applying expansion of $\hat{p}$ at p, we have

$$\hat{p} = p + \frac{\partial \hat{p}}{\partial \mu_X}(\bar{X} - \mu_X) + \frac{\partial \hat{p}}{\partial \mu_Y}(\bar{Y} - \mu_Y) + \frac{\partial \hat{p}}{\partial V_X}(\hat{V}_X - V_X) + \frac{\partial \hat{p}}{\partial V_Y}(\hat{V}_Y - V_Y)$$

$$+ \frac{1}{2}\left[\frac{\partial^2 \hat{p}}{\partial \mu_X^2}(\bar{X} - \mu_X)^2 + \frac{\partial^2 \hat{p}}{\partial \mu_Y^2}(\bar{Y} - \mu_Y)^2 + \frac{\partial^2 \hat{p}}{\partial V_X^2}(\hat{V}_X - V_X)^2 + \frac{\partial^2 \hat{p}}{\partial V_Y^2}(\hat{V}_Y - V_Y)^2\right] + \ldots$$

The other second-order partial derivatives are not considered because they will lead to expected values of order $O(n^{-2})$ or higher. Taking expectation,

$$E(\hat{p}) = p + \frac{1}{2}\left[\frac{\partial^2 \hat{p}}{\partial \mu_X^2}\frac{V_X}{n_X} + \frac{\partial^2 \hat{p}}{\partial \mu_Y^2}\frac{V_Y}{n_Y} + \frac{\partial^2 \hat{p}}{\partial V_X^2}\left(\frac{2V_X^2}{n_X}\right) + \frac{\partial^2 \hat{p}}{\partial V_Y^2}\left(\frac{2V_Y^2}{n_Y}\right)\right] + O(n^{-2})$$

and

$$\mathrm{var}(\hat{p}) = \left[\left(\frac{\partial\hat{p}}{\partial\mu_X}\right)^2\frac{V_X}{n_X} + \left(\frac{\partial\hat{p}}{\partial\mu_Y}\right)^2\frac{V_Y}{n_Y} + \left(\frac{\partial\hat{p}}{\partial V_X}\right)^2\left(\frac{2V_X^2}{n_X}\right) + \left(\frac{\partial\hat{p}}{\partial V_Y}\right)^2\left(\frac{2V_Y^2}{n_Y}\right)\right] + O(n^{-2})$$

Therefore,

$$B(p) = \frac{1}{2}\left[\frac{\partial^2 \hat{p}}{\partial \mu_X^2}\frac{V_X}{n_X} + \frac{\partial^2 \hat{p}}{\partial \mu_Y^2}\frac{V_Y}{n_Y} + \frac{\partial^2 \hat{p}}{\partial V_X^2}\left(\frac{2V_X^2}{n_X}\right) + \frac{\partial^2 \hat{p}}{\partial V_Y^2}\left(\frac{2V_Y^2}{n_Y}\right)\right] \tag{8.4}$$

and

$$C(p) = \left[\left(\frac{\partial\hat{p}}{\partial\mu_X}\right)^2\frac{V_X}{n_X} + \left(\frac{\partial\hat{p}}{\partial\mu_Y}\right)^2\frac{V_Y}{n_Y} + \left(\frac{\partial\hat{p}}{\partial V_X}\right)^2\left(\frac{2V_X^2}{n_X}\right) + \left(\frac{\partial\hat{p}}{\partial V_Y}\right)^2\left(\frac{2V_Y^2}{n_Y}\right)\right]. \tag{8.5}$$

For the sake of simplicity, denote

$$z_1 = \frac{\log(1-\delta) - (\mu_X - \mu_Y)}{\sqrt{V_X + V_Y}},$$

$$z_2 = \frac{-\log(1-\delta) - (\mu_X - \mu_Y)}{\sqrt{V_X + V_Y}}$$

and

$$\phi(z) = \frac{1}{\sqrt{2\pi}}\exp\left(-\frac{z^2}{2}\right).$$

Then, after some algebra, the partial derivatives are given as

$$\frac{\partial\hat{p}}{\partial\mu_X} = -\frac{\partial\hat{p}}{\partial\mu_Y} = \left(\frac{-1}{\sqrt{V_X + V_Y}}\right)[\phi(z_2) - \phi(z_1)],$$

Statistical Test for Consistency

$$\frac{\partial \hat{p}}{\partial V_X} = \frac{\partial \hat{p}}{\partial V_Y} = \left(\frac{-1}{2\sqrt{V_X + V_Y}}\right)[z_2\phi(z_2) - z_1\phi(z_1)],$$

$$\frac{\partial^2 \hat{p}}{\partial \mu_X^2} = \frac{\partial^2 \hat{p}}{\partial \mu_Y^2} = \left(\frac{-1}{V_X + V_Y}\right)[z_2\phi(z_2) - z_1\phi(z_1)],$$

and

$$\frac{\partial^2 \hat{p}}{\partial V_X^2} = \frac{\partial^2 \hat{p}}{\partial V_Y^2} = \frac{1}{4(V_X + V_Y)^{3/2}}\left[\left(2z_2 - z_2^3\right)\phi(z_2) - \left(2z_1 - z_1^3\right)z_1\phi(z_1)\right].$$

This completes the proof. ∎

On the basis of the result of Theorem 8.1, an approximate $(1 - \alpha) \times 100\%$ confidence interval for p, i.e., $[LL(\hat{p}), UL(\hat{p})]$, can be obtained. As follows,

$$LL(\hat{p}) = \hat{p} - B(\hat{p}) - z_{\alpha/2}\sqrt{C(\hat{p})}, \quad \text{and} \quad UL(\hat{p}) = \hat{p} - B(\hat{p}) + z_{\alpha/2}\sqrt{C(\hat{p})}. \quad (8.6)$$

where z_α is the upper α-percentile of a standard normal distribution.

8.3 Statistical Quality Control for Consistency

For a valid statistical quality control process, a testing procedure is necessarily performed according to some pre-specified acceptance criteria under a sampling plan. In this section, we propose a statistical quality control (QC) method for assessing consistency of raw materials and/or final product of TCM. The idea is to construct a 95 percent confidence interval for a proposed consistency index described above under a sampling plan. If the constructed 95 percent confidence lower limit is greater than a pre-specified QC lower limit, then we claim that the raw material or final product has passed the QC and hence can be released for further processing or use. Otherwise, the raw materials and/or final product should be rejected. For a given component (the most active component if possible), a sampling plan is derived to ensure that there is a desired probability for establishing consistency between sites when truly there is no difference in raw materials or final products between sites. In what follows, details regarding the choice of acceptance criteria, sampling plan and the corresponding testing procedure are briefly outlined.

8.3.1 Acceptance Criteria

In terms of consistency, we propose the following QC criterion. If the probability that the lower limit $LL(\hat{p})$ of the constructed $(1 - \alpha) \times 100\%$ confidence interval of p is greater than or equal to a pre-specified quality control lower limit, say, QC_L, exceeds a pre-specified number β (say $\beta = 80\%$), then we claim that U and W are consistent or similar. In other words, U and W are consistent or similar if $P(QC_L \leq LL(\hat{p})) \geq \beta$, where β is a pre-specified constant.

8.3.2 Sampling Plan

In practice, it is necessary to select a sample size to ensure that there is a high probability, say β, of consistency between U and W when, in fact, U and W are consistent. It is suggested that the sample size is chosen such that there is more than 80 percent chance that the lower confidence limit of p is greater than or equal to the QC lower limit, i.e., $\beta = 0.8$. In other words, the sample size is determined such that

$$P\{QC_L \leq LL(\hat{p})\} \geq \beta. \tag{8.7}$$

Using Equation 8.7, this leads to

$$P\{QC_L \leq \hat{p} - B(\hat{p}) - z_{\alpha/2}\sqrt{\mathrm{var}(\hat{p})}\} \geq \beta.$$

Thus,

$$P\{QC_L + z_{\alpha/2}\sqrt{\mathrm{var}(\hat{p})} - p \leq \hat{p} - p - B(p)\} \geq \beta.$$

This gives

$$P\left\{ \frac{QC_L - p}{\sqrt{\mathrm{var}(\hat{p})}} + z_{\alpha/2} \leq \frac{\hat{p} - p - B(p)}{\sqrt{\mathrm{var}(\hat{p})}} \right\} \geq \beta.$$

Therefore, the sample size required for achieving a probability higher than β can be obtained by solving the following equation:

$$\frac{QC_L - p}{\sqrt{\mathrm{var}(\hat{p})}} + z_{\alpha/2} \leq -z_{1-\beta}. \tag{8.8}$$

Assuming that $n_X = n_Y = n$, then the common sample size is given by

$$n \geq \frac{(z_{1-\beta} + z_{\alpha/2})^2}{(p - QC_L)^2} \left\{ \left(\frac{\partial \hat{p}}{\partial \mu_X} \right)^2 V_X + \left(\frac{\partial \hat{p}}{\partial \mu_Y} \right)^2 V_Y + \left(\frac{\partial \hat{p}}{\partial V_X} \right)^2 (2V_X^2) + \left(\frac{\partial \hat{p}}{\partial V_Y} \right)^2 (2V_Y^2) \right\}. \tag{8.9}$$

The above result suggests that the required sample size will depend on the choices of α, β, V_X, V_Y, $\mu_X - \mu_Y$, and $p - QC_L$. It is clear from the expression in Equation 8.9 that larger sample size is required for smaller α and larger β, i.e., the interval is expected to have high confidence level $(1 - \alpha)$ and high chance that the lower confidence limit is larger than QC_L. Furthermore, if we require the QC_L to be close to p, i.e., $p - QC_L$ is small, a relatively large sample size is required. The dependence of the sample size n on the other parameters V_X, V_Y and $\mu_X - \mu_Y$ is relatively unclear because these parameters are linked to the corresponding partial derivatives. A numerical study is conducted to explore the pattern. Given the large number of parameters involved in Equation 8.9, it is impractical to list the value of n for all the parameter combinations. However, for illustrative purpose, we only consider a certain combination of parameter values in an attempt to explore the pattern of dependence of n on the parameters. For the sake of simplicity, define

$$S = \frac{1}{(p - QC_L)^2} \left\{ \left(\frac{\partial \hat{p}}{\partial \mu_X} \right)^2 V_X + \left(\frac{\partial \hat{p}}{\partial \mu_Y} \right)^2 V_Y + \left(\frac{\partial \hat{p}}{\partial V_X} \right)^2 (2V_X^2) + \left(\frac{\partial \hat{p}}{\partial V_Y} \right)^2 (2V_Y^2) \right\}.$$

Then, for given choices of α and β, the required sample size n is equal to $(z_{1-\beta} + z_{\alpha/2})^2 S$. In particular, in our study, $\delta = 0.10, 0.15$, and 0.20; $\mu_X - \mu_Y = 0.5$, 1.0, and 1.5; $p - QC_L = 0.02, 0.05$, and 0.08. V_X is chosen to be 1, and $V_Y = 0.2$, $0.5, 1.0, 2.0$, and 5.0. For each combination of these parameters values, the corresponding value of S is listed in Table 8.1. Given the number of parameters involved and the complexity of the mathematical expression of S, it is not easy to detect a general pattern. However, in general, the results suggest that S increases as $\mu_X - \mu_Y$ decreases; and as the variances V_x and V_y differ more from each other. In other words, smaller sample size is required if the difference between the population means is large or the variability of the two sites is of similar magnitude.

As an illustration, if for a study with $\delta = 0.2$, $V_X = 1$, $V_Y = 0.5$, $\mu_X - \mu_Y = 1.0$, and an experiment expect $p - QC_L$ to be not larger than 0.05, then results in Table 8.1 suggests that $S = 3.024$. Suppose a probability higher than $\beta = 0.8$ at the $\alpha = 0.05$ level of significance is required, the corresponding required sample size is given by

$$n \geq (z_{1-0.8} + z_{0.05/2})^2 S = (0.842 + 1.96)^2 (3.024) = 23.74,$$

i.e., a sample of size at least 24 is required.

TABLE 8.1

Values of $n/(z_{1-\beta} + z_{\alpha/2})^2$

	V_Y	$\delta = 0.10$			$\delta = 0.15$			$\delta = 0.20$		
		$\Delta = 0.5$	$\Delta = 1.0$	$\Delta = 1.5$	$\Delta = 0.5$	$\Delta = 1.0$	$\Delta = 1.5$	$\Delta = 0.5$	$\Delta = 1.0$	$\Delta = 1.5$
D = 0.02	0.2	5.693	5.376	4.955	13.403	12.681	11.702	24.861	23.594	21.810
	0.5	4.518	4.289	4.196	10.655	10.134	9.921	19.820	18.901	18.520
	1.0	3.939	3.336	3.237	9.310	7.894	7.662	17.370	14.761	14.333
	2.0	4.231	2.962	2.226	10.020	7.021	5.280	18.756	13.163	9.906
	5.0	5.728	4.159	2.469	13.595	9.876	5.866	25.534	18.558	11.032
D = 0.05	0.2	0.911	0.860	0.793	2.144	2.029	1.872	3.978	3.775	3.490
	0.5	0.723	0.686	0.671	1.705	1.622	1.587	3.171	3.024	2.963
	1.0	0.630	0.534	0.518	1.490	1.263	1.226	2.779	2.362	2.293
	2.0	0.677	0.474	0.356	1.603	1.123	0.845	3.001	2.106	1.585
	5.0	0.916	0.666	0.395	2.175	1.580	0.939	4.085	2.969	1.765
D = 0.08	0.2	0.356	0.336	0.310	0.838	0.793	0.731	1.554	1.475	1.363
	0.5	0.282	0.268	0.262	0.666	0.633	0.620	1.239	1.181	1.158
	1.0	0.246	0.208	0.202	0.582	0.493	0.479	1.086	0.923	0.896
	2.0	0.264	0.185	0.139	0.626	0.439	0.330	1.172	0.823	0.619
	5.0	0.358	0.260	0.154	0.850	0.617	0.367	1.596	1.160	0.690

Note: The value n is the required sample size. Notation: $\Delta = \mu_X - \mu_Y$, $D = p - QC_L$.

Statistical Test for Consistency

8.3.3 Testing Procedure

Hypotheses testing of the consistency index p can also be conducted based on the asymptotic normality of $\hat{p}$. Consider the following hypotheses:

$$H_0: p \leq p_0 \text{ versus } H_1: p > p_0.$$

We would reject the null hypothesis in favor of the alternative hypothesis of consistency. Under H_0, we have

$$\frac{\hat{p} - p_0 - B(\hat{p})}{\sqrt{\text{var}(\hat{p})}} \sim N(0, 1) \tag{8.10}$$

Thus, we reject the null hypothesis H_0 at the α level of significance if

$$\frac{\hat{p} - p_0 - B(\hat{p})}{\sqrt{\text{var}(\hat{p})}} > Z_{\alpha}.$$

This is equivalent to rejecting the null hypothesis H_0 when

$$\hat{p} > p_0 + B(\hat{p}) + Z_{\alpha}\sqrt{\text{var}(\hat{p})}.$$

Again, for illustrative purposes, Table 8.2 provides critical values of the proposed test for consistency index for various combinations of the parameters. In particular, $\alpha = 0.1$; $p_0 = 0.75, 0.85,$ and 0.9; $\delta = 0.10$ and 0.20; $\mu_X - \mu_Y = 0.5, 1.0,$ and 1.5. V_X is chosen to be 1 and $V_Y = 0.2, 0.5, 1.0, 2.0$ and 5.0. Note that the critical value is closer to the corresponding p_0 either for larger sample size n, smaller δ or smaller $\mu_X - \mu_Y$.

8.3.4 Strategy for Statistical Quality Control

In practice, raw materials, in-process materials, and/or final products at different sites are manufactured sequentially in batches or lots. As a result, it is important to perform statistical quality control on batches. A typical approach is to randomly select samples from several (consecutive) batches for testing. In this case, observations from the study would be subject to batch-to-batch variability. For the sake of administrative convenience, it is common to have an equal number of observations from the batches. Consider the following model:

$$X_{ij} = \mu_X + A_i^X + \varepsilon_{ij}^X, i = 1, \ldots, m_X; j = 1, \ldots, n_X,$$

TABLE 8.2

Critical Values of the Proposed Test for Consistency Index p_0

			$\Delta = 0.5$			$\Delta = 1.0$			$\Delta = 1.5$		
p_0	δ	V_Y	$n = 15$	$n = 30$	$n = 50$	$n = 15$	$n = 30$	$n = 50$	$n = 15$	$n = 30$	$n = 50$
0.75	0.10	0.2	0.7695	0.7640	0.7609	0.7683	0.7632	0.7604	0.7680	0.7629	0.7601
		0.5	0.7673	0.7624	0.7597	0.7665	0.7619	0.7593	0.7665	0.7619	0.7593
		1.0	0.7662	0.7616	0.7590	0.7646	0.7605	0.7582	0.7645	0.7604	0.7581
		2.0	0.7668	0.7620	0.7594	0.7639	0.7600	0.7578	0.7620	0.7586	0.7567
		5.0	0.7697	0.7640	0.7609	0.7667	0.7619	0.7593	0.7628	0.7592	0.7572
	0.20	0.2	0.7907	0.7791	0.7727	0.7884	0.7777	0.7717	0.7878	0.7771	0.7712
		0.5	0.7863	0.7760	0.7703	0.7846	0.7749	0.7695	0.7847	0.7749	0.7695
		1.0	0.7839	0.7743	0.7689	0.7807	0.7721	0.7673	0.7805	0.7719	0.7671
		2.0	0.7853	0.7753	0.7697	0.7793	0.7710	0.7664	0.7754	0.7682	0.7642
		5.0	0.7915	0.7797	0.7731	0.7853	0.7752	0.7697	0.7771	0.7694	0.7651
0.85	0.10	0.2	0.8695	0.8640	0.8609	0.8683	0.8632	0.8604	0.8680	0.8629	0.8601
		0.5	0.8673	0.8624	0.8597	0.8665	0.8619	0.8593	0.8665	0.8619	0.8593
		1.0	0.8662	0.8616	0.8590	0.8646	0.8605	0.8582	0.8645	0.8604	0.8581
		2.0	0.8668	0.8620	0.8594	0.8639	0.8600	0.8578	0.8620	0.8586	0.8567
		5.0	0.8697	0.8640	0.8609	0.8667	0.8619	0.8593	0.8628	0.8592	0.8572
	0.20	0.2	0.8907	0.8791	0.8727	0.8884	0.8777	0.8717	0.8878	0.8771	0.8712
		0.5	0.8863	0.8760	0.8703	0.8846	0.8749	0.8695	0.8847	0.8749	0.8695
		1.0	0.8839	0.8743	0.8689	0.8807	0.8721	0.8673	0.8805	0.8719	0.8671
		2.0	0.8853	0.8753	0.8697	0.8793	0.8710	0.8664	0.8754	0.8682	0.8642
		5.0	0.8915	0.8797	0.8731	0.8853	0.8752	0.8697	0.8771	0.8694	0.8651
0.90	0.10	0.2	0.9195	0.9140	0.9109	0.9183	0.9132	0.9104	0.9180	0.9129	0.9101
		0.5	0.9173	0.9124	0.9097	0.9165	0.9119	0.9093	0.9165	0.9119	0.9093
		1.0	0.9162	0.9116	0.9090	0.9146	0.9105	0.9082	0.9145	0.9104	0.9081
		2.0	0.9168	0.9120	0.9094	0.9139	0.9100	0.9078	0.9120	0.9086	0.9067
		5.0	0.9197	0.9140	0.9109	0.9167	0.9119	0.9093	0.9128	0.9092	0.9072
	0.20	0.2	0.9407	0.9291	0.9227	0.9384	0.9277	0.9217	0.9378	0.9271	0.9212
		0.5	0.9363	0.9260	0.9203	0.9346	0.9249	0.9195	0.9347	0.9249	0.9195
		1.0	0.9339	0.9243	0.9189	0.9307	0.9221	0.9173	0.9305	0.9219	0.9171
		2.0	0.9353	0.9253	0.9197	0.9293	0.9210	0.9164	0.9254	0.9182	0.9142
		5.0	0.9415	0.9297	0.9231	0.9353	0.9252	0.9197	0.9271	0.9194	0.9151

Note: Notation: $\Delta = \mu_X - \mu_Y$.

where A_i^X accounts for the batch-to-batch variability for the observations collected in site 1 and is normally distributed with mean 0 and variance σ_{b1}^2; m_X is the number of batches collected in the study at site 1 and ε_{ij}^X are normal random variables with mean 0 and variance σ_1^2. Similarly,

$$Y_{ij} = \mu_Y + A_i^Y + \varepsilon_{ij}^Y, i = 1, \ldots, m_Y; j = 1, \ldots, n_Y,$$

Statistical Test for Consistency 181

where A_i^Y accounts for the batch-to-batch variability for the observations collected in site 2 and is normally distributed with mean 0 and variance σ_{b2}^2; m_Y is the number of batches collected in the study at site 2 and ε_{ij}^Y are normal random variables with mean 0 and variance σ_2^2. Therefore, the total variability of the most active component at the two sites is given by var $X = V_X = \sigma_{b1}^2 + \sigma_1^2$ and var $Y = V_Y = \sigma_{b2}^2 + \sigma_2^2$, respectively.

Furthermore, let $\bar{X}_{i.} = \dfrac{1}{n_X} \sum_{j=1}^{n_X} X_{ij}$ and $\bar{X} = \dfrac{1}{m_X} \sum_{i=1}^{m_X} \bar{X}_{i.}$. Then, the observed sums of squares are $SSA_1 = n_X \sum_{i=1}^{m_X} (\bar{X}_{i.} - \bar{X})^2$, $SSE_1 = \sum_{i=1}^{m_X} \sum_{j=1}^{n_X} (X_{ij} - \bar{X}_{i.})^2$ and $SST_1 = SSA_1 + SSE_1$. Following the results of Chow and Tse (1991), the MLE of σ_{b1}^2 and σ_1^2 are

$$
\hat{\sigma}_{b1}^2 = \begin{cases} \dfrac{1}{n_X}\left(\dfrac{1}{m_X} SSA_1 - \dfrac{1}{m_X(n_X - 1)} SSE_1\right) & \dfrac{1}{m_X} SSA_1 \geq \dfrac{1}{m_X(n_X - 1)} SSE_1 \\[4mm] & \text{if} \\[2mm] 0 & \dfrac{1}{m_X} SSA_1 < \dfrac{1}{m_X(n_X - 1)} SSE_1 \end{cases}
$$

(8.11)

and

$$
\hat{\sigma}_1^2 = \begin{cases} \dfrac{1}{m_X(n_X - 1)} SSE_1 & \dfrac{1}{m_X} SSA_1 \geq \dfrac{1}{m_X(n_X - 1)} SSE_1 \\[4mm] & \text{if} \\[2mm] \dfrac{1}{n_X m_X} SST_1 & \dfrac{1}{m_X} SSA_1 < \dfrac{1}{m_X(n_X - 1)} SSE_1. \end{cases}
$$

(8.12)

Furthermore, the MLE of the total variability V_X is given by $\hat{V}_X = \dfrac{1}{n_X m_X} SST_1$. The MLE of σ_{b2}^2, σ_2^2, and V_Y, denoted by $\hat{\sigma}_{b2}^2$, $\hat{\sigma}_2^2$, and $\hat{V}_Y$ respectively, can be obtained in a similar way using observations Y_{ij}. Comparison of the estimates $\hat{\sigma}_{b2}^2$ and $\hat{\sigma}_{b1}^2$ would give an idea of the magnitude of the batch-to-batch variability at the two sites.

8.3.5 An Example

To illustrate the proposed statistical quality control process for testing consistency, consider test for raw materials of a traditional Chinese medicine (TCM) that is intended for treating patients with rheumatoid arthritis. The TCM contains three active components, namely, *Herba Epimedii* (HE) extract (the most active component) and the other two components B extract and C extract. HE is the dried aerial parts of herbaceous perennial plants of

182 *Quantitative Methods for Traditional Chinese Medicine Development*

berberidaceae family. The botanical for medical use is harvested in summer or autumn when foliage branch growing luxuriantly. The TCM contains multiherb substance that is prepared by combining individually processed botanical substances. That is, HE, B, and C contain 0.6 kg of HE solid extract, 0.25 kg of B solid extract, and 0.25 kg of C solid extract, respectively, while the HE extract is standardized and quality controlled to contain at least 2 percent of icariin, the B extract is standardized and controlled to contain at least 20 percent of naringin, and the C is standardized to contain 0.06 to 0.08% of triptolide, respectively. The component of HE is mainly distributed in Shianxi, Sichuan, Hubei, Shanxi, and Guangxi provinces of China. Each of these three components has been used as herbal remedies since ancient China. These components are well documented in the recent edition of *Chinese Pharmacopoeia*. The formulation of the TCM is summarized in Table 8.3.

Suppose the sponsor of the TCM is interested in testing the consistency of the raw materials, based mainly on the most active component of HE, from Shianxi, Sichuan, and Hubei. Suppose that three batches from each site will be tested and eight samples from each batch will be randomly selected. Therefore, in each site, there are a total of 24 samples are selected for testing. Also suppose that δ is equal to 0.2. Furthermore, the acceptance criterion for testing consistency is chosen such that the probability of the lower limit $LL(\hat{p})$ of the 95 percent confidence interval of p is greater than the quality control lower limit QC_L has to be at least 0.8.

To assess the consistency of the active component from the three sites, test results (in percent of label claim) of the test samples selected from the three provinces are log-transformed. The corresponding summary statistics are

TABLE 8.3

Formulation of a Given TCM

Component	TCM Formulation	Standardized for QC
HE	60 mg	1.2 mg of icarium
B	25 mg	5 mg of naringin
C	25 mg	1.5–2.0 mg of triptolide
Excipient	90 mg	Not applicable
Total	200 mg	

TABLE 8.4

Summary Statistics

Site	Sample Mean	Sample Standard Deviation
Shianxi	4.537	0.032
Sichuan	4.445	0.045
Hubei	4.258	0.061

TABLE 8.5

Pairwise Comparisons among the Three Provinces

Sites	$\bar{X} - \bar{Y}$	var($\hat{p}$)	Estimated Consistency Index	$P\left\{\dfrac{QC_L - p}{\sqrt{\mathrm{var}(\hat{p})}} + z_{\alpha/2} < Z\right\}$
Shianxi vs. Sichuan	0.092	0.00455	0.99	$P\{-20.01 < Z\} = 1.00$
Shianxi vs. Hubei	0.279	0.05728	0.21	$P\{0.214 < Z\} = 0.417$
Sichuan vs. Hubei	0.187	0.07116	0.68	$P\{0.555 < Z\} = 0.288$

given in Table 8.4. For illustrative purposes, QC_L is selected in such a way that $p - QC_L < 0.1$. The results for the comparison among the three provinces are: given in Table 8.5. As can be seen from Table 8.5, we claim that raw materials of HE component obtained from the Shianxi and Sichuan are consistent because the corresponding probability $P\left\{\dfrac{QC_L - p}{\sqrt{\mathrm{var}(\hat{p})}} + z_{\alpha/2} < Z\right\}$ is larger than the required value β (= 0.8); whilst those from Hubei is not consistent with Shianxi and Sichuan because the corresponding probabilities are less than 0.8.

8.4 Tolerance Region Approach

Instead of assessing the consistency of the materials from two sites as described in the previous section, Lai and Hsiao (2013) proposed a tolerance region approach to manage the quality of the materials from different locations simultaneously. If the materials do not pass the tolerance region (derived from a random effects model) for the purpose of quality control, Lai and Hsiao suggested that pairwise comparisons be performed in order to extract the failed one in order to reduce the cost of materials. In what follows, Lai and Hsiao's tolerance region approach under a multivariate random effects model is briefly introduced.

8.4.1 A Multivariate Random Effects Model

The concept of tolerance region for a multivariate normal population has been well studied in the literature. For example, Wald (1942) proposed a general parametric method, applicable to any given density function, to construct tolerance limits for large samples. However, it is not clear whether Wald's approach for small samples is adequate. Alternatively, John (1963) provided theoretical formulation for the problem of constructing tolerance region for multivariate normal distributions. Many approximate methods for construction of tolerance regions for multivariate normal distributions

184 *Quantitative Methods for Traditional Chinese Medicine Development*

have been proposed in the literature since then. See, for example, Siotani (1964), Chew (1966), Guttman (1970), Fuchs and Kenett (1987), Hall and Sheldon (1979), Krishnamoorthy and Mathew (1999), and Krishnamoorthy and Mondal (2006).

Because TCMs often contain multiple components, we will first introduce the multivariate random effects model. Following the approach given by John (1963), a tolerance region of the multivariate random effects model can be derived. Denote by p vector y_{ijk} the measurement of the p active components from the kth sample of the jth batch from the ith region. The random p vectors A_i and B_{ij} stand for the random effects of the ith region and the jth batch nested in the ith region, respectively. Now, consider the following multivariate random effects model:

$$y_{ijk} = \mu + A_i + B_{ij} + \varepsilon_{ijk}, \ i = 1, \ \ldots, \ I; j = 1, \ \ldots, \ J; k = 1, \ \ldots, \ K, \qquad (8.13)$$

where the constant vector μ is the true mean of y_{ijk} and the random vectors A_i, B_{ij}, and ε_{ijk} are independent and multivariate normally distributed with mean zero and covariance matrices $\sum_A$, $\sum_B$, and $\sum_e$, respectively. That is,

$$A_i \sim N_p(0, \textstyle\sum_A), \ B_{ij} \sim N_p(0, \textstyle\sum_B), \ \varepsilon_{ijk} \sim N_p(0, \textstyle\sum_e).$$

According to model (Equation 8.13), it can be verified that y_{ijk} follows $N_p(0, \sum_A + \sum_B + \sum_e)$ distribution. Under model (Equation 8.13), John (1963) derived tolerance region based on a general multivariate normal distribution as follows. Let y be a $N_p(\mu, \sum_y)$ distributed random vector with unknown mean vector μ and covariance matrix $\sum_y$. On the basis of a random sample $y_1, \ldots, y_N$ from $N_p(\mu, \sum_y)$, a β-content, γ-confidence tolerance region $T(\beta, \gamma)$ of y is defined to be a subset of R^p such that

$$P_{y_1, y_2, \ldots, y_N} \{ P_y(y \in T(\beta, \gamma) | y_1, y_2, \ldots, y_N) \geq \beta \} = \gamma. \qquad (8.14)$$

Denote the sample mean and the sample covariance matrix as $\bar{y}$ and $\hat{\Sigma}_y$, respectively. Moreover, the sample covariance matrix follows a Wishart distribution with certain scale matrix Λ and degree of freedom v. On the basis of a random sample $y_1, \ldots, y_N$ from $N_p(\mu, \sum_y)$. John (1963) showed that the tolerance ellipsoid, with $100\gamma\%$ confidence level, includes at least $100\beta\%$ of the population, which satisfies the following inequality:

$$(y - \bar{y})' \hat{\Sigma}_y (y - \bar{y}) \leq \frac{\chi'^2_{1-\beta, p, p/(2N)}}{\chi^2_{\gamma, vp}/p},$$

where denotes the upper $(1 - \beta) \times 100\%$ point of the noncentral chi-square distribution with p degree of freedom p and noncentrality parameter $p/(2N)$,

Statistical Test for Consistency 185

and $\chi^2_{\gamma,vp}$ denotes the upper $100\gamma\%$ point of chi-squared distribution with vp degree of freedom. The tolerance region $T(\beta, \gamma)$ is then given by

$$T(\beta,\gamma) = \left\{ y : (y - \bar{y})' \hat{\Sigma}_y (y - \bar{y}) \le \frac{\chi'^2_{1-\beta,p,p/(2N)}}{\chi^2_{\gamma,vp}/p} \right\}. \tag{8.15}$$

The upper bound in Equation 8.15 is usually referred to as the tolerance factor of the tolerance region $T(\beta, \gamma)$. Under model Equation 8.13, to obtain the tolerance region $T(\beta, \gamma)$ as given in Equation 8.15, we need to calculate the degree of freedom of $\hat{\Sigma}_y$. Thus, on the basis of the random samples, y_{ijk}, $i = 1, \ldots, I; j = 1, \ldots, J; k = 1, \ldots, K$, the following averages and sum of squares can be obtained:

$$\bar{y} = \sum_{i=1}^{I} \sum_{j=1}^{J} \sum_{k=1}^{K} \frac{y_{ijk}}{IJK},$$

$$\bar{y}_{i\cdot} = \sum_{j=1}^{J} \sum_{k=1}^{K} \frac{y_{ijk}}{JK}, \text{ for } i = 1, \ldots, I,$$

$$\bar{y}_{ij} = \sum_{k=1}^{K} \frac{y_{ijk}}{K}, \text{ for } i = 1, \ldots, I \text{ and } j = 1, \ldots, J, \tag{8.16}$$

$$\text{SSA} = JK \sum_{i=1}^{I} (\bar{y}_{i\cdot} - \bar{y})(\bar{y}_{i\cdot} - \bar{y})',$$

$$\text{SSB} = K \sum \sum (\bar{y}_{ij\cdot} - \bar{y}_{i\cdot})(\bar{y}_{ij\cdot} - \bar{y}_{i\cdot})',$$

$$\text{SSE} = \sum_{i=1}^{I} \sum_{j=1}^{J} \sum_{k=1}^{K} (y_{ijk} - \bar{y}_{ij\cdot})(y_{ijk} - \bar{y}_{ij\cdot})'.$$

The mean squares and expected mean squares are then given by

$$S_A = \frac{\text{SSA}}{I-1}, S_B = \frac{\text{SSB}}{I(J-1)}, S_e = \frac{\text{SSE}}{IJ(K-1)},$$

$$\Lambda_A = E(S_A) = JK \Sigma_A + K \Sigma_B + \Sigma_e,$$

$$\Lambda_B = E(S_B) = K \Sigma_B + \Sigma_e,$$

$$\Lambda_e = E(S_e) = \Sigma_e.$$

TABLE 8.6

Multivariate Analysis of Variance Table of Model (Equation 8.13)

Source	Degree of Freedom	Sum of Squares	Mean Squares	Expected Mean Squares
Region	$I-1$	SSA	S_A	Λ_A
Batch	$I(J-1)$	SSB	S_B	Λ_B
Error	$IJ(K-1)$	SSE	S_e	Λ_e

The above results are summarized in Table 8.6. By Equation 8.16, it can be verified that S_A, S_B, and S_e follow Wishart distributions $W_p(\Lambda_A, I-1)$, $W_p(\Lambda_B, I(J-1))$, and $W_p(\Lambda_e, IJ(K-1))$, respectively, where $W_p\Lambda, k$ denotes the Wishart distribution with the scale matrix Λ and degrees of freedom k.

Under the normality assumption of model (Equation 8.13), the random vectors y and $\bar{y}$ follow $N_p(\mu, \Sigma_y)$ and $N_p(\mu, \Sigma_{\bar{y}})$ distributions, respectively, where $\Sigma_y = \Sigma_A + \Sigma_B + \Sigma_e$, and $\Sigma_{\bar{y}} = \dfrac{\Sigma_A}{I} + \dfrac{\Sigma_B}{IJ} + \dfrac{\Sigma_e}{IJK}$. Thus, the covariance matrix Σ_y can be expressed as follows:

$$\Sigma_y = \frac{1}{JK}\Lambda_A + \frac{J-1}{JK}\Lambda_B + \frac{K-1}{K}\Lambda_e = c_A\Lambda_A + c_B\Lambda_B + \frac{K-1}{K}\Lambda_e,$$

where

$$c_A S_A \sim W_p\left(\frac{c_A\Lambda_A}{I-1}, I-1\right),$$

$$c_B S_B \sim W_p\left(\frac{c_B\Lambda_B}{I(J-1)}, I(J-1)\right),$$

$$c_e S_e \sim W_p\left(\frac{c_e\Lambda_e}{IJ(K-1)}, IJ(K-1)\right).$$

Applying the modified multivariate Satterthwaite approximation for the distribution of a linear combination of independent Wishart matrices by Nel and van der Merwe (1986), the sample covariance matrix $\hat{\Sigma}_y$ follows $W_p(\Sigma_y/v, v)$ distribution with the degree of freedom:

$$v = \frac{tr[(\Sigma_y)^2] + [tr(\Sigma_y)]^2}{\displaystyle\sum_{i=1}^{I}\frac{1}{m_i}\{tr[(c_i\Lambda_i)^2] + [tr(c_i\Lambda_i)]^2\}}, \tag{8.17}$$

Statistical Test for Consistency

where $m_A = I - 1$, $m_B = I(J - 1)$, $m_e = IJ(K - 1)$. Note that when $\sum_A$, $\sum_B$, and $\sum_e$ are unknown, the unknown degree of freedom v can be estimated simply by replacing Λ_i with S_i. However, such an estimated degree of freedom is not invariant under nonsingular transformation. As an alternative, Krishnamoorthy and Yu (2004) suggested considering the Wishart approximation to the distribution of $\sum_y^{-1/2} \sum_{sy} \sum_y^{-1/2}$. That is, replacing $\sum_i$ with $\sum_y^{-1/2} \sum_y \sum_y^{-1/2}$. As a result, the resulting degree of freedom becomes

$$\tilde{v} = \frac{p + p^2}{\sum_{i=1}^{I} \frac{1}{m_i} \left\{ tr\left[\left(c_i S_i \hat{\Sigma}_i^{-1} \right)^2 \right] + \left[tr\left(c_i S_i \hat{\Sigma}_i^{-1} \right) \right]^2 \right\}}. \tag{8.18}$$

8.4.2 An Example

To illustrate the tolerance region approach proposed by Lai and Hsiao (2013), consider the synthetic data from Lu et al. (2007). The TCM intended for treating patients with rheumatoid arthritis contains two active components, namely, extract A and B. Each of these two active components has been used as a herbal remedy since ancient China. We are interested in testing the consistency of the raw materials, based on the two active components, from

TABLE 8.7

Tolerance Factor Defined in Equation 8.15 with $\tilde{v} = 2.970581$ and $\tilde{v} = 3.127606$ Corresponding to Specific Content Proportion β and Confidence Level γ

	$\gamma = 0.8$	$\gamma = 0.85$	$\gamma = 0.9$	$\gamma = 0.95$
$\tilde{v} = 2.970581$ (Krishnamoorthy and Yu 2004)				
$\beta = 0.8$	2.123451	2.451901	2.964166	4.003442
$\beta = 0.85$	2.497194	2.883454	3.485881	4.708076
$\beta = 0.9$	3.026625	3.494776	4.224924	5.706237
$\beta = 0.95$	3.941354	4.550993	5.501812	7.460819
$\tilde{v} = 3.127606$ (Nel and van der Merwe 1986)				
$\beta = 0.8$	1.971383	2.265580	2.721244	3.635920
$\beta = 0.85$	2.318361	2.664338	3.200203	4.285868
$\beta = 0.9$	2.809877	3.229206	3.878679	5.182396
$\beta = 0.95$	3.659099	4.205161	5.050992	6.748659

Source: Lai, Y.H. and Hsiao, C.F., Using a tolerance region approach as a statistical quality control process for traditional Chinese medicine. The 3rd International Conference on Applied Mathematics and Pharmaceutical Sciences, April 29–30, 2013, Singapore, pp. 346–349, 2013.

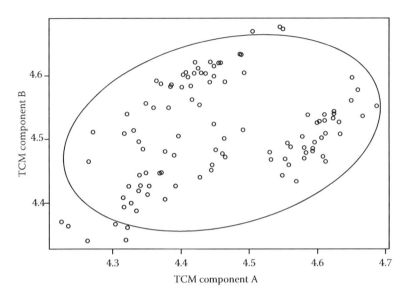

FIGURE 8.1
Tolerance region of TCM data with content proportion $\beta = 0.8$, confidence level $\gamma = 0.9$, and the degree of freedom $\tilde{v} = 2.970581$.

three different sites. Suppose that four batches from each site will be tested and nine samples from each batch will be randomly selected. Multivariate analysis of variance (MANOVA) table is given in Table 8.6. By Equation 8.18, the degree of freedom of $\hat{\Sigma}_y$ is given by $\tilde{v} = 2.970581$.

Thus, based on the values of $\tilde{v}$ estimated by the approaches described by Krishnamoorthy and Yu (2004) and Nel and van der Merwe (1986), the tolerance factors given in Equation 8.15 can be obtained. The results are summarized in Table 8.7 for various content proportion and confidence level. The ellipsoid of the tolerance region (Figure 8.1) indicates that the tolerance region of data with content proportion $\beta = 0.8$, confidence level $\gamma = 0.9$ and the degree of freedom $\tilde{v} = 2.970581$.

8.5 Concluding Remarks

In this chapter, statistical quality control for raw material inspection of a TCM with multiple components is discussed. Tse et al. (2006) proposed the idea is to construct a 95 percent confidence interval for a proposed consistency index under a sampling plan. If the constructed 95 percent confidence lower limit is greater than a pre-specified QC lower limit, then we claim that the raw materials has passed the QC and hence can be released for

Statistical Test for Consistency 189

further processing. Otherwise, the raw materials should be rejected. For a given component (the most active component if possible), a sampling plan is derived to ensure that there is a desired probability for establishment of consistency between sites when truly there is no difference in raw materials between sites. The results can be similarly extended to in-process materials and final products. In practice, if other individual components can be identified, the procedure discussed in the above can be applied in a similar fashion to establish limits for these individual components.

When there is more than one active ingredient in a particular TCM, under certain assumptions, the above proposed method can be modified and extended to test the following consistency index:

$$p = P\left(1 - \delta_k < \frac{U_k}{W_k} < \frac{1}{1 - \delta_k} ; k = 1, 2, \dots, K\right),$$

where $0 < \delta_k < 1$ and is the limit that allows for consistency for the kth components of U_k and W_k from the two sites. Suppose that the components are acting independently, then

$$p = P\left(1 - \delta_k < \frac{U_k}{W_k} < \frac{1}{1 - \delta_k} ; k = 1, 2, \dots, K\right)$$

$$= \prod_{k=1}^{K} P\left(1 - \delta_k < \frac{U_k}{W_k} < \frac{1}{1 - \delta_k}\right)$$

$$= \prod_{k=1}^{K} p_k$$

where p_k can be estimated using Equation 8.2 based on the observations obtained from the kth component. In particular,

$$\hat{p} = \prod_{k=1}^{K} \Phi\left(\frac{-\log(1 - \delta_k) - (\bar{X}_k - \bar{Y}_k)}{\sqrt{\hat{V}_{k,X} + \hat{V}_{k,Y}}}\right) - \Phi\left(\frac{\log(1 - \delta_k) - (\bar{X}_k - \bar{Y}_k)}{\sqrt{\hat{V}_{k,X} + \hat{V}_{k,Y}}}\right),$$

where $\bar{X}_k, \bar{Y}_k, \hat{V}_{k,X}, \hat{V}_{k,Y}$ are the sample means and sample variances based on the kth component of the TCM from the two sites respectively.

Alternatively, Lai and Hsiao (2013) proposed a flexible approach for assessing the consistency of raw materials and/or final products of TCM. They considered the use of the tolerance region of the multivariate random effects model to assess the quality of TCM. If the tolerance region is within the permitted range, then the product is considered passing the QC; otherwise, it should be rejected and further comparisons should be carried out. It should be noted, however that TCMs generally contain more than two active components. Lai and Hsiao's approach provides a quality control assessment to make sure that all the materials meet the requirement of quality simultaneously. This property provides the flexibility for assessing the consistency over high-dimensional data corresponding to multiple components from different locations.

9

Statistical Process for Quality Control/Assurance

9.1 Introduction

As indicated in Chapter 1, as more and more innovator drug products are going off patent protection, the search for new medicines for treating critical and/or life-threatening diseases has become the center of attention of many investigators from either research organizations or pharmaceutical companies. As a result, the Westernization of TCM has attracted much attention in pharmaceutical/clinical research and development. A TCM typically consists of multiple components or active ingredients (e.g., extracts from herbs). In practice, the pharmacological activities of these components are usually unknown. However, it is believed that each component is targeted for a specific organ. Chinese doctors believe that all organs within a healthy subject should reach global dynamic balance or harmony among organs (see, also Chow et al. 2006). Thus, a flexible dose consisting of several components with different relative proportions of these components is usually prescribed. On the basis of the fact that each component may come from different locations and/or be manufactured (or processed) at different sites, the consistency such as content uniformity and weight variation from location to location (or from site to site) is a concern for quality control and assurance of the resultant TCM especially when the TCM is used in humans.

For a given component such as the most active component among these components, Tse et al. (2006) proposed the concept of consistency to test for content uniformity across different study sites. The idea is to construct a 95 percent confidence interval for a proposed consistency index under a sampling plan. If the constructed 95 percent confidence lower limit is greater than a pre-specified quality control (QC) lower limit, then we claim that the TCM has passed the QC and hence can be released for human use. Otherwise, the TCM should be rejected. Tse et al. (2006) focused on the construction of a consistency index for TCM based on a single component, assuming that it is the most active component of the TCM. Following a similar idea, Lu et al. (2007) extended Tse et al.'s (2006) results to the case of two correlative components.

192   *Quantitative Methods for Traditional Chinese Medicine Development*

In Section 9.2, the consistency index for two correlative components of a TCM proposed by Lu et al. (2007) is described. Acceptance criteria and the corresponding testing procedure for the hypotheses on consistency index are discussed in Section 9.3. Also included in this section is the issue of sample size calculation. Results are developed for the determination of sample size required to ensure that there is a high probability of consistency between formulations from different places. In Section 9.4, an example concerning a TCM for treating patients with rheumatoid arthritis is presented to illustrate the proposed method. Some concluding remarks are given in Section 9.5.

9.2 Statistical Model

Let (U_1, U_2) and (W_1, W_2) be the characteristics of the two most active ingredients among the multiple components of a TCM from two different places, respectively. Suppose that $(X_1, X_2) = (\log U_1, \log U_2)$ follows a bivariate normal distribution with mean vector $\left(\mu_{X_1}, \mu_{X_2}\right)$ and covariance matrix Σ_1; similarly, $(Y_1, Y_2) = (\log W_1, \log W_2)$ follows a bivariate normal distribution with mean vector $\left(\mu_{Y_1}, \mu_{Y_2}\right)$ and covariance matrix Σ_2. In particular, denote

$$
\Sigma_1 = \begin{pmatrix} V_{X_1} & \rho_X \left(V_{X_1} V_{X_2} \right)^{\frac{1}{2}} \\ \rho_X \left(V_{X_1} V_{X_2} \right)^{\frac{1}{2}} & V_{X_2} \end{pmatrix}
$$

and

$$
\Sigma_2 = \begin{pmatrix} V_{Y_1} & \rho_Y \left(V_{Y_1} V_{Y_2} \right)^{\frac{1}{2}} \\ \rho_Y \left(V_{Y_1} V_{Y_2} \right)^{\frac{1}{2}} & V_{Y_2} \end{pmatrix}.
$$

Suppose that two random samples of observations $(X_{1i}, X_{2i}) = (\log U_{1i}, \log U_{2i})$, $i = 1, \ldots, n_X$ and $(Y_{1i}, Y_{2i}) = (\log W_{1i}, \log W_{2i})$, $i = 1, \ldots, n_Y$ are collected in an assay study. For the sake of simplicity, we assume $n_X = n_Y = n$. Following the idea of using $P(X < Y)$ to assess reliability in a strength-stress relationship (Enis and Geisser 1971), Tse et al. (2006) proposed an index to assess the consistency of raw materials and/or final products from two different sites when there is only one active component. Let p_1 and p_2 denote the consistency indices, as defined in Tse et al. (2006), of the two most active components of a TCM from two different sites. We propose to define the consistency index

Statistical Process for Quality Control/Assurance 193

of a TCM with two correlative components by $\min(p_1, p_2)$ and denote it by p, where

$$p_i = P\left(1 - \delta_i < \frac{U_i}{W_i} < \frac{1}{1 - \delta_i}\right), \ 0 < \delta_i < 1, \ i = 1, 2$$

and δ_i is a limit that allows for consistency. Therefore, the consistency index p is a function of the parameters

$$\theta = \left(\mu_{X_1}, \mu_{X_2}, \mu_{Y_1}, \mu_{Y_2}, V_{X_1}, V_{X_2}, V_{Y_1}, V_{Y_2}\right),$$

i.e., $p = h(\theta)$. By invariance principle, the maximum likelihood estimators (MLE) of p_1 and p_2 are given by

$$\hat{p}_i = \Phi\left(\frac{-\log(1 - \delta_i) - (\bar{X}_i - \bar{Y}_i)}{\sqrt{\hat{V}_{X_i} + \hat{V}_{Y_i}}}\right) - \Phi\left(\frac{\log(1 - \delta_i) - (\bar{X}_i - \bar{Y}_i)}{\sqrt{\hat{V}_{X_i} + \hat{V}_{Y_i}}}\right), \tag{9.1}$$

where $\Phi(z_0) = P(Z < z_0)$ with Z being a standard normal random variable,

$$\bar{X}_i = \frac{1}{n}\sum_{j=1}^{n} X_{ij}, \bar{Y}_i = \frac{1}{n}\sum_{j=1}^{n} Y_{ij}, \hat{V}_{X_i} = \frac{1}{n}\sum_{j=1}^{n}\left(X_{ij} - \bar{X}_i\right)^2 \text{ and } \hat{V}_{Y_i} = \frac{1}{n}\sum_{j=1}^{n}\left(Y_{ij} - \bar{Y}_i\right)^2,$$

$i = 1, 2$. Thus, the maximum likelihood estimator (MLE) of the proposed consistency index p is given by $\hat{p} = \min(\hat{p}_1, \hat{p}_2)$. Furthermore, it can be easily verified that the following asymptotic result holds.

Lemma 9.1

The $\left(\log \hat{p}_1, \log \hat{p}_2\right)$ is asymptotically distributed as $N\left(E\left(\log \hat{p}_1, \log \hat{p}_2\right), \frac{1}{s_1^2 s_2^2} A\right)$, where $A = (a_{ij})_{2\times2}$. The detailed expressions of a_{ij}, s_1, s_2 are given in expressions A1.1 through A1.5 in the Appendix. ∎

Proof

Details of the arguments can be found in Section 9.6.1. ∎

Lemma 9.2

$$\text{(A)} \quad E(\log \hat{p}) = \begin{cases} E(\log \hat{p}_2) + o(n^{-1}) & \text{if } \quad p_1 > p_2 \\ E(\log \hat{p}_1) + o(n^{-1}) & p_1 \leq p_2; \end{cases} \tag{9.2}$$

194   *Quantitative Methods for Traditional Chinese Medicine Development*

and

$$(B) \quad \text{Var}(\log \hat{p}) = \begin{cases} \text{Var}(\log \hat{p}_2) + o(n^{-1}) \\ \text{Var}(\log \hat{p}_1) + o(n^{-1}) \end{cases} \text{if} \quad \begin{matrix} p_1 > p_2 \\ p_1 \le p_2. \end{matrix} \tag{9.3}$$

∎

Proof

Details of the arguments can be found in Section 9.6.2.   ∎

Theorem 9.1

The $\log \hat{p}$ as given in Equation 9.1 is with mean $E(\log \hat{p})$ and variance $\text{Var}(\log \hat{p})$, where $E(\log \hat{p}) = \log p + B(p) + o(n^{-1})$ and $\text{Var}(\log \hat{p}) = C(p) + o(n^{-1})$. The detailed expressions of $B(p)$ and $C(p)$ are given in the Appendix. Furthermore,

$$\frac{\log \hat{p} - \log p - B(\hat{p})}{\sqrt{C(\hat{p})}} \to N(0, 1) \tag{9.4}$$

where $B(\hat{p})$ and $C(\hat{p})$ are estimates of $B(p)$ and $C(p)$ with the unknown population parameters $\theta = \left(\mu_{X_1}, \mu_{X_2}, \mu_{Y_1}, \mu_{Y_2}, V_{X_1}, V_{X_2}, V_{Y_1}, V_{Y_2} \right)$ estimated by their corresponding MLEs $\hat{\theta} = \left(\bar{X}_1, \bar{X}_2, \bar{Y}_1, \bar{Y}_2, \hat{V}_{X_1}, \hat{V}_{X_2}, \hat{V}_{Y_1}, \hat{V}_{Y_2} \right)$. ∎

Proof

The details of the derivation of $B(p)$ and $C(p)$ are given in the Appendix. In particular,

$$B(p) = \frac{1}{np_k} \frac{\partial^2 \hat{p}_k}{\partial V_{X_k}^2} \left(V_{X_k}^2 + V_{Y_k}^2 \right) - \frac{1}{2np_k^2} \left[\left(\frac{\partial \hat{p}_k}{\partial \mu_{X_k}} \right)^2 \left(V_{X_k} + V_{Y_k} \right) \right.$$

$$\left. + 2 \left(\frac{\partial \hat{p}_k}{\partial V_{X_k}} \right)^2 \left(V_{X_k}^2 + V_{Y_k}^2 \right) \right]$$

and $C(p) = \frac{1}{np_k^2} \left[\left(\frac{\partial \hat{p}_k}{\partial \mu_{X_k}} \right)^2 \left(V_{X_n} + V_{Y_n} \right) + 2 \left(\frac{\partial \hat{p}_k}{\partial V_{X_k}} \right)^2 \left(V_{X_k}^2 + V_{Y_k}^2 \right) \right]$; where the subscript k is defined by $k = j$ if $\hat{p} = \hat{p}_j, j = 1$ or 2.

Note that $B(p)$ converges to 0 as n tend to infinity. Thus, $\hat{p}$ is asymptotically unbiased. Since $\hat{\theta} = \left(\bar{X}_1, \bar{X}_2, \bar{Y}_1, \bar{Y}_2, \hat{V}_{X_1}, \hat{V}_{X_2}, \hat{V}_{Y_1}, \hat{V}_{Y_2} \right)$ is asymptotically multivariate normally distributed and $\hat{p}$ is a function of $\hat{\theta}$, it follows from Serfling (1980) that

$$\frac{\log \hat{p} - E(\log \hat{p})}{\sqrt{\text{var}(\log \hat{p})}} \to N(0, 1).$$

Using Slutsky's theorem, it can be shown that

$$\frac{\log \hat{p} - \log p - B(\hat{p})}{\sqrt{C(\hat{p})}}$$

is asymptotically normal since $B(\hat{p})$ and $C(\hat{p})$ are consistent estimates of $B(p)$ and $C(p)$, respectively.

On the basis of the results given in Theorem 9.1, for a given level $0 < \alpha < 1$, an approximate $(1 - \alpha) \times 100\%$ confidence interval for $\log p$, denoted by $(LL(\log \hat{p}), UL(\log \hat{p}))$, can be obtained based on Equation 9.4. In particular,

$$LL(\log \hat{p}) = \log \hat{p} - B(\hat{p}) - z_{\alpha/2} \sqrt{C(\hat{p})}, \tag{9.5}$$

and

$$UL(\log \hat{p}) = \log \hat{p} - B(\hat{p}) + z_{\alpha/2} \sqrt{C(\hat{p})}, \tag{9.6}$$

where $z_{\alpha/2}$ is the upper $\alpha/2$-percentile of the standard normal distribution. Consequently, an approximate $(1 - \alpha) \times 100\%$ confidence interval for p, denoted by $(LL(\hat{p}), UL(\hat{p}))$, is given as

$$\left(e^{LL(\log \hat{p})}, e^{UL(\log \hat{p})} \right). \tag{9.7}$$

■

9.3 Assessing Consistency for QC/QA

9.3.1 Sample Size Determination

The following criterion is proposed to assess the consistency of two formulations with two correlative active components manufactured from two different sites. If the probability that the lower limit $LL(\hat{p})$ of the constructed

$(1 - \alpha) \times 100\%$ confidence interval of p is greater than or equal to a pre-specified quality control lower limit, say, QC_L exceeds a pre-specified number β (say $\beta = 80\%$), then $U = (U_1, U_2)$ and $W = (W_1, W_2)$ are claimed to be consistent or similar. In other words, U and W are consistent or similar if $P(QC_L \leq LL(\hat{p})) \geq \beta$, where β is a pre-specified constant. Thus, for a given value of β, a practical question is to determine the required sample size n to ensure that there is at least with probability β that the lower confidence limit of p is greater than or equal to the QC lower limit. In other words, the sample size can be determined such that

$$P\{QC_L \leq LL(\hat{p})\} \geq \beta. \tag{9.8}$$

Using the results from Equations 9.4 and 9.5, Equation 9.8 becomes

$$P\left(\log QC_L \leq \log \hat{p} - B(\hat{p}) - z_{\alpha/2}\sqrt{C(\hat{p})}\right) \geq \beta. \tag{9.9}$$

Therefore,

$$P\left(\frac{\log QC_L - \log p}{\sqrt{C(\hat{p})}} + z_{\alpha/2} \leq \frac{\log \hat{p} - B(p) - \log p}{\sqrt{C(\hat{p})}}\right) \geq \beta. \tag{9.10}$$

Since, on the basis of Equation 9.1, $\dfrac{\log \hat{p} - B(p) - \log p}{\sqrt{C(\hat{p})}}$ is asymptotically distributed as a standard normal random variable, the required sample size can be obtained by solving the following inequality:

$$\frac{\log QC_L - \log p}{\sqrt{C(\hat{p})}} + z_{\alpha/2} \leq -z_{1-\beta}, \tag{9.11}$$

In particular, the required sample size n is given by

$$n \geq \frac{(z_{\alpha/2} + z_{1-\beta})^2}{p^2(\log QC_L - \log p)^2}\left[\left(\frac{\partial \hat{p}_k}{\partial \mu_{X_k}}\right)^2(V_{X_k} + V_{Y_k}) + 2\left(\frac{\partial \hat{p}_k}{\partial V_{X_k}}\right)^2(V_{X_k}^2 + V_{Y_k}^2)\right], \tag{9.12}$$

where the subscript k is defined by $k = j$ if $\hat{p} = \hat{p}_j, j = 1, 2$.

The above inequality (Equation 9.8) suggests that the required sample size n depends on the parameters α, β, V_{X_i}, V_{Y_i}, $\mu_{X_i} - \mu_{Y_i}$ and $\log QC_L - \log p_i$. From Equation 9.8, it can be seen that a larger sample size is required for

Statistical Process for Quality Control/Assurance 197

larger β and smaller α. Equivalently, in order to assure that the lower limit of a confidence interval is greater than QC_L with a higher confidence level, a larger sample size is required. Similarly, a relatively large sample size is required when $\log QC_L - \log p_i$ is small, i.e., when the consistency index is close to the quality control limit QC_L. However, the pattern of the required sample size on the other parameters such as V_{X_i}, V_{Y_i} and $\mu_{X_i} - \mu_{Y_i}$ is not easy to track as these parameters are involved in the partial derivatives and consistency indices.

Thus, a numerical study is conducted in order to gain more insight about the pattern of the required sample size for different combinations of parameters. For the sake of simplicity, define

$$S = \frac{1}{p_i^2}\left[\left(\frac{\partial \hat{p}_i}{\partial \mu_{X_i}}\right)^2 \left(V_{X_i} + V_{Y_i}\right) + 2\left(\frac{\partial \hat{p}_i}{\partial V_{X_i}}\right)^2 \left(V_{X_i}^2 + V_{Y_i}^2\right)\right]. \tag{9.13}$$

Then, for given values of α, β, and $\log p - \log QC_L$, the required sample size n is equal to $[(z_\alpha + z_{1-\beta})^2 S/(\log p - \log QC_L)^2]$, where $[x]$ denotes the smallest integer greater than or equal to x. In our study, $\delta_1 = 0.15$ and 0.20; $\delta_2 = 0.10$, 0.15 and 0.20; $\mu_{X_1} - \mu_{Y_1} = 0.03$ and 0.05; $\mu_{X_2} - \mu_{Y_2} = 0.00, 0.05$, and 0.10; V_{X_1} is chosen to be 0.02, $V_{Y_1} = 0.01, 0.03$, and 0.05; $V_{X_2} = 0.01$ and 0.03; $V_{Y_2} = 0.02$, 0.04, and 0.06. For each combination of the above parameter values, the corresponding value of S is listed in Table 9.1. The results suggest that S increases as $\mu_{X_1} - \mu_{Y_1}$, $\mu_{X_2} - \mu_{Y_2}$ increases or δ_1, δ_2 decreases.

On the basis of the results given in Table 9.1, the required sample size can be determined for a given combination of parameters. However, these results are based on asymptotic approximation. To assess the accuracy of these results, a simulation study is conducted to check whether the corresponding power based on simulated data is close to the nominal power level for the combinations considered. For each of the parameter combinations considered in Table 9.1, 5000 samples were simulated and the corresponding powers based on the simulated data are listed in Table 9.2. In particular, the simulated power is the proportion of the number of simulated samples with $LL(\log \hat{p}) > \log QC_L$. It can be noted that most of the cases listed in Table 9.2 are in general with simulated power close to the nominal power value 0.8. Further investigation reveals that for those cases with simulated power much smaller than 0.8 are those with p_1 being very close to p_2. In summary, the finite sample performance of the sample size determination is satisfactory in term of achieved the desired power level.

9.3.2 Hypotheses Testing

The idea of the consistency index can be further extended for the control of quality of TCM manufactured at different sites. In practice, to assess the

TABLE 9.1

Table of S Values

| | | | | V_{Y_2} | $V_{X_2} = 0.01$ | | | | | | | | | $V_{X_2} = 0.03$ | | | | | | | | |
					$V_{Y_1} = 0.01$			$V_{Y_1} = 0.03$			$V_{Y_1} = 0.05$			$V_{Y_1} = 0.01$			$V_{Y_1} = 0.03$			$V_{Y_1} = 0.05$		
					0.02	0.04	0.06	0.02	0.04	0.06	0.02	0.04	0.06	0.02	0.04	0.06	0.02	0.04	0.06	0.02	0.04	0.06
$\delta_1 = 0.15$	$\delta_2 = 0.10$	$\Delta_1 = 0.03$	$\Delta_2 = 0.00$		0.2164	0.2929	0.3395	0.2164	0.2929	0.3395	0.2164	0.2929	0.3395	0.2240	0.2294	0.2558	0.2240	0.2294	0.2558	0.2240	0.2294	0.2558
			0.05		0.2510	0.3095	0.3490	0.2510	0.3095	0.3490	0.2510	0.3095	0.3490	0.2468	0.2462	0.2679	0.2468	0.2462	0.2679	0.2468	0.2462	0.2679
			0.10		0.3687	0.3669	0.3823	0.3687	0.3669	0.3823	0.3687	0.3669	0.3823	0.3211	0.3000	0.3065	0.3211	0.3000	0.3065	0.3211	0.3000	0.3065
		$\Delta_1 = 0.05$	$\Delta_2 = 0.00$		0.2164	0.2929	0.3395	0.2164	0.2929	0.3395	0.2430	0.2929	0.3395	0.2240	0.2294	0.2558	0.2240	0.2294	0.2558	0.2240	0.2294	0.2558
			0.05		0.2510	0.3095	0.3490	0.2510	0.3095	0.3490	0.2510	0.3095	0.3490	0.2468	0.2462	0.2679	0.2468	0.2462	0.2679	0.2468	0.2462	0.2679
			0.10		0.3687	0.3669	0.3823	0.3687	0.3669	0.3823	0.3687	0.3669	0.3823	0.3211	0.3000	0.3065	0.3211	0.3000	0.3065	0.3211	0.3000	0.3065
	$\delta_2 = 0.15$	$\Delta_1 = 0.03$	$\Delta_2 = 0.00$		0.1621	0.2376	0.2927	0.1890	0.1890	0.2927	0.2342	0.2342	0.2342	0.1817	0.1977	0.2280	0.1890	0.1977	0.2280	0.2342	0.2342	0.2280
			0.05		0.1806	0.2535	0.3024	0.1890	0.2535	0.3024	0.2342	0.2342	0.3024	0.2021	0.2133	0.2395	0.2021	0.2133	0.2395	0.2342	0.2133	0.2395
			0.10		0.2735	0.3062	0.3351	0.1890	0.3062	0.3351	0.2342	0.2342	0.3351	0.2671	0.2624	0.2759	0.2671	0.2624	0.2759	0.2342	0.2624	0.2759
		$\Delta_1 = 0.05$	$\Delta_2 = 0.00$		0.1806	0.2376	0.2927	0.2021	0.2021	0.2927	0.2430	0.2430	0.2430	0.1817	0.1977	0.2280	0.2021	0.1977	0.2280	0.2430	0.2430	0.2280
			0.05		0.1806	0.2535	0.3024	0.2021	0.2535	0.3024	0.2430	0.2430	0.3024	0.2021	0.2133	0.2395	0.2021	0.2133	0.2395	0.2430	0.2133	0.2395
			0.10		0.2735	0.3062	0.3351	0.2021	0.3062	0.3351	0.2430	0.2430	0.3351	0.2671	0.2624	0.2759	0.2671	0.2624	0.2759	0.2430	0.2624	0.2759

(Continued)

TABLE 9.1 (CONTINUED)

Table of S Values

δ_1	δ_2	Δ_1	Δ_2 / V_{Y_2}	$V_{X_2}{=}0.01$; $V_{Y_1}{=}0.01$; 0.02	0.04	0.06	$V_{Y_1}{=}0.03$; 0.02	0.04	0.06	$V_{Y_1}{=}0.05$; 0.02	0.04	0.06	$V_{X_2}{=}0.03$; $V_{Y_1}{=}0.01$; 0.02	0.04	0.06	$V_{Y_1}{=}0.03$; 0.02	0.04	0.06	$V_{Y_1}{=}0.05$; 0.02	0.04	0.06
0.20	0.20	0.03	0.00	0.1621	0.1621	0.2324	0.1890	0.1890	0.1890	0.2342	0.2342	0.2342	0.1621	0.1570	0.1908	0.1890	0.1890	0.1890	0.2342	0.2342	0.2342
0.20	0.20	0.03	0.05	0.1621	0.1621	0.2421	0.1890	0.1890	0.1890	0.2342	0.2342	0.2342	0.1621	0.1707	0.2014	0.1890	0.1890	0.1890	0.2342	0.2342	0.2342
0.20	0.20	0.03	0.10	0.1621	0.2311	0.2732	0.1890	0.1890	0.1890	0.2342	0.2342	0.2342	0.2006	0.2132	0.2344	0.1890	0.1890	0.1890	0.2342	0.2342	0.2342
0.20	0.20	0.05	0.00	0.1806	0.1806	0.2324	0.2021	0.2021	0.2021	0.2430	0.2430	0.2430	0.1806	0.1570	0.1908	0.2021	0.2021	0.2021	0.2430	0.2430	0.2430
0.20	0.20	0.05	0.05	0.1806	0.1806	0.2421	0.2021	0.2021	0.2021	0.2430	0.2430	0.2430	0.1806	0.1707	0.2014	0.2021	0.2021	0.2021	0.2430	0.2430	0.2430
0.20	0.20	0.05	0.10	0.1806	0.1806	0.2732	0.2021	0.2021	0.2021	0.2430	0.2430	0.2430	0.1806	0.2132	0.2344	0.2021	0.2021	0.2021	0.2430	0.2430	0.2430
0.20	0.10	0.03	0.00	0.2164	0.2929	0.3395	0.2164	0.2929	0.3395	0.2164	0.2929	0.3395	0.2240	0.2294	0.2558	0.2240	0.2294	0.2558	0.2240	0.2294	0.2558
0.20	0.10	0.03	0.05	0.2510	0.3095	0.3490	0.2510	0.3095	0.3490	0.2510	0.3095	0.3490	0.2468	0.2462	0.2679	0.2468	0.2462	0.2679	0.2468	0.2462	0.2679
0.20	0.10	0.03	0.10	0.3687	0.3669	0.3823	0.3687	0.3669	0.3823	0.3687	0.3669	0.3823	0.3211	0.3000	0.3065	0.3211	0.3000	0.3065	0.3211	0.3000	0.3065
0.20	0.10	0.05	0.00	0.2164	0.2929	0.3395	0.2164	0.2929	0.3395	0.2164	0.2929	0.3395	0.2240	0.2294	0.2558	0.2240	0.2294	0.2558	0.2240	0.2294	0.2558
0.20	0.10	0.05	0.05	0.2510	0.3095	0.3490	0.2510	0.3095	0.3490	0.2510	0.3095	0.3490	0.2468	0.2462	0.2679	0.2468	0.2462	0.2679	0.2468	0.2462	0.2679
0.20	0.10	0.05	0.10	0.3687	0.3669	0.3823	0.3687	0.3669	0.3823	0.3687	0.3669	0.3823	0.3211	0.3000	0.3065	0.3211	0.3000	0.3065	0.3211	0.3000	0.3065
0.20	0.15	0.03	0.00	0.1519	0.2376	0.2927	0.1866	0.2376	0.2927	0.1866	0.2376	0.2927	0.1817	0.1977	0.2280	0.1817	0.1977	0.2280	0.1817	0.1977	0.2280
0.20	0.15	0.03	0.05	0.1806	0.2535	0.3024	0.1866	0.2535	0.3024	0.1866	0.2535	0.3024	0.2021	0.2133	0.2395	0.2021	0.2133	0.2395	0.2021	0.2133	0.2395
0.20	0.15	0.03	0.10	0.2735	0.3062	0.3351	0.2735	0.3062	0.3351	0.2735	0.3062	0.3351	0.2671	0.2624	0.2759	0.2671	0.2624	0.2759	0.2671	0.2624	0.2759

(Continued)

TABLE 9.1 (CONTINUED)

Table of S Values

			$V_{X_2} = 0.01$									$V_{X_2} = 0.03$								
			$V_{Y_1} = 0.01$			$V_{Y_1} = 0.03$			$V_{Y_1} = 0.05$			$V_{Y_1} = 0.01$			$V_{Y_1} = 0.03$			$V_{Y_1} = 0.05$		
		V_{Y_2}	0.02	0.04	0.06	0.02	0.04	0.06	0.02	0.04	0.06	0.02	0.04	0.06	0.02	0.04	0.06	0.02	0.04	0.06
$\Delta_1 = 0.05$	$\Delta_2 = 0.00$		0.1519	0.2376	0.2927	0.1519	0.2376	0.2927	0.1945	0.2376	0.2927	0.1817	0.1977	0.2280	0.1817	0.1977	0.2280	0.1817	0.1977	0.2280
		0.05	0.1806	0.2535	0.3024	0.1806	0.2535	0.3024	0.1945	0.2535	0.3024	0.2021	0.2133	0.2395	0.2021	0.2133	0.2395	0.2021	0.2133	0.2395
		0.10	0.2735	0.3062	0.3351	0.2735	0.3062	0.3351	0.2735	0.3062	0.3351	0.2671	0.2624	0.2759	0.2671	0.2624	0.2759	0.2671	0.2624	0.2759
$\delta_2 = 0.20$ $\Delta_1 = 0.03$	$\Delta_2 = 0.00$		0.0941	0.1714	0.2324	0.1371	0.1371	0.2324	0.1866	0.1866	0.1866	0.1310	0.1570	0.1908	0.1371	0.1570	0.1908	0.1866	0.1866	0.1908
		0.05	0.1073	0.1857	0.2421	0.1371	0.1857	0.2421	0.1866	0.1866	0.2421	0.1479	0.1707	0.2014	0.1479	0.1707	0.2014	0.1866	0.1707	0.2014
		0.10	0.1719	0.2311	0.2732	0.1371	0.2311	0.2732	0.1866	0.1866	0.2732	0.2006	0.2132	0.2344	0.2006	0.2132	0.2344	0.1866	0.2132	0.2344
$\Delta_1 = 0.05$	$\Delta_2 = 0.00$		0.1073	0.1714	0.2324	0.1479	0.1479	0.2324	0.1945	0.1945	0.1945	0.1310	0.1570	0.1908	0.1479	0.1570	0.1908	0.1945	0.1945	0.1908
		0.05	0.1073	0.1857	0.2421	0.1479	0.1857	0.2421	0.1945	0.1945	0.2421	0.1479	0.1707	0.2014	0.1479	0.1707	0.2014	0.1945	0.1707	0.2014
		0.10	0.1719	0.2311	0.2732	0.1479	0.2311	0.2732	0.1945	0.1945	0.2732	0.2006	0.2132	0.2344	0.2006	0.2132	0.2344	0.1945	0.2132	0.2344

Note: $V_{X_1} = 0.02$; $\Delta_1 = \mu_{X_1} - \mu_{Y_1}$, $\Delta_2 = \mu_{X_2} - \mu_{Y_2}$.

TABLE 9.2

Simulated Power Based on 5000 Samples

| | | | $V_{X_2} = 0.01$ | | | | | | | | | | $V_{X_2} = 0.03$ | | | | | | | | |
| | | | $V_{Y_1} = 0.01$ | | | $V_{Y_1} = 0.03$ | | | $V_{Y_1} = 0.05$ | | | $V_{Y_1} = 0.01$ | | | $V_{Y_1} = 0.03$ | | | $V_{Y_1} = 0.05$ | | |
δ_2	Δ_1	V_{Y_2}	0.02	0.04	0.06	0.02	0.04	0.06	0.02	0.04	0.06	0.02	0.04	0.06	0.02	0.04	0.06	0.02	0.04	0.06
$\delta_1 = 0.15$																				
0.10	0.03	$\Delta_2 =$ 0.00	0.7912	0.7922	0.7980	0.7862	0.7902	0.8014	0.6472	0.7862	0.7976	0.7860	0.7844	0.7932	0.7996	0.7940	0.7882	0.7988	0.7962	0.7900
		0.05	0.7790	0.7832	0.7916	0.7900	0.7984	0.7882	0.7890	0.7936	0.7850	0.7896	0.7952	0.7920	0.7896	0.7858	0.7890	0.7768	0.7886	0.7998
		0.10	0.7836	0.7900	0.7922	0.7890	0.7998	0.7906	0.7820	0.8014	0.7916	0.7788	0.7880	0.8020	0.7826	0.7830	0.7954	0.7902	0.7850	0.7886
	0.05	$\Delta_2 =$ 0.00	0.7872	0.7886	0.7866	0.7846	0.7862	0.7988	0.7060	0.7902	0.7926	0.8008	0.7830	0.7966	0.7958	0.7912	0.7802	0.7868	0.8068	0.7922
		0.05	0.7888	0.7776	0.7930	0.7868	0.7980	0.8030	0.7494	0.7874	0.7844	0.7984	0.7936	0.7806	0.7888	0.7882	0.7932	0.8038	0.7922	0.7800
		0.10	0.7926	0.7870	0.7872	0.7748	0.7934	0.7828	0.7894	0.7918	0.7874	0.7924	0.7934	0.7912	0.7868	0.7946	0.7840	0.7936	0.7906	0.7836
0.15	0.03	$\Delta_2 =$ 0.00	0.6914	0.7860	0.7886	0.7932	0.6218	0.7982	0.7748	0.7884	0.6134	0.7912	0.7988	0.7906	0.6952	0.7870	0.7930	0.7956	0.7112	0.7848
		0.05	0.7398	0.7838	0.7896	0.7874	0.7560	0.7994	0.7874	0.7942	0.7534	0.7924	0.7904	0.7876	0.7042	0.7768	0.7802	0.7858	0.6734	0.7856
		0.10	0.7738	0.7856	0.7934	0.7796	0.7846	0.7910	0.7990	0.7778	0.7922	0.7746	0.7888	0.7776	0.7826	0.7950	0.7790	0.7698	0.7866	0.7858
	0.05	$\Delta_2 =$ 0.00	0.7570	0.7910	0.7918	0.7860	0.7014	0.7916	0.7982	0.7880	0.6542	0.7878	0.7930	0.7890	0.7468	0.7862	0.7902	0.7854	0.7416	0.7936
		0.05	0.6216	0.7944	0.7958	0.7836	0.7162	0.7934	0.7918	0.7798	0.6970	0.7774	0.7882	0.7884	0.6438	0.7814	0.7780	0.7802	0.6128	0.7832
		0.10	0.7854	0.7820	0.7782	0.7840	0.7882	0.7926	0.7832	0.7874	0.7920	0.7884	0.7836	0.7942	0.7918	0.7866	0.7874	0.7912	0.7896	0.7890

(Continued)

TABLE 9.2 (CONTINUED)

Simulated Power Based on 5000 Samples

δ_2	Δ_1	Δ_2	V_{y_2}	$V_{x_2}=0.01$									$V_{x_2}=0.03$								
				$V_{y_1}=0.01$			$V_{y_1}=0.03$			$V_{y_1}=0.05$			$V_{y_1}=0.01$			$V_{y_1}=0.03$			$V_{y_1}=0.05$		
				0.02	0.04	0.06	0.02	0.04	0.06	0.02	0.04	0.06	0.02	0.04	0.06	0.02	0.04	0.06	0.02	0.04	0.06
0.20	0.03	$\Delta_2=$	0.00	0.7780	0.7664	0.7856	0.7852	0.7926	0.7942	0.7874	0.7898	0.7942	0.7732	0.7840	0.7854	0.7940	0.7896	0.7468	0.7836	0.7860	0.7854
			0.05	0.7750	0.7358	0.7878	0.7858	0.7888	0.7814	0.7844	0.7894	0.7860	0.7638	0.7876	0.7850	0.7792	0.7948	0.6968	0.7816	0.7834	0.7942
			0.10	0.7850	0.7568	0.7906	0.7810	0.7912	0.7670	0.7920	0.7844	0.7878	0.7484	0.7786	0.7888	0.7878	0.7818	0.7598	0.7840	0.7840	0.7878
	0.05	$\Delta_2=$	0.00	0.7844	0.7718	0.7750	0.7952	0.7854	0.7840	0.7976	0.7804	0.7804	0.7722	0.7596	0.7836	0.7894	0.7930	0.7708	0.7846	0.7864	0.7878
			0.05	0.7780	0.7658	0.7802	0.7766	0.7804	0.7792	0.7858	0.7836	0.7858	0.7804	0.7772	0.7862	0.7804	0.7934	0.7526	0.7754	0.7810	0.7942
			0.10	0.7746	0.5896	0.7952	0.7896	0.7830	0.7852	0.7868	0.7836	0.7776	0.6298	0.7754	0.7860	0.7788	0.7878	0.7048	0.7824	0.7826	0.7946

$\delta_1 = 0.20$

δ_2	Δ_1	Δ_2	V_{y_2}	$V_{x_2}=0.01$									$V_{x_2}=0.03$								
				$V_{y_1}=0.01$			$V_{y_1}=0.03$			$V_{y_1}=0.05$			$V_{y_1}=0.01$			$V_{y_1}=0.03$			$V_{y_1}=0.05$		
				0.02	0.04	0.06	0.02	0.04	0.06	0.02	0.04	0.06	0.02	0.04	0.06	0.02	0.04	0.06	0.02	0.04	0.06
0.10	0.03	$\Delta_2=$	0.00	0.7860	0.7868	0.7942	0.7774	0.7924	0.7924	0.7896	0.7882	0.7884	0.7848	0.7896	0.8024	0.7908	0.7924	0.7886	0.7896	0.7978	0.7898
			0.05	0.7892	0.7878	0.7940	0.7854	0.7872	0.8086	0.7814	0.7798	0.7830	0.7906	0.7962	0.7824	0.7882	0.7834	0.7880	0.7870	0.7928	0.7942
			0.10	0.7830	0.7826	0.7954	0.7880	0.7916	0.7870	0.7822	0.7848	0.7930	0.7854	0.7908	0.7874	0.7910	0.7758	0.7846	0.7828	0.7830	0.7974
	0.05	$\Delta_2=$	0.00	0.7904	0.7972	0.8018	0.7708	0.7930	0.8006	0.7816	0.7866	0.7960	0.7886	0.7862	0.7978	0.7984	0.7944	0.7938	0.7978	0.7842	0.7976
			0.05	0.7942	0.7908	0.7920	0.7774	0.7886	0.7946	0.7914	0.7932	0.7956	0.7846	0.7920	0.7974	0.7894	0.7892	0.7946	0.7948	0.7884	0.8002
			0.10	0.7876	0.7808	0.7912	0.7788	0.7820	0.7910	0.7840	0.7890	0.7994	0.7788	0.7836	0.7932	0.7850	0.7848	0.7834	0.7870	0.7874	0.7806

(Continued)

TABLE 9.2 (CONTINUED)

Simulated Power Based on 5000 Samples

| δ_2 | Δ_1 | V_{Y_2} | $V_{X_2} = 0.01$ | | | | | | | | | $V_{X_2} = 0.03$ | | | | | | | | |
| | | | $V_{Y_1} = 0.01$ | | | $V_{Y_1} = 0.03$ | | | $V_{Y_1} = 0.05$ | | | $V_{Y_1} = 0.01$ | | | $V_{Y_1} = 0.03$ | | | $V_{Y_1} = 0.05$ | | |
			0.02	0.04	0.06	0.02	0.04	0.06	0.02	0.04	0.06	0.02	0.04	0.06	0.02	0.04	0.06	0.02	0.04	0.06
0.15	0.03	$\Delta_2 =$ 0.00	0.7822	0.7846	0.8008	0.7698	0.7858	0.7970	0.7880	0.7864	0.7794	0.7858	0.7812	0.7902	0.7872	0.7816	0.7862	0.7780	0.7848	0.7822
		0.05	0.7808	0.7856	0.7852	0.7852	0.7946	0.7952	0.7874	0.7832	0.7840	0.7868	0.7844	0.7880	0.7866	0.7916	0.7796	0.7848	0.7916	0.7868
		0.10	0.7918	0.7940	0.7790	0.7906	0.7916	0.7928	0.7806	0.7850	0.7930	0.7752	0.7804	0.7866	0.7772	0.7836	0.7870	0.7980	0.7846	0.7834
	0.05	$\Delta_2 =$ 0.00	0.7822	0.7856	0.7812	0.7408	0.7818	0.7976	0.7778	0.7934	0.8028	0.7936	0.7862	0.7874	0.7846	0.7962	0.7898	0.7870	0.7810	0.7836
		0.05	0.7692	0.7882	0.8002	0.7826	0.7780	0.7858	0.7738	0.7882	0.7968	0.7844	0.7942	0.7992	0.7784	0.7978	0.7950	0.7852	0.7744	0.7880
		0.10	0.7816	0.7826	0.7946	0.7762	0.7906	0.7912	0.7658	0.7772	0.7944	0.7812	0.7854	0.7828	0.7844	0.7914	0.7984	0.7922	0.7818	0.7890
0.20	0.03	$\Delta_2 =$ 0.00	0.6590	0.7824	0.7826	0.7812	0.6106	0.7768	0.7758	0.7970	0.6080	0.7714	0.7884	0.7836	0.6676	0.7842	0.7708	0.7838	0.7062	0.7774
		0.05	0.7020	0.7846	0.7758	0.7778	0.7442	0.7952	0.7832	0.7782	0.7514	0.7700	0.7778	0.7922	0.6966	0.7734	0.7888	0.7922	0.6668	0.7860
		0.10	0.7704	0.7802	0.7920	0.7700	0.7878	0.7892	0.7826	0.7692	0.7850	0.7718	0.7742	0.7828	0.7720	0.7706	0.7806	0.7712	0.7814	0.7832
	0.05	$\Delta_2 =$ 0.00	0.7364	0.7730	0.7896	0.7762	0.6740	0.7870	0.7762	0.7842	0.6530	0.7696	0.7796	0.7894	0.7412	0.7932	0.7828	0.7846	0.7378	0.7922
		0.05	0.6216	0.7838	0.7886	0.7794	0.6814	0.7786	0.7728	0.7896	0.7102	0.7710	0.7776	0.7834	0.6320	0.7838	0.7820	0.7772	0.6154	0.7896
		0.10	0.7626	0.7806	0.7858	0.7760	0.7860	0.7844	0.7800	0.7770	0.7874	0.7726	0.7808	0.7824	0.7790	0.7734	0.7834	0.7680	0.7748	0.7876

204   *Quantitative Methods for Traditional Chinese Medicine Development*

uniformity of a TCM manufactured at different sites, a minimum baseline value for the consistency index, say p_0, can be set up to monitor the consistency of the products from different sites. Thus, in order to test whether the performance of a TCM manufactured at two different sites is consistent, it can be done by considering the following hypotheses

$$H_0: p \le p_0 \text{ versus } H_1: p > p_0,$$

where p_0 is a limit of consistency, $0 < p_0 < 1$. If the null hypothesis H_0 is rejected, then the TCM is considered to be consistent.

From Theorem 9.1, if $p = p_0$, we have

$$\frac{\log \hat{p} - \log p_0 - B(p_0)}{\sqrt{C(p_0)}} \to N(0,1). \tag{9.14}$$

where $B(p_0)$ and $C(p_0)$ are the values of $B(p)$ and $C(p)$ evaluated at $p = p_0$. Therefore, the hypothesis H_0 is rejected at a level of significance α if

$$\frac{\log \hat{p} - \log p_0 - B(p_0)}{\sqrt{C(p_0)}} > z_\alpha. \tag{9.15}$$

In other words, the null hypothesis H_0 is rejected if $\log \hat{p} > \log p_0 + B(p_0) + z_\alpha \sqrt{C(p_0)}$. For illustration purpose, a numerical study is conducted to find critical values of the above test for various combinations of the parameters. In our study, $\alpha = 0.1$, $p_0 = 0.50, 0.65,$ and 0.80; $\delta_1 = 0.20$; $\delta_2 = 0.15$ and 0.20; $\mu_{X_1} - \mu_{Y_1}$ is chosen to be 0.05; $\mu_{X_2} - \mu_{Y_2} = 0.00, 0.05,$ and 0.10, V_{X_1} is chosen to be 0.02, $V_{Y_1} = 0.01$ and 0.03; $V_{X_2} = 0.01$; $V_{Y_2} = 0.02, 0.04,$ and 0.06. For each combination of those parameters values, the critical value of the test is listed in Table 9.3. The results suggest that the difference between the critical value and p_0 is smaller for smaller V_{Y_1} and V_{Y_2}, larger δ_2, larger n or smaller $\mu_{X_2} - \mu_{Y_2}$.

9.4 An Example

To illustrate the proposed ideas for testing consistency, consider a test for raw materials of a traditional Chinese medicine (TCM), which is intended for treating patients with rheumatoid arthritis. The TCM contains two active components, namely, A extract and B extract. The botanical substance for medical use is harvested in summer or autumn when foliage is growing luxuriantly. The TCM contains a multiherb substance, which is prepared by combining individually processed botanical substances. Each of these two

TABLE 9.3

Critical Values of the Proposed Test for Consistency Index p_0

p_0	δ_2	V_{Y_1}	V_{Y_2}	$\Delta = 0.00$			$\Delta = 0.05$			$\Delta = 0.10$		
				$n = 15$	$n = 30$	$n = 50$	$n = 15$	$n = 30$	$n = 50$	$n = 15$	$n = 30$	$n = 50$
0.50	0.15	0.01	0.02	0.5742	0.5503	0.5381	0.5795	0.5542	0.5412	0.5940	0.5649	0.5496
			0.04	0.5967	0.5648	0.5487	0.5984	0.5662	0.5499	0.6040	0.5708	0.5537
			0.06	0.6097	0.5730	0.5547	0.6102	0.5736	0.5553	0.6122	0.5756	0.5571
		0.03	0.02	0.5742	0.5503	0.5381	0.5795	0.5542	0.5412	0.5940	0.5649	0.5496
			0.04	0.5967	0.5648	0.5487	0.5984	0.5662	0.5499	0.6040	0.5708	0.5537
			0.06	0.6097	0.5730	0.5547	0.6102	0.5736	0.5553	0.6122	0.5756	0.5571
	0.20	0.01	0.02	0.5591	0.5407	0.5311	0.5591	0.5407	0.5311	0.5738	0.5511	0.5391
			0.04	0.5794	0.5537	0.5406	0.5818	0.5555	0.5421	0.5890	0.5608	0.5463
			0.06	0.5952	0.5639	0.5481	0.5963	0.5648	0.5488	0.5997	0.5676	0.5511
		0.03	0.02	0.5717	0.5489	0.5372	0.5717	0.5489	0.5372	0.5717	0.5489	0.5372
			0.04	0.5717	0.5489	0.5372	0.5818	0.5555	0.5421	0.5890	0.5608	0.5463
			0.06	0.5952	0.5639	0.5481	0.5963	0.5648	0.5488	0.5997	0.5676	0.5511
0.65	0.15	0.01										
			0.02	0.7465	0.7154	0.6996	0.7534	0.7204	0.7035	0.7722	0.7343	0.7145
			0.04	0.7757	0.7342	0.7133	0.7780	0.7361	0.7149	0.7852	0.7420	0.7198
			0.06	0.7926	0.7449	0.7211	0.7932	0.7456	0.7218	0.7958	0.7483	0.7243
		0.03	0.02	0.7465	0.7154	0.6996	0.7534	0.7204	0.7035	0.7722	0.7343	0.7145
			0.04	0.7757	0.7342	0.7133	0.7780	0.7361	0.7149	0.7852	0.7420	0.7198
			0.06	0.7926	0.7449	0.7211	0.7932	0.7456	0.7218	0.7958	0.7483	0.7243
	0.20	0.01	0.02	0.7268	0.7029	0.6904	0.7268	0.7029	0.6904	0.7459	0.7164	0.7008
			0.04	0.7532	0.7198	0.7028	0.7564	0.7222	0.7047	0.7656	0.7291	0.7102
			0.06	0.7738	0.7330	0.7125	0.7752	0.7342	0.7135	0.7796	0.7378	0.7165

(Continued)

TABLE 9.3 (CONTINUED)

Critical Values of the Proposed Test for Consistency Index p_0

p_0	δ_2	V_{Y_1}	V_{Y_2}	$\Delta = 0.00$			$\Delta = 0.05$			$\Delta = 0.10$		
				$n = 15$	$n = 30$	$n = 50$	$n = 15$	$n = 30$	$n = 50$	$n = 15$	$n = 30$	$n = 50$
		0.03	0.02	0.7432	0.7136	0.6983	0.7432	0.7136	0.6983	0.7432	0.7136	0.6983
			0.04	0.7432	0.7136	0.6983	0.7564	0.7222	0.7047	0.7656	0.7291	0.7102
			0.06	0.7738	0.7330	0.7125	0.7752	0.7342	0.7135	0.7796	0.7378	0.7165
0.80	0.15	0.01	0.02	0.9188	0.8805	0.8610	0.9272	0.8867	0.8658	0.9505	0.9038	0.8793
			0.04	0.9547	0.9036	0.8780	0.9575	0.9059	0.8799	0.9664	0.9133	0.8859
			0.06	0.9755	0.9168	0.8875	0.9763	0.9177	0.8884	0.9795	0.9210	0.8914
		0.03	0.02	0.9188	0.8805	0.8610	0.9272	0.8867	0.8658	0.9505	0.9038	0.8793
			0.04	0.9547	0.9036	0.8780	0.9575	0.9059	0.8799	0.9664	0.9133	0.8859
			0.06	0.9755	0.9168	0.8875	0.9763	0.9177	0.8884	0.9795	0.9210	0.8914
	0.20	0.01	0.02	0.8945	0.8651	0.8498	0.8945	0.8651	0.8498	0.9181	0.8817	0.8626
			0.04	0.9270	0.8860	0.8650	0.9309	0.8889	0.8673	0.9423	0.8973	0.8740
			0.06	0.9524	0.9022	0.8769	0.9541	0.9036	0.8781	0.9595	0.9081	0.8818
		0.03	0.02	0.9147	0.8783	0.8595	0.9147	0.8783	0.8595	0.9147	0.8783	0.8595
			0.04	0.9147	0.8783	0.8595	0.9309	0.8889	0.8673	0.9423	0.8973	0.8740
			0.06	0.9524	0.9022	0.8769	0.9541	0.9036	0.8781	0.9595	0.9081	0.8818

Note: $V_{X_1} = 0.02$, $V_{X_2} = 0.01$, $\mu_{X_1} - \mu_{Y_1} = 0.05$, $\delta_1 = 0.20$; $\Delta = \mu_{X_2} - \mu_{Y_2}$.

Statistical Process for Quality Control/Assurance 207

active components A and B has been used as a herbal remedy since ancient China.

Suppose the sponsor of the TCM is interested in testing the consistency of the raw materials, based on the two active components, from three different sites. Suppose that four batches from each site will be tested and nine samples from each batch will be randomly selected. Therefore, in each site, there are a total of 36 samples selected for testing. Suppose that δ_1 and δ_2 are equal to 0.2. Furthermore, the acceptance criterion for testing consistency is chosen such that the probability of the lower limit $LL(\hat{p})$ of the 95 percent confidence interval of p is greater than the quality control lower limit QC_L has to be at least 0.8; i.e., $\beta = 0.8$.

To assess the consistency of the active component from the three sites, test results (in percent of label claim) of the selected samples are log transformed. The corresponding summary statistics are listed in Table 9.4. The results of the comparison among the three sites are given in Table 9.5. Thus, in this example, it is very likely that the components from sites 1 and 3 are inconsistent because the consistency index is only 0.464. For illustrative purposes, suppose $QC_L = 0.65$. In order to ensure that there is a 0.80 probability of claiming consistency between raw materials from sites 1 and 2, the sample size is determined as

$$n = \frac{(z_{0.20} + z_{0.975})^2 nC(\hat{p})}{(\log QC_L - \log \hat{p})^2} = \frac{2.8016^2 \times 0.1129}{0.2493^2} \approx 15.$$

TABLE 9.4

Summary Statistics of Three Sites

Site	Sample Mean		Sample Standard Deviation	
	A	B	A	B
1	4.6002	4.5001	0.0365	0.0367
2	4.4408	4.6103	0.0546	0.0423
3	4.3703	4.4408	0.0671	0.0542

TABLE 9.5

Results of Pairwise Comparisons among the Three Sites

Sites	$\bar{X}_1 - \bar{Y}_1$	$\bar{X}_2 - \bar{Y}_2$	$\hat{p}_1$	$\hat{p}_2$	$\hat{p} = \min(\hat{p}_1, \hat{p}_2)$	$nC(\hat{p})$
1 vs 2	0.1594	−0.1102	0.834	0.978	0.834	0.1129
1 vs 3	0.2299	0.0593	0.464	0.993	0.464	0.7330
2 vs 3	0.0705	0.1695	0.961	0.782	0.782	0.1643

208   *Quantitative Methods for Traditional Chinese Medicine Development*

Similarly, in order to ensure that there is a 0.80 probability of claiming consistency between raw materials from sites 2 and 3, the sample size is determined as

$$n = \frac{(z_{0.20} + z_{0.975})^2 nC(\hat{p})}{(\log QC_L - \log \hat{p})^2} = \frac{2.8016^2 \times 0.1643}{0.1849^2} \approx 38.$$

9.5 Discussion

In this study, we investigated the problem of controlling the quality of raw materials and/or final products of traditional Chinese medicine. We proposed an index to assess the consistency of raw materials and/or final products processed or manufactured from different locations or sites. In particular, if the TCM considered has two active components, the consistency index of this TCM is defined as the minimum of the consistency indices of the corresponding two active components. Though the discussion in this paper is focused on only two active components, the idea can easily be extended to more than two active components. In general, if a TCM contains more than two active components, say k, a natural extension is to use the minimum of the k consistency indices p_i corresponding to the k active components to be the consistency index p of the TCM, i.e., $p = \min(p_1, p_2, \ldots, p_k)$.

Note that the corresponding MLE of p is given by $\hat{p} = \min(\hat{p}_1, \hat{p}_2, \ldots, \hat{p}_k)$, where $\hat{p}_i$ is the MLE of p_i, $i = 1, 2, \ldots, k$. Define j to be the index such that $p_j = \min(p_1, p_2, \ldots, p_k)$. It can be shown by following the similar arguments used in Equations 9.2 through 9.4 that

$$E(\log \hat{p}) = E\left(\log \hat{p}_j\right), \ \mathrm{Var}(\log \hat{p}) = \mathrm{Var}(\log \hat{p}_j)$$

and

$$\frac{\log \hat{p} - E\left(\log \hat{p}\right)}{\sqrt{\mathrm{Var}\left(\hat{p}\right)}} \to N(0, 1).$$

Thus, the construction of an acceptance criterion can be done in a similar way. However, a question of interest is the performance of this measure when the number of active components k is relatively large, which may lead to a rather conservative measure. One may explore alternative approaches to assess the consistency of TCM when the number of active components is

Statistical Process for Quality Control/Assurance 209

relatively large. More research efforts are certainly needed in this issue in order to provide useful insights for practical applications.

In connection to applications of this proposed procedure in practice, the characteristics of the components are usually measured as the percentage of the labeled claim for each component. In other words, if a TCM contains quantities $q_1, \ldots, q_k$ for components $1, \ldots, k$ and $c_1, c_2, \ldots, c_k$ are the theoretical values of the active components in the TCM under consideration, the characteristics U_i are usually given in terms of the percentages $\dfrac{q_i}{c_i}$. Thus, as suggested in this study, it is reasonable to assume the corresponding logarithmic transformation of U_i to be normally distributed. In fact, it should be noted that the use of percentages $\dfrac{q_i}{c_i}$ conforms to the suggestion by FDA.

9.6 Appendix: Proof of Theorem

9.6.1 Appendix I. Proof of Lemma 9.1

Note that the parameters $\theta = \left(\mu_{X_1}, \mu_{X_2}, \mu_{Y_1}, \mu_{Y_2}, V_{X_1}, V_{X_2}, V_{Y_1}, V_{Y_2} \right)$ are estimated by their corresponding MLEs $\hat{\theta} = \left(\bar{X}_1, \bar{X}_2, \bar{Y}_1, \bar{Y}_2, \hat{V}_{X_1}, \hat{V}_{X_2}, \hat{V}_{Y_1}, \hat{V}_{Y_2} \right)$. It is easy to verify that $\hat{\theta}$ is asymptotically multivariate normal distributed with mean $E(\hat{\theta})$ and covariance matrix $\mathrm{Cov}(\hat{\theta})$. It follows easily that

$$E(\hat{\theta}) = \left(\mu_{X_1}, \mu_{X_2}, \mu_{Y_1}, \mu_{Y_2}, \frac{n-1}{n} V_{X_1}, \frac{n-1}{n} V_{X_2}, \frac{n-1}{n} V_{Y_1}, \frac{n-1}{n} V_{Y_2} \right).$$ Note that only

terms of order up to $o(n^{-1})$ are derived for the various entries of the covariance matrix $\mathrm{Cov}(\hat{\theta})$. In particular, terms of only up to order $o(n^{-1})$ of the first moments and the second order central moments of the components of the MLE $\hat{\theta}$ are given as follows:

a. $\mathrm{Cov}(\bar{X}_i, \bar{Y}_j) = \mathrm{Cov}(\bar{X}_i, \hat{V}_{Y_j}) = \mathrm{Cov}(\hat{V}_{X_i}, \bar{Y}_j) = \mathrm{Cov}(\hat{V}_{X_i}, \hat{V}_{Y_j}) = 0,\, i = 1, 2;\, j = 1, 2.$

b. $\mathrm{Var}(\bar{X}_1) = \dfrac{1}{n} V_{X_1} + o(n^{-1}),\ \mathrm{Var}(\bar{X}_2) = \dfrac{1}{n} V_{X_2} + o(n^{-1}),\ \mathrm{Var}(\bar{Y}_1) = \dfrac{1}{n} V_{Y_1} + o(n^{-1}),$

$\mathrm{Var}(\bar{Y}_2) = \dfrac{1}{n} V_{Y_2} + o(n^{-1}).$

c. $\mathrm{Var}(\hat{V}_{X_1}) = \dfrac{2}{n} V_{X_1}^2 + o(n^{-1}),\ \mathrm{Var}(\hat{V}_{X_2}) = \dfrac{2}{n} V_{X_2}^2 + o(n^{-1}),$

$\mathrm{Var}(\hat{V}_{Y_1}) = \dfrac{2}{n} V_{Y_1}^2 + o(n^{-1}),\ \mathrm{Var}(\hat{V}_{Y_2}) = \dfrac{2}{n} V_{Y_2}^2 + o(n^{-1}).$

d. $\text{Cov}(\bar{X}_1, \hat{V}_{X_1}) = \dfrac{4}{n}\mu_{X_1}V_{X_1} + o(n^{-1}),\ \text{Cov}(\bar{X}_2, \hat{V}_{X_2}) = \dfrac{4}{n}\mu_{X_2}V_{X_2} + o(n^{-1}),$

$\text{Cov}(\bar{Y}_1, \hat{V}_{Y_1}) = \dfrac{4}{n}\mu_{Y_1}V_{Y_1} + o(n^{-1}),\ \text{Cov}(\bar{Y}_2, \hat{V}_{Y_2}) = \dfrac{4}{n}\mu_{Y_2}V_{Y_2} + o(n^{-1}).$

e. $\text{Cov}(\bar{X}_1, \bar{X}_2) = \dfrac{1}{n}\rho_X(V_{X_1}V_{X_2})^{\frac{1}{2}} + o(n^{-1}),\ \text{Cov}(\bar{Y}_1, \bar{Y}_2) = \dfrac{1}{n}\rho_Y(V_{Y_1}V_{Y_2})^{\frac{1}{2}} + o(n^{-1}).$

f. $\text{Cov}(\hat{V}_{X_1}, \hat{V}_{X_2}) = \dfrac{2}{n}\left[\rho_X^2 V_{X_1}V_{X_2} + \dfrac{1}{3}\rho_X\mu_{X_1}\mu_{X_2}(V_{X_1}V_{X_2})^{\frac{1}{2}}\right] + o(n^{-1}),$

$\text{Cov}(\hat{V}_{Y_1}, \hat{V}_{Y_2}) = \dfrac{2}{n}\left[\rho_Y^2 V_{Y_1}V_{Y_2} + \dfrac{1}{3}\rho_Y\mu_{Y_1}\mu_{Y_2}(V_{Y_1}V_{Y_2})^{\frac{1}{2}}\right] + o(n^{-1}).$

g. $\text{Cov}(\bar{X}_1, \hat{V}_{X_2}) = \dfrac{1}{n}\rho_X\mu_{X_2}(V_{X_1}V_{X_2})^{\frac{1}{2}} + o(n^{-1}),$

$\text{Cov}(\bar{X}_2, \hat{V}_{X_1}) = \dfrac{1}{n}\rho_X\mu_{X_1}(V_{X_1}V_{X_2})^{\frac{1}{2}} + o(n^{-1}),$

$\text{Cov}(\bar{Y}_1, \hat{V}_{Y_2}) = \dfrac{1}{n}\rho_Y\mu_{Y_2}(V_{Y_1}V_{Y_2})^{\frac{1}{2}} + o(n^{-1}),$

$\text{Cov}(\bar{Y}_2, \hat{V}_{Y_1}) = \dfrac{1}{n}\rho_Y\mu_{Y_1}(V_{Y_1}V_{Y_2})^{\frac{1}{2}} + o\left(n^{-1}\right).$

For the sake of simplicity, denote

$$z_1 = \frac{\log(1-\delta_1) - (\mu_{X_1} - \mu_{Y_1})}{\sqrt{V_{X_1} + V_{Y_1}}},$$

$$z_2 = \frac{-\log(1-\delta_1) - (\mu_{X_1} - \mu_{Y_1})}{\sqrt{V_{X_1} + V_{Y_1}}},$$

$$z_3 = \frac{\log(1-\delta_2) - (\mu_{X_2} - \mu_{Y_2})}{\sqrt{V_{X_2} + V_{Y_2}}},$$

$$z_4 = \frac{-\log(1-\delta_2) - (\mu_{X_2} - \mu_{Y_2})}{\sqrt{V_{X_2} + V_{Y_2}}},$$

$$t_{11} = \phi(z_2) - \phi(z_1),\ t_{12} = \phi(z_4) - \phi(z_3),$$

Statistical Process for Quality Control/Assurance

$$t_{21} = z_2\phi(z_2) - z_1\phi(z_1),$$

$$t_{22} = z_4\phi(z_4) - z_3\phi(z_3);$$

where ϕ and Φ are the probability density function and cumulative distribution function of a standard normal distribution, respectively. In particular, denote

$$s_1 = \Phi(z_2) - \Phi(z_1), \tag{9.16}$$

$$s_2 = \Phi(z_4) - \Phi(z_3). \tag{9.17}$$

Denote $\hat{p}_1 = g_1(\hat{\theta})$, $\hat{p}_2 = g_2(\hat{\theta})$ and $g(\hat{\theta}) = (g_1(\hat{\theta}), g_2(\hat{\theta})) = (\hat{p}_1, \hat{p}_2)$. The first-order partial derivatives with respect to the parameters $\theta = (\mu_{X_1}, \mu_{X_2}, \mu_{Y_1}, \mu_{Y_2}, V_{X_1}, V_{X_2}, V_{Y_1}, V_{Y_2})$ are given by

$$\frac{\partial g_1(\hat{\theta})}{\partial \mu_{X_1}} = -\frac{\partial g_1(\hat{\theta})}{\partial \mu_{Y_1}} = \frac{-t_{11}}{\sqrt{V_{X_1} + V_{Y_1}}},$$

$$\frac{\partial g_2(\hat{\theta})}{\partial \mu_{X_2}} = -\frac{\partial g_2(\hat{\theta})}{\partial \mu_{Y_2}} = \frac{-t_{12}}{\sqrt{V_{X_2} + V_{Y_2}}},$$

$$\frac{\partial g_1(\hat{\theta})}{\partial V_{X_1}} = \frac{\partial g_1(\hat{\theta})}{\partial V_{Y_1}} = \frac{-t_{21}}{2(V_{X_1} + V_{Y_1})},$$

$$\frac{\partial g_2(\hat{\theta})}{\partial V_{X_2}} = \frac{\partial g_2(\hat{\theta})}{\partial V_{Y_2}} = \frac{-t_{22}}{2(V_{X_2} + V_{Y_2})},$$

and the other first-order derivatives are equal to 0.

By delta's method, the covariance matrix of $g(\hat{\theta})$ can be approximated by $A = (a_{ij})_{2\times 2}$, where a_{ij} are the terms of order $o(n^{-1})$ and, in particular,

$$a_{11} = \frac{1}{n}t_{11}^2 + \frac{4t_{11}t_{21}\left(\mu_{X_1}V_{X_1} - \mu_{Y_1}V_{Y_1}\right)}{n\left(V_{X_1} + V_{Y_1}\right)^{\frac{3}{2}}} + \frac{t_{21}^2\left(V_{X_1}^2 + V_{Y_1}^2\right)}{2n\left(V_{X_1} + V_{Y_1}\right)^2}, \tag{9.18}$$

$$a_{22} = \frac{1}{n}t_{12}^2 + \frac{4t_{12}t_{22}\left(\mu_{X_2}V_{X_2} - \mu_{Y_2}V_{Y_2}\right)}{n\left(V_{X_2} + V_{Y_2}\right)^{\frac{3}{2}}} + \frac{t_{22}^2\left(V_{X_2}^2 + V_{Y_2}^2\right)}{2n\left(V_{X_2} + V_{Y_2}\right)^2}, \tag{9.19}$$

$$a_{12} = a_{21} = \frac{t_{11}t_{12}\left[\rho_X\left(V_{X_1}V_{X_2}\right)^{\frac{1}{2}} + \rho_Y\left(V_{Y_1}V_{Y_2}\right)^{\frac{1}{2}}\right]}{n\left(V_{X_2} + V_{Y_2}\right)^{\frac{1}{2}}\left(V_{X_1} + V_{Y_1}\right)^{\frac{1}{2}}}$$

$$+ \frac{t_{12}t_{21}\left[\rho_X\mu_{X_1}\left(V_{X_1}V_{X_2}\right)^{\frac{1}{2}} - \rho_Y\mu_{Y_1}\left(V_{Y_1}V_{Y_2}\right)^{\frac{1}{2}}\right]}{2n\left(V_{X_2} + V_{Y_2}\right)^{\frac{1}{2}}\left(V_{X_1} + V_{Y_1}\right)}$$

$$+ \frac{t_{11}t_{22}\left[\rho_X\mu_{X_2}\left(V_{X_1}V_{X_2}\right)^{\frac{1}{2}} - \rho_Y\mu_{Y_2}\left(V_{Y_1}V_{Y_2}\right)^{\frac{1}{2}}\right]}{2n\left(V_{X_2} + V_{Y_2}\right)\left(V_{X_1} + V_{Y_1}\right)^{\frac{1}{2}}}$$

$$+ \frac{t_{21}t_{22}\left[\rho_X^2 V_{X_1}V_{X_2} + \frac{1}{3}\mu_{X_1}\mu_{X_2}(V_{X_1}V_{X_2})^{\frac{1}{2}} + \rho_Y^2 V_{Y_1}V_{Y_2} + \frac{1}{3}\mu_{Y_1}\mu_{Y_2}(V_{Y_1}V_{Y_2})^{\frac{1}{2}}\right]}{2n(V_{X_2} + V_{Y_2})(V_{X_1} + V_{Y_1})}. \quad (9.20)$$

Note that $\hat{\theta} \sim N\left(E(\hat{\theta}), \mathrm{Cov}(\hat{\theta})\right)$ asymptotically. By Slutsky theorem, $g(\hat{\theta})$ is $\sim N\left(E(\hat{p}_1, \hat{p}_2), A\right)$ asymptotically. Again, because log transform is a continuous function, it follows easily that the joint distribution of $\left(\log \hat{p}_1, \log \hat{p}_2\right)$ is asymptotically normally distributed as $N\left(E(\log \hat{p}_1, \log \hat{p}_2), \frac{1}{s_1^2 s_2^2} A\right)$.

9.6.2 Appendix II. Proof of Lemma 9.2

Define $Z_1 = \log \hat{p}_1 - \log \hat{p}_2$ and $Z_2 = \log \hat{p}_1$. Then, (Z_1, Z_2) is asymptotically normally distributed as

$$N\left(E\left(Z_1, Z_2\right), \frac{1}{s_1^2 s_2^2} B\right),$$

where

$$B = \begin{pmatrix} a_{11} + a_{22} - 2a_{12} & a_{11} - a_{12} \\ a_{11} - a_{12} & a_{11} \end{pmatrix}.$$

Thus, from Johnson and Kotz (1970), it can be shown easily that $Z_1 | Z_1 > 0$ is asymptotically normal with mean

Statistical Process for Quality Control/Assurance

$$\xi + \frac{\phi\left(\dfrac{-\xi}{\sigma}\right)}{1 - \Phi\left(\dfrac{-\xi}{\sigma}\right)}\sigma$$

and variance

$$\left[1 - \frac{\phi^2\left(\dfrac{-\xi}{\sigma}\right)}{\left(1 - \Phi\left(\dfrac{-\xi}{\sigma}\right)\right)^2} - \frac{\xi\phi\left(\dfrac{-\xi}{\sigma}\right)}{\sigma\left(1 - \Phi\left(\dfrac{-\xi}{\sigma}\right)\right)}\right]\sigma^2,$$

where

$$\xi = E\left(\log \hat{p}_1 - \log \hat{p}_2\right)$$

and

$$\sigma^2 = \frac{1}{s_1^2 s_2^2}\left(a_{11} + a_{22} - 2a_{12}\right).$$

Note that $\xi = E\left(\log \hat{p}_1 - \log \hat{p}_2\right) = \log p_1 - \log p_2 + o(n^{-1})$, where p_1 and p_2 are given in Equation 9.1. Furthermore, it is easy to see that

$$\sigma^2 = \frac{1}{s_1^2 s_2^2}\left(a_{11} + a_{22} - 2a_{12}\right) = o(n^{-1}).$$

Therefore, $\xi/\sigma = o(\sqrt{n})$.

Note for all integers k, $\phi(x)/x^{-k} \to 0$ as $x \to \infty$. Thus, $\phi(-\xi/\sigma)$ is of order $o(n^{-1})$. Consider

$$P(Z_1 > 0) = 1 - P\left(\log \hat{p}_1 - \log \hat{p}_2 < 0\right) = 1 - E\Phi\left[-\left(\log \hat{p}_1 - \log \hat{p}_2\right)/\hat{\sigma}\right] + o(n^{-1}),$$

where $\hat{\sigma}$ is the MLE of σ. Expanding the above expression at $\hat{\theta} = \theta$, we have

$$E\Phi\left[-\left(\log \hat{p}_1 - \log \hat{p}_2\right)/\hat{\sigma}\right] = \Phi\left[-\left(\log p_1 - \log p_2\right)/\sigma\right] + \left.\frac{\partial \Phi}{\partial \hat{\theta}}\right|_{\hat{\theta}=\theta} [E(\hat{\theta} - \theta)] + \dots$$

$$(9.21)$$

Note that in Equation 9.21, except the leading term $\Phi[-(\log p_1 - \log p_2)/\sigma]$, all the other terms are at least of order $o(n^{-1})$, since $\left.\dfrac{\partial \Phi}{\partial \theta}\right|_{\hat{\theta}=\theta}$ and all the other higher-order partial derivatives involves the factor $\phi[(\log p_1 - \log p_2)/\sigma]$, which is of order $o(n^{-1})$.

Note that $\log \hat{p}$ and $(\log \hat{p})^2$ can be expressed in the following forms:

$$\log \hat{p} = \log \hat{p}_1 - (\log \hat{p}_1 - \log \hat{p}_2) I (\log \hat{p}_1 - \log \hat{p}_2 > 0) = Z_2 - Z_1 I(Z_1 > 0) \tag{9.22}$$

and

$$(\log \hat{p})^2 = Z_2^2 + (Z_1^2 - 2Z_1 Z_2) I(Z_1 > 0). \tag{9.23}$$

Consider the following two cases:

Case 1: $\log p_1 - \log p_2 > 0$

Note that from Feller (1968),

$$\phi(x)\left(\frac{1}{x} - \frac{1}{x^3}\right) \le (1 - \Phi(x)) \le \phi(x)\frac{1}{x}.$$

But, for integer value k,

$$\frac{\phi(x)x^{-1}}{x^{-k}} \to 0$$

and

$$\frac{\phi(x)(x^{-1} - x^{-3})}{x^{-k}} \to 0,$$

as $x \to \infty$.

Hence, $[1 - \Phi(x)]$ is of order $o(x^{-k})$. Because $(\log p_1 - \log p_2)/\sigma$ is of order $o(\sqrt{n})$,

then

$$(1 - \Phi((\log p_1 - \log p_2)/\sigma))$$

Statistical Process for Quality Control/Assurance

is of order $o(n^{-1})$. This leads to

$$P(Z_1 > 0) = 1 - E\Phi\left[-\left(\log\hat{p}_1 - \log\hat{p}_2\right)/\hat{\sigma}\right] = 1 - o(n^{-1}).$$

Case 2: $\log p_1 - \log p_2 > 0$

Following similar arguments as above, it can be showed that $P(Z_1 > 0) = o(n^{-1})$.

Therefore, from Equation 9.22,

$$E(\log\hat{p}) = E(Z_2) - E(Z_1 | Z_1 > 0)P(Z_1 > 0)$$

$$= E(\log p_1) - \left[\xi + \frac{\phi\left(\dfrac{-\xi}{\sigma}\right)}{1 - \Phi\left(\dfrac{-\xi}{\sigma}\right)}\sigma\right]P(Z_1 > 0)$$

$$= E(\log p_1) - \xi P(Z_1 > 0) + o(n^{-1})$$

$$= \begin{cases} E(\log\hat{p}_1) - \xi = E\log\hat{p}_2 & \text{if} & p_1 > p_2 \\ E(\log\hat{p}_1) & & p_1 \le p_2. \end{cases}$$

Note that

$$E\left(Z_2^2\right) = \frac{a_{11}}{s_1^2 s_2^2} + \left(E\left(\log(\hat{p}_1)\right)\right)^2$$

and

$$E\left(Z_1^2 | Z_1 > 0\right) = \xi^2 + \frac{\xi\phi(-\xi/\sigma)}{\sigma(1 - \Phi(-\xi/\sigma))} + \sigma^2.$$

On the basis of the results of a truncated normal distribution (Johnson and Kotz 1970),

$$E(Z_1 Z_2 | Z_1 > 0) = E(Z_1)E(Z_2) + \text{Cov}(Z_1, Z_2)\left(1 - \frac{\xi\phi(-\xi/\sigma)}{\sigma(1 - \Phi(-\xi/\sigma))}\right)$$

$$+ (\sigma_1 E(Z_1) + \rho\sigma_2 E(Z_2))\frac{\phi(-\xi/\sigma)}{1 - \Phi(-\xi/\sigma)}$$

$$(9.24)$$

and

$$2E(Z_1Z_2 \mid Z_1 > 0)P(Z_1 > 0)$$

$$= 2\left[E(Z_1)E(Z_2) + \rho\sigma_1\sigma_2\left(1 - \frac{\xi\phi(-\xi/\sigma)}{\sigma(1 - \Phi(-\xi/\sigma))} \right) \right.$$

$$\left. + (\sigma_1 E(Z_1) + \rho\sigma_2 E(Z_2)) \frac{\phi(-\xi/\sigma)}{1 - \Phi(-\xi/\sigma)} \right] P(Z_1 > 0) \qquad (9.25)$$

$$= 2(E(Z_1)E(Z_2) + \text{Cov}(Z_1, Z_2))P(Z_1 > 0) + o(n^{-1})$$

$$= 2E(Z_1Z_2)P(Z_1 > 0) + o(n^{-1})$$

Therefore, combining Equations 9.23 through 9.25,

$$E(\log \hat{p})^2 = E(Z_2^2) + [E(Z_1^2 \mid Z_1 > 0) - 2E(Z_1Z_2 \mid Z_1 > 0)]P(Z_1 > 0)$$

$$= E(Z_2^2) + (\xi^2 + \sigma^2)P(Z_1 > 0) - 2E(Z_1Z_2)P(Z_1 > 0) + o(n^{-1})$$

$$= E(Z_2^2) + E(Z_1^2)P(Z_1 > 0) - 2E(Z_1Z_2)P(Z_1 > 0) + o(n^{-1})$$

$$= \begin{cases} E(Z_1 - Z_2)^2 + o(n^{-1}) & \text{if} & p_1 > p_2 \\ E(Z_2^2) + o(n^{-1}) & & p_1 \leq p_2 \end{cases}$$

$$= \begin{cases} E(\log \hat{p}_2)^2 + o(n^{-1}) & \text{if} & p_1 > p_2 \\ E(\log \hat{p}_1)^2 + o(n^{-1}), & & p_1 \leq p_2 \end{cases}$$

Therefore, combining the above results, we have

$$E(\log \hat{p}) = \begin{cases} E(\log \hat{p}_2) + o\left(n^{-1}\right) & \text{if } p_1 > p_2 \\ E(\log \hat{p}_1) + o\left(n^{-1}\right) & \text{if } p_1 < p_2 \end{cases}$$

and

$$\text{Var}(\log \hat{p}) = \begin{cases} \text{Var}(\log \hat{p}_2) + o\left(n^{-1}\right) & \text{if } p_1 > p_2 \\ \text{Var}(\log \hat{p}_1) + o\left(n^{-1}\right) & \text{if } p_1 < p_2. \end{cases}$$

Statistical Process for Quality Control/Assurance 217

In particular, apply expansion of $\hat{p}_i$ at p_i and take expectation, it can be shown easily that

$$E(\log(\hat{p}_i)) = \log p_i + B(p_i) + o(n^{-1})$$

and

$$\text{Var}(\log(\hat{p}_i)) = \frac{1}{p_i^2} \text{Var}(\hat{p}_i) + o(n^{-1}) = C(p_i) + o(n^{-1}),$$

where

$$B(p_i) = \frac{1}{np_i} \frac{\partial^2 \hat{p}_i}{\partial V_{X_i}^2} \left(V_{X_i}^2 + V_{Y_i}^2 \right) - \frac{1}{2np_i^2} \left[\left(\frac{\partial \hat{p}_i}{\partial \mu_{X_i}} \right)^2 \left(V_{X_i} + V_{Y_i} \right) + 2 \left(\frac{\partial \hat{p}_i}{\partial V_{X_i}} \right)^2 \left(V_{X_i}^2 + V_{Y_i}^2 \right) \right]$$

and

$$C(p_i) = \frac{1}{np_i^2} \left[\left(\frac{\partial \hat{p}_i}{\partial \mu_{X_i}} \right)^2 \left(V_{X_i} + V_{Y_i} \right) + 2 \left(\frac{\partial \hat{p}_i}{\partial V_{X_i}} \right)^2 \left(V_{X_i}^2 + V_{Y_i}^2 \right) \right].$$

10

Bioavailability and Bioequivalence

10.1 Introduction

In 1984, the US Congress passed the *Drug Price Competition and Patent Term Restoration Act*, which allows a regulatory framework for a low-cost pathway for generic drug products to enter the market. This Act gives the FDA the authority to approve a generic drug product via an Abbreviated New Drug Application (ANDA). As a result, when an innovative (brand name) drug product is going off patent, pharmaceutical or generic companies can file an ANDA for generic approval. For approval of a generic drug product, most regulatory agencies require evidence of average bioavailability (in terms of extent and rate of drug absorption) be provided through the conduct of bioequivalence studies. As indicated by a survey conducted by the Association of American Retired People (AARP) in 2002, about 22 percent of the responders considered that generic drug products are less effective or of poor quality than the innovator drug products. This shows that a sizable portion of the public in United States still lacks of confidence in generic drug products even if they are approved by the FDA. Therefore, in May 2007, the FDA added generic drugs in the critical path opportunities to use the latest breakthroughs in technique to assure that the efficacy and safety of the generic drug products are same as those of the innovator drug products. However, the FDA critical path opportunities for generic drugs do not cover all important emerging challenges for generic drugs.

In Section 10.2, the concept of bioavailability and bioequivalence is briefly introduced. Statistical design and analysis for assessment of bioequivalence are described in Section 10.3. Drug interchangeability in terms of drug prescribability and drug switchability are discussed in Section 10.4. Section 10.5 presents some controversial issues that are commonly encountered when conducting bioequivalence studies for assessment of average bioequivalence. These controversial issues include, but are not limited to, (1) challenge of the Fundamental Bioequivalence Assumption, (2) adequacy of one-size-fits-all criterion, and (3) appropriateness of log-transformation. Some frequently asked questions during the ANDA submission for generic approval are

219

220 *Quantitative Methods for Traditional Chinese Medicine Development*

given in Section 10.6. Section 10.7 raises scientific/statistical issues for assessing biosimilarity and interchangeability of follow-on biologics. Section 10.8 provides brief concluding remarks to end the chapter.

10.2 What Is Bioavailability/Bioequivalence?

As indicated in 21 Codes of Federal Regulations (CFR) Part 320.1, bioavailability of a drug is defined as the extent and rate to which the active drug ingredient or active moiety from the drug product is absorbed and becomes available at the site of drug action. The extent and rate of drug absorption are usually measured by the area under the blood or plasma concentration-time curve (AUC) and the maximum concentration (C_{max}), respectively. For drug products that are not intended to be absorbed into the bloodstream, bioavailability may be assessed by measurements intended to reflect the rate and extent to which the active ingredient or active moiety is absorbed and becomes available at the site of action. A comparative bioavailability study refers to the comparison of bioavailabilities of different formulations of the same drug or different drug products. As indicated by Chow and Liu (2008), the definition of bioavailability has evolved over time with different meanings by different individuals and organizations. For example, differences are evident in the definitions by Academy of Pharmaceutical Sciences in 1972, the Office of Technology Assessment (OTA) of the Congress of the United States in 1974, Wagner (1975), and the 1984 *Drug Price Competition and Patent Restoration* amendments to the Food, Drug, and Cosmetic Act. For more discussion regarding the definition of bioavailability, see Balant (1991) and Chen et al. (2001).

When two formulations of the same drug or two drug products are claimed bioequivalent, it is assumed that they will provide the same therapeutic effect or that they are therapeutically equivalent and they can be used interchangeably. Two drug products are considered pharmaceutical equivalents if they contain identical amounts of the same active ingredient. Two drugs are identified as pharmaceutical alternatives to each other if both contain an identical therapeutic moiety, but not necessarily in the same amount or dosage form or as the same salt or ester. Two drug products are said to be bioequivalent if they are pharmaceutical equivalents (i.e., similar dosage forms made, perhaps, by different manufacturers) or pharmaceutical alternatives (i.e., different dosage forms) and if their rates and extents of absorption do not show a significant difference to which the active ingredient or active moiety in pharmaceutical equivalents or pharmaceutical alternatives become available at the site of action when administered at the same molar dose under similar conditions in an appropriately designed study.

Bioavailability and Bioequivalence 221

When an innovative (or brand name) drug product is going off patient, pharmaceutical companies may file an ANDA for generic approval. Generic drug products are defined as drug products that are identical to an innovative drug that is the subject of an approved NDA with regard to active ingredient(s), route of administration, dosage form, strength, and conditions of use. Because ANDA submissions for generic applications do not require lengthy clinical evaluation of the generic drugs under investigation (see Table 10.1), the price of generics is usually much lower than that of the originals. On average, it is about 20 percent of the price of the brand name originals. In 1984, the FDA was authorized to approve generic drug products under the Drug Price Competition and Patent Term Restoration Act. The purpose is to make less expensive, safe, and equally efficacious generics available to the general public after the expiration of patent protection of expensive brand name drugs. For approval of generic drug products, the FDA requires that evidence of average bioequivalence in drug absorption be provided through the conduct of bioavailability and bioequivalence studies. Bioequivalence assessment is considered as a surrogate for clinical evaluation of the therapeutic equivalence of drug products.

A typical process for bioequivalence assessment is to conduct a bioavailability/bioequivalence study with healthy volunteers under the assumption that bioavailability of the drug product under investigation is predictive of clinical outcomes of the drug product in clinical trials (see, e.g., Purich 1980; FDA 1992, 1995, 2001a, 2003b). A bioequivalence study is often conducted utilizing a crossover design that allows comparison within individual subjects, i.e., each subject is at his/her own control. On the basis of pharmacokinetic (PK) data collected, bioequivalence can then be assessed using valid statistical methods according to some pre-specified regulatory criteria for bioequivalence. As indicated by the FDA, an approved generic drug product can be used as a substitute for the brand name drug.

TABLE 10.1

NDA versus ANDA

NDA	ANDA
1. Chemistry	1. Chemistry
2. Manufacturing	2. Manufacturing
3. Controls	3. Controls
4. Testing	4. Testing
5. Labeling	5. Labeling
6. PK/bioavailability	6. PK/bioavailability
7. Animal studies	–
8. Clinical safety and efficacy trials	–

Note: ANDA, Abbreviated New Drug Application; NDA, New Drug Application.

10.3 Bioequivalence Assessment for Generic Approval

For approval of generic drug products, the FDA requires that evidence of average bioequivalence in drug absorption in terms of some pharmacokinetic parameters such as the AUC and peak concentration (C_{max}) be provided through the conduct of bioequivalence studies. We claim that a test drug product is bioequivalent to a reference (innovative) drug product if the 90 percent confidence interval for the geometric mean ratio (GMR) of means of the primary PK parameter between the test product and the reference product is totally within the bioequivalence limit of (80.00 percent, 125.00 percent). The confidence interval for the ratio of means of the primary PK parameter is obtained based on log-transformed data. In what follows, basic considerations, study designs, statistical methods that are commonly considered in bioequivalence studies, and limitations of average bioequivalence are briefly introduced.

10.3.1 Basic Considerations

10.3.1.1 Sample Size

For pivotal fasting studies, FDA suggests that sample size be determined for achieving an 80 percent power for establishment of average bioequivalence based on Schuirmann's two one-sided tests procedure (see, e.g., Phillips 1990; Hauschke et al. 1992; Liu and Chow 1992; Chow et al. 2002b). In practice, 24 to 36 subjects are usually considered depending upon the intrasubject coefficient of variation (CV) of the reference product (see Table 10.2). As can be seen from Table 10.2, if there is no difference in mean average bioavailability between the test product and the reference product, a total of 24 subjects are required for achieving an 80 percent power for establishing average bioequivalence when the intrasubject CV or relative standard deviation is about 22 percent. Required sample size will increase as the intrasubject CV increases

TABLE 10.2

Sample Size for Pivotal Fasting Studies

Power (%)	CV (%)	Differences			
		0%	5%	10%	15%
80%	20	20	24	52	200
	22	24	28	62	242
	24	28	34	74	288
	26	32	40	86	336
	28	36	46	100	390
	30	40	52	114	448

Note: CV, intrasubject coefficient of variation of the reference product.

Bioavailability and Bioequivalence 223

(i.e., the reference product is more variable). Note that a drug product is considered a highly variable drug by the FDA if its intrasubject CV is greater than or equal to 30 percent. On the other hand, if there is a difference in average bioavailability between the test product and the reference product, a much larger sample size is required for demonstrating average bioequivalence.

On the other hand, for limited fasting food studies, FDA suggests that a minimum of 12 subjects be considered.

10.3.1.2 Subject Selection

In practice, for bioavailability/bioequivalence studies, male healthy volunteers aged 18 to 50 years old whose body weight is within 10 percent of ideal body weight are considered for accurate and reliable characterization of the drug absorption profile of the test product under investigation. Other types of populations such as females, elderly, and/or patients may also be considered. In cases where other types of populations are considered, there may be special considerations. For example, if female subjects are to be included in bioavailability/bioequivalence studies, ethical considerations, liability for undetected pregnancy, and possible pharmacokinetic effects of hormonal variation (especially during the monthly period) should be carefully addressed. For an elderly population, subjects' stress, blood loss, the status of chronic disease, and pharmacokinetic effects of altered organ function should be taken into consideration as these factors may alter the drug absorption profiles under study. Similarly, the factors of stress, blood loss, pharmacokinetic effects of disease states, concurrent medications, and special diets should be considered when the bioavailability/bioequivalence studies are intended to be conducted with a patient population as these factors may inflate both the intrasubject and intersubject variabilities and consequently result in a more heterogeneous population under study.

10.3.1.3 Washout

In bioavailability/bioequivalence studies utilizing crossover design, a sufficient length of washout period between dosing periods is necessary to wear off the possible residual effect from the previous dose that may be carried over to the next dosing period. For pivotal fasting studies, FDA requires that at least 5.5 half-lives be considered to ensure there is a sufficient length of washout for immediate release (IR) products. For controlled release (CR) products, on the other hand, FDA indicates that at least 8.5 half-lives should be considered to limit the chance of possible carryover residual effect.

10.3.1.4 Blood Sampling

In practice, it is undesirable to draw too much blood and/or too frequently from subjects under study. However, sufficient blood should be drawn at

224   *Quantitative Methods for Traditional Chinese Medicine Development*

different sampling intervals in order to accurately and reliably characterize the blood concentration-time curve and consequently the drug absorption profile. For this purpose, it is suggested that more blood sampling around C_{max} should be taken and sampling intervals should cover at least three half-lives of the drug product.

10.3.1.5 IR Product versus CR Products

For IR products, FDA indicates that a single dose fasting study is required, while a limited food effect study may be required when needed. For CR products, on the other hand, single dose fasting studies, multiple dose fasting studies, and limited food effect studies are required. Other single/multiple dose studies can be used as deemed necessary.

10.3.2 Study Design

As indicated in the *Federal Register* (Vol. 42 No. 5 Sec. 320.26[b] and Sec. 320.27[b], 1977), a bioavailability study single dose or multidose should be crossover in design, unless a parallel or other design is more appropriate for valid scientific reasons. Thus, in practice, a standard two-sequence, two-period (or 2 × 2) crossover design is often considered for a bioavailability/bioequivalence study (see, also Jones and Kenward 1989). Denote T and R as the test product and the reference product, respectively. The standard 2 × 2 crossover design can be expressed as (TR, RT), where TR is the first sequence of treatments and RT denotes the second sequence of treatments. Under the (TR, TR) design, qualified subjects who are randomly assigned to sequence 1 (TR) will receive the test product (T) first and then receive the reference product (R) after a sufficient length of wash out period. Similarly, subjects who are randomly assigned to sequence 2 (RT) will receive the reference product (R) first and then receive the test product (T) after a sufficient length of wash out period.

One of the limitations of the standard 2 × 2 crossover design is that it does not provide independent estimates of intrasubject variabilities since each subject will only receive the same treatment once. In the interest of assessing intrasubject variabilities, the following alternative designs for comparing two drug products are often considered:

1. Balaam's design – (TT, RR, RT, TR);
2. Two-sequence, three-period dual design – (TRR, RTT);
3. Four-sequence, four-period design – (TTRR, RRTT, TRTR, RTTR).

Note that the above study designs are also referred to as higher-order crossover designs. A higher-order crossover design is defined as a design with the number of sequences or the number of periods greater than the number of treatments to be compared.

Bioavailability and Bioequivalence 225

For comparing more than two drug products, a Williams' design is often considered. For example, for comparing three drug products, a six-sequence, three-period (6 × 3) Williams' design is usually considered, while a 4 × 4 Williams' design is employed for comparing four drug products. Williams' design is a variance stabilizing design. More information regarding the construction and good design characteristics of Williams' designs can be found in the work of Chow and Liu (2008).

In the interest of assessing population and/or individual bioequivalence, the FDA recommends that a replicate design be considered for obtaining independent estimates of intrasubject variabilities and variability due to subject-by-drug product interaction. A commonly considered replicate crossover design is the replicate of a 2 × 2 crossover design, which is given by (TRTR, RTRT).

In some cases, an incomplete block design or an extra-reference design such as (TRR, RTR) may be considered depending upon the study objectives of the bioavailability/bioequivalence studies.

10.3.3 Statistical Methods

As indicated earlier, bioequivalence is claimed if the ratio of average bioavailabilities between test and reference products is within the bioequivalence limit of (80.00 percent, 125.00 percent) with 90 percent assurance based on log-transformed data. Along this line, commonly employed statistical methods are the confidence interval approach and the method of interval hypotheses testing.

For the confidence interval approach, a 90 percent confidence interval for the ratio of means of the primary pharmacokinetic response such as AUC or C_{max} is obtained under an analysis of variance model. We claim bioequivalence if the obtained 90 percent confidence interval is totally within the bioequivalence limit of (80.00 percent, 125.00 percent). For the method of interval hypotheses testing, the interval hypotheses that H_0: Bioinequivalence versus H_a: Bioequivalence was decomposed into two sets of one-sided hypotheses. The first set of hypotheses is to verify that the average bioavailability of the test product is not too low, whereas the second set of hypotheses is to verify that average bioavailability of the test product is not too high. Schuirmann's two one-sided tests procedure is commonly employed to for interval hypotheses testing for average bioequivalence (ABE) (Schuirmann 1987).

In practice, other statistical methods such as Westlake's symmetric confidence interval approach, confidence interval based on Fieller's theorem, Chow and Shao's joint confidence region approach (Chow and Shao 1990), Bayesian methods (e.g., Rodda and Davis' method and Mandallaz and Mau's method), and nonparametric methods (e.g., Wilcoxon-Mann-Whitney two one-sided tests procedure, distribution-free confidence interval based on the Hodges-Lehmann estimator, and bootstrap confidence interval) are sometimes considered.

10.3.4 Limitations of Average Bioequivalence

Chen (1997) pointed out that the current ABE approach for bioequivalence assessment has limitations for addressing drug interchangeability especially for drug switchability. These limitations include (1) ABE focuses only on the comparison of population averages between the test and reference drug products, (2) ABE does not provide independent estimation of the intrasubject variances of the drug products under study, and (3) ABE ignores the subject-by-formulation interaction, which may have an impact on drug switchability. As a result, Chen (1997) suggested that current regulation of ABE be switched to the approach of population bioequivalence (PBE) and individual bioequivalence (IBE) to overcome these disadvantages.

Chow and Liu (1997) proposed to perform a meta-analysis for an overview of ABE. The proposed meta-analysis provides an assessment of bioequivalence among generic copies of a brand name drug that can be used as a tool to monitoring the performance of the approved generic copies of the brand name drug. In addition, it provides more accurate estimates of intersubject and intrasubject variabilities of the drug product.

Although the assessment of ABE for generic approval has been in practice for years. Many authors criticize that the assessment of ABE does not address the question of drug interchangeability and it may penalize drug products with less variability. Note that for assessment of bioequivalence for highly variable drug products, Haidar et al. (2008a,b) suggested that a scaled average bioequivalence (SABE) criterion be used in order to account for reference products with huge variability (see, also Davit et al. 2008; Tothfalusi et al. 2009).

10.4 Drug Interchangeability

Under current FDA regulation, two formulations of the same drug or two drug products are said to be bioequivalent if the ratio of means of the primary PK responses such as AUC and C_{max} between the two formulations of the same drug or the two drug products is within (80.00 percent, 125.00 percent) with 90 percent assurance (FDA 1992, 2003a). A generic drug product can serve as the substitute of its brand name drug product if it has been shown to be bioequivalent to the brand name drug. The FDA, however, does not indicate that a generic drug can be substituted by another generic drug even though both of the generic drugs have been shown to be bioequivalent to the same brand name drug. Bioequivalence among generic copies of the same brand name drug is not required. As more generic drugs become available in the marketplace, it is very likely that a patient may switch from one generic drug to another. Therefore, an interesting question for the physicians and the patients is whether the brand name drug and its generic copies can be used safely and interchangeably (see Figure 10.1).

Bioavailability and Bioequivalence

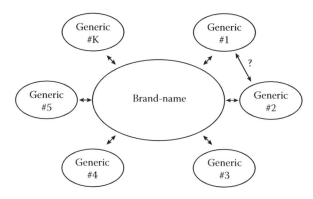

FIGURE 10.1
Drug interchangeability.

10.4.1 Drug Prescribability and Drug Switchability

Basically, drug interchangeability can be classified as drug prescribability or drug switchability. Drug prescribability is defined as the physician's choice for prescribing an appropriate drug product for his/her new patients between a brand name drug product and a number of generic drug products of the brand name drug product that have been shown to be bioequivalent to the brand name drug product. The underlying assumption of drug prescribability is that the brand name drug product and its generic copies can be used interchangeably in terms of the efficacy and safety of the drug product. Drug prescribability, therefore, is the interchangeability for the new patient.

Drug switchability, on the other hand, is related to the switch from a drug product (e.g., a brand name drug product) to an alternative drug product (e.g., a generic copy of the brand name drug product) within the same subject, whose concentration of the drug product has been titrated to a steady, efficacious, and safe level. As a result, drug switchability is considered more critical than drug prescribability in the study of drug interchangeability for patients who have been on medication for a while. Drug switchability, therefore, is exchangeability within the same subject.

10.4.2 Population and Individual Bioequivalence

As indicated by Chow and Liu (2008), ABE can guarantee neither drug prescribability nor drug switchability. Therefore, it is suggested that the assessment of bioequivalence should take into consideration drug prescribability and drug switchability for drug interchangeability. To address drug interchangeability, it is recommended that PBE and IBE be considered for testing drug prescribability and drug switchability, respectively. More specifically, the FDA recommends that PBE be applied to new formulations, additional strengths, or new dosage forms in NDAs, while IBE should be considered for ANDA or Abbreviated Antibiotic Drug Application (AADA) for generic drugs.

To address drug prescribability, the FDA proposed the following population bioequivalence criterion (PBC), which is an aggregated, scaled, moment-based, one-sided criterion:

$$\text{PBC} = \frac{(\mu_T - \mu_R)^2 + \left(\sigma_{TT}^2 - \sigma_{TR}^2\right)}{\max\left(\sigma_{TR}^2, \sigma_{T0}^2\right)} \leq \theta_P,$$

where μ_T and μ_R are the mean of the test drug product and the reference drug product, respectively, σ_{TT}^2 and σ_{TR}^2 are the total variance of the test drug product and the reference drug product, respectively, σ_{T0}^2 is a constant that can be adjusted to control the probability of passing PBE, and θ_P is the bioequivalence limit for PBE. The numerator on the left-hand side of the criterion is the sum of the squared difference of the population averages and the difference in total variance between the test and reference drug products, which measures the similarity for the marginal population distribution between the test and reference drug products. The denominator on the left-hand side of the criterion is a scaled factor that depends on the variability of the drug class of the reference drug product. The FDA guidance suggests that θ_P be chosen as

$$\theta_P = \frac{(\log 1.25)^2 + \varepsilon_P}{\sigma_{T0}^2},$$

where ε_P is guided by the consideration of the variability term $\sigma_{TT}^2 - \sigma_{TR}^2$ added to the ABE criterion. As suggested by the FDA guidance, it may be appropriate that ε_P chosen to be 0.02. For the determination of σ_{T0}^2, the guidance suggests the use of so-called population difference ratio (PDR), which is defined as

$$\text{PDR} = \left[\frac{E(T-R)^2}{E(R-R')^2} \right]^{1/2}$$
$$= \left[\frac{(\mu_T - \mu_R)^2 + \sigma_{TT}^2 + \sigma_{TR}^2}{2\sigma_{TR}^2} \right]^{1/2}$$
$$= \left[\frac{\text{PBC}}{2} + 1 \right]^{1/2}.$$

Therefore, assuming that the maximum allowable PDR is 1.25, substitution of $(\log 1.25)^2/\sigma_{T0}^2$ for PBC without adjustment of the variance term approximately yield $\sigma_{T0} = 0.2$.

Bioavailability and Bioequivalence 229

Similarly, to address drug switchability, the FDA recommended the following individual bioequivalence criterion (IBC), which is an aggregated, scaled, moment-based, one-sided criterion:

$$IBC = \frac{(\mu_T - \mu_R)^2 + \sigma_D^2 + \left(\sigma_{WT}^2 - \sigma_{WR}^2\right)}{\max\left(\sigma_{WR}^2, \sigma_{W0}^2\right)} \leq \theta_I,$$

where σ_{WT}^2 and σ_{WR}^2 are the within subject variance of the test drug product and the reference drug product, respectively, σ_D^2 is the variance due to subject-by-drug interaction, σ_{W0}^2 is a constant that can be adjusted to control the probability of passing IBE, and θ_I is the bioequivalence limit for IBE. The FDA guidance suggests that θ_I be chosen as

$$\theta_I = \frac{(\log 1.25)^2 + \varepsilon_I}{\sigma_{W0}^2},$$

where ε_I is the variance allowance factor, which can be adjusted for sample size control. As indicated in the FDA guidance, ε_I may be fixed between 0.04 and 0. For the determination of σ_{W0}^2, the guidance suggests the use of individual difference ratio (IDR), which is defined as

$$\begin{aligned} IDR &= \left[\frac{E(T-R)^2}{E(R-R')^2}\right]^{1/2} \\ &= \left[\frac{(\mu_T - \mu_R)^2 + \sigma_D^2 + \left(\sigma_{WT}^2 + \sigma_{WR}^2\right)}{2\sigma_{WR}^2}\right]^{1/2} \\ &= \left[\frac{IBC}{2} + 1\right]^{1/2}. \end{aligned}$$

Therefore, assuming that the maximum allowable IDR is 1.25, substitution of $(\log 1.25)^2/\sigma_{W0}^2$ for IBC without adjustment of the variance term approximately yield $\sigma_{W0} = 0.2$.

10.4.3 A Review of the FDA Guidance on Population/Individual Bioequivalence

As indicated earlier, the 2001 FDA draft guidance on Statistical Approaches to Establishing Bioequivalence is intended to address drug interchangeability. As a result, the guidance for assessment of PBE and IBE has a significant impact on pharmaceutical research and development. In what follows, we provide a comprehensive review of the FDA 2001 guidance on population and individual bioequivalence from both scientific/statistical and practical points of view (see also Chow 1999). Without loss of generality, we will only focus on IBE.

10.4.3.1 Aggregated Criteria versus Disaggregated Criteria

The 2001 FDA guidance recommends aggregated criteria as described earlier for assessment of IBE. The IBE criterion takes into account average of bioavailability, variability of bioavailability, and variability due to subject-by-formulation interaction. Under the proposed aggregated criteria, however, it is not clear whether IBE criterion is superior to ABE criterion for assessment of drug interchangeability. In other words, it is not clear whether or not IBE implies ABE under aggregate criteria. Hence, the question of particular interest to pharmaceutical scientists is whether the proposed aggregated criterion can really address drug interchangeability?

Liu and Chow (1997) suggested disaggregated criteria be implemented for assessment of drug interchangeability. The concept of disaggregated criteria for assessment of IBE is described below. In addition to ABE, we may consider the following hypotheses testing for equivalence in variability of bioavailabilities and variability due to subject-by-formulation interaction:

$$H_0 : \sigma_{WT}^2/\sigma_{WR}^2 \geq \Delta_v$$
$$\text{versus } H_a : \sigma_{WT}^2/\sigma_{WR}^2 < \Delta_v$$

and

$$H_0 : \sigma_D^2 \geq \Delta_s$$
$$\text{versus } H_a : \sigma_D^2 < \Delta_s$$

where Δ_v is bioequivalence limit for the ratio of intrasubject variabilities and Δ_s is an acceptable limit for variability due to subject-by-formulation interaction. We conclude IBE if both $(1 - \alpha) \times 100\%$ upper confidence limit for $\sigma_{WT}^2/\sigma_{WR}^2$ is less than Δ_v and $(1 - \alpha) \times 100\%$ upper confidence limit for σ_D^2 is less than Δ_s. Under the above disaggregated criteria, it is clear that IBE implies ABE.

In practice, it is of interest to examine the relative merits and disadvantages between the FDA recommended aggregated criteria and the disaggregated criteria described above for assessment of drug interchangeability. In addition, it is also of interest to compare the aggregated and disaggregated criteria of IBE with the current ABE criterion in terms of the consistencies and inconsistencies in concluding bioequivalence for regulatory approval.

Bioavailability and Bioequivalence 231

10.4.3.2 Masking Effect

The goal for evaluation of bioequivalence is to assess the similarity of the distributions of the PK metrics obtained either from the population or from individuals in the population. However, under the aggregated criteria, different combinations of values for the components of the aggregated criterion can yield the same value. In other words, bioequivalence can be reached by two totally different distributions of PK metrics. This is another artifact of the aggregated criteria. For example, at the 1996 Advisory Committee meeting, it was reported that the data sets from the FDA's files showed that a 14 percent increase in the average (ABE only allow 80.00 to 125.00 percent) is offset by a 48 percent decrease in the variability and the test passes IBE but fails ABE.

10.4.3.3 Power and Sample Size Determination

For the proposed aggregated criterion, it is desirable to have sufficient statistical power to declare IBE if the value of the aggregated criterion is small. On the other hand, we would not want to declare IBE if the value is large. In other words, a desirable property for assessment of bioequivalence is that the power function of the statistical procedure is a monotone decreasing function. However, because different combinations of values of the components in the aggregated criteria may reach the same value, the power function for any statistical procedure based on the proposed aggregated criteria is not a monotone decreasing function. The experience for implementing the aggregated criteria in regulatory approval of generic drugs is lacking.

Another major concern is how the proposed criteria for IBE will affect the sample size determination based on power analysis. Unlike ABE, there exists no closed form for the power function of the proposed statistical procedure for IBE. As a result, the sample size may be determined through a Monte Carlo simulation study. Chow et al. (2002c, 2003) provided formulas (based on normal approximation) for sample size calculation for assessment of PBE and IBE under a 2×4 replicated crossover design. Sample sizes calculated from the formulas were shown to be consistent with those obtained from simulation studies.

10.4.3.4 Two-Stage Test Procedure

To apply the proposed criteria for assessment of IBE, the FDA 2001 guidance suggests the constant scale be used if the observed estimator of σ_{TR} or σ_{WR} is smaller than σ_{T0} or σ_{W0}. However, statistically, the observed estimator of σ_{TR} or σ_{WR} being smaller than σ_{T0} or σ_{W0} does not mean that σ_{TR} or σ_{WR} is smaller than σ_{T0} or σ_{W0}. A test on the null hypothesis that σ_{TR} or σ_{WR} is smaller than

232   *Quantitative Methods for Traditional Chinese Medicine Development*

σ_{T0} or σ_{W0} is necessarily performed. As a result, the proposed statistical procedure for assessment of IBE becomes a two-stage test procedure. It is then recommended that the overall type I error rate and the calculation of power be adjusted accordingly.

10.4.3.5 Replicated Crossover Design

The 2001 FDA draft guidance recommends a 2×4 replicated designs, i.e., (TRTR, RTRT) be used for assessment of IBE without any scientific and/or statistical justification (FDA 2001a). As an alternative to the 2×4 replicated design, the 2001 FDA guidance indicates that a 2×3 replicated crossover design, i.e., (TRT, RTR) may be considered. Several questions are raised. First, it is not clear whether the two replicated crossover designs the optimal design (in terms of power) among all 2×4 and 2×3 replicated crossover designs with respect to the aggregated criterion? Second, it is not clear what the relative efficiency of the two designs is if the total number of observations is fixed. Third, it is not clear how these two designs compare to other 2×4 and 2×3 replicated designs such as (TRRT, RTTR) and (TTRR, RRTT) designs and (TRR, RTT) and (TTR, RRT) designs. Finally, it may be of interest to study the relative merits and disadvantages of these two designs as compared to other designs such as Latin square designs and four-sequence and four-period designs.

Other issues regarding the proposed replicated designs include (1) it will take longer to complete, (2) subject's compliance may be a concern, (3) it is likely to have a higher dropout rate and missing values especially in 2×4 designs, and (4) there is little literature on statistical methods dealing with dropouts and missing values in a replicated crossover design setting.

Note that the 2001 FDA draft guidance provides detailed statistical procedures for assessment of PBE and IBE under the recommended 2×4 replicated design (Hyslop et al. 2000; FDA 2001a). However, no details regarding statistical procedures for assessment of PBE and IBE under the alternative 2×3 replicated design are given. Chow et al. (2002c, 2003) provided detailed statistical procedures for assessment of IBE and PBE, respectively. Note that Chow et al. (2003) pointed out that the statistical procedure for assessment of PBE under the recommended 2×4 replicated design as described in the 2001 FDA guidance (FDA 2001a) was inappropriate owing to the violation of the primary assumption of independence.

10.4.3.6 Outlier Detection

The procedure suggested for detection of outliers is not appropriate for the standard 2×2, the 2×3, or the 2×4 replicated crossover designs because the observed PK metrics from the same subject are correlated. For a valid statistical assessment, the procedures proposed by Chow and Tse (1990) and Liu and Weng (1991) should be used. These proposed statistical procedures

Bioavailability and Bioequivalence 233

for outlier detection in bioequivalence studies were derived under crossover designs, which incorporate the correlations within the same subject. The 2001 FDA draft guidance provides little or no discussion regarding the treatment of identified outliers.

10.5 Controversial Issues

In this section, we will focus on controversial issues related to Fundamental Bioequivalence Assumption, one-fits-all criterion, and issues related to log-transformation of pharmacokinetic data prior to analysis. These controversial issues are briefly described.

10.5.1 Fundamental Bioequivalence Assumption

As indicated by Chow and Liu (2008), bioequivalence studies are performed under the so-called Fundamental Bioequivalence Assumption, which constitutes the legal basis for regulatory approval of generic drug products. Fundamental Bioequivalence Assumption states that

> If two drug products are shown to be bioequivalent, it is assumed that they will reach the same therapeutic effect or they are therapeutically equivalent.

Under the assumption, many investigators interpret it as "If two drug products are shown to be bioequivalent, it is assumed that they will reach the same therapeutic effect or they are therapeutically equivalent, and hence can be used *interchangeably*." Thus, one of the controversial issues is that bioequivalence in a drug absorption profile may not necessarily imply therapeutic equivalence and therapeutic equivalence does not guarantee bioequivalence either. The verification of the Fundamental Bioequivalence Assumption is often difficult, if not impossible, without conducting clinical trials. For some drug products, the Fundamental Bioequivalence Assumption may be verified through the study of *in vitro* and *in vivo* correlation (IVIVC). It should be noted that the Fundamental Bioequivalence Assumption is for drug products with identical active ingredient(s). In practice, there are four possible scenarios when assessing bioequivalence for generics approval:

1. Drug absorption profiles are similar and they are therapeutically equivalent.
2. Drug absorption profiles are not similar but they are therapeutically equivalent.

234   *Quantitative Methods for Traditional Chinese Medicine Development*

3. Drug absorption profiles are similar but they are not therapeutically equivalent.

4. Drug absorption profiles are not similar and they are not therapeutically equivalent.

Scenario 1 is the Fundamental Bioequivalence Assumption, which works if the drug absorption (in terms of the rate and extent of absorption) is predictive of clinical outcomes. In this case, PK responses such as AUC and C_{max} serve as surrogate endpoints for clinical endpoints for assessment of efficacy and safety of the test product under investigation. Scenario 2 is the case where generic companies argue for generic approval of their drug products especially when their products fail to meet regulatory requirements for bioequivalence. In this case, it is doubtful that there is a relationship between PK responses and clinical endpoints. The innovator companies usually argue with the regulatory agency against generic approval with scenario 3. However, more studies are necessarily conducted in order to verify scenario 3. There are no arguments with respect to scenario 4. Under the Fundamental Bioequivalence Assumption, the assessment of average bioequivalence for generic approval has been criticized in that it is based on legal/political deliberations rather than scientific considerations. In the past several decades, many sponsors/researchers have made an attempt to challenge this assumption with no success.

To protect the exclusivity of a brand name drug product, the sponsors of the innovator drug products will make every attempt to prevent generic drug products from being approved by the regulatory agencies such as the FDA. One of the strategies is to challenge the Fundamental Bioequivalence Assumption by filing a *citizen petition* with scientific/clinical justification. Upon the receipt of a citizen petition, the FDA has a legal obligation to respond within 180 days. It should be noted, however, that the FDA will not suspend the review/approval process of generic submission of a given brand name drug even if a citizen petition is under review within the FDA. In practice, whether the Fundamental Bioequivalence Assumption is applicable to drug products with similar but different active ingredient(s) then becomes an interesting but controversial question.

10.5.2 One-Size-Fits-All Criterion

For assessment of average bioequivalence, the FDA adopted a one-fits-all criterion. That is, a test drug product is said to be bioequivalent to a reference drug product if the obtained 90 percent confidence interval for the ratio of means of the primary study endpoint such as AUC or C_{max} is totally within the bioequivalence limit of (80.00 percent, 125.00 percent). The one-fits-all criterion does not take into consideration individual therapeutic window and intrasubject variability, which have been identified to have non-negligible

Bioavailability and Bioequivalence

TABLE 10.3

Classification of Drugs

Class	ITW	ISV	Example
A	Narrow	High	Cyclosporine
B	Narrow	Low	Theophylline
C	Wide	Low to moderate	Most drugs
D	Wide	High	Chlorpromazine or topical corticosteroids

Source: Chen, M.L., Individual bioequivalence. Invited presentation at International Workshop: Statistical and Regulatory Issues on the Assessment of Bioequivalence. Dusseldorf, Germany, October 19–20, 1995.

Note: ISV, intrasubject variability; ITW, individual therapeutic window.

impact on safety and efficacy of generic drug products as compared to the innovative drug products.

In the past several decades, this one-fits-all criterion has been challenged and criticized by many researchers (see, e.g., Chow and Liu 1994). It is suggested flexible criteria in terms of safety (upper bioequivalence limit) and efficacy (lower bioequivalence limit) should be developed based on individual therapeutic window (ITW) and intrasubject variability (ISV) according to the nature of the drug class under study (Table 10.3). However, the one-fits-all criterion is still considered by most regulatory agencies. This is probably because no (documented) evidence of safety issues is raised for those generic drug products approved based on the one-fits-all criterion.

10.5.3 Issues Related to Log Transformation

In practice, bioequivalence is assessed either based on raw data or log-transformed data depending on whether the data are normally distributed. This has raised a controversial issue regarding which model should be used for a fair assessment of bioequivalence. The sponsors often choose the model that serves their purposes (e.g., demonstration of bioequivalence). In many cases, a raw data model may reach a different conclusion regarding bioequivalence than a log-transformation model. This controversial issue has been discussed extensively until guidance on bioequivalence published by the FDA, which recommends a log transformation be performed prior to the assessment of bioequivalence (FDA 2001a).

The 2001 FDA draft guidance provides a rationale for use of logarithmic transformation of exposure measures. The guidance emphasizes that the limited sample size in a typical BE study precludes a reliable determination of the distribution of the data. For some unknown reasons, the guidance does not encourage sponsors to test for normality of error distribution after log transformation nor to use normality of error distribution as a reason for carrying out statistical analysis on the original scale.

With respect to the (pharmacokinetic) rationale, deterministic multiplicative pharmacokinetic models are used to justify the routine use of logarithmic transformation for AUC$(0-\infty)$ and C_{max}. However, the deterministic pharmacokinetic (PK) models are theoretical derivations of AUC$(0-\infty)$ and C_{max} for a single object. The guidance suggest that AUC$(0-\infty)$ be calculated from the observed plasma–blood concentration–time curve using the trapezoidal rule and that C_{max} be obtained directly from the curve, without interpolation. It is not known whether the observed AUC$(0-\infty)$ and C_{max} can provide good approximations to those under the theoretical models if the models are correct.

It should be noted that the AUC$(0-\infty)$ and C_{max} are calculated from the observed plasma-blood concentrations. Therefore, the distributions of the observed AUC$(0-\infty)$ and C_{max} depend on the distributions of plasma-blood concentrations. Liu and Weng (1994) showed that the log-transformed AUC$(0-\infty)$ and C_{max} do not generally follow a normal distribution, even when either the plasma concentrations or log-plasma concentrations are normally distributed. This argues against the routine use of the logarithmic transformation in assessment of bioequivalence. Moreover, Patel (1994) also pointed out that performing a routine log transformation of data and then applying normal, theory-based methods is not a scientific approach. In addition, the sample size of a typical BE study is generally too small to allow an adequate large-sample normal approximation.

Because current statistical methods for evaluation of bioequivalence are based on the normality assumption on the intersubject and intrasubject variabilities, the examination of the normal probability plots for the studentized intersubject and intrasubject residuals should always be carried out for the scale intended to be used in the analysis. In addition, formal statistical tests for normality of the intersubject and intrasubject variabilities can also be carried out through the Shapiro-Wilk's method. Contrary to the misconception of many people, the Shapiro-Wilk's method is an exact method for small samples, such as bioequivalence studies. It is then scientifically imperative that tests for normality be routinely performed for the scale used in analysis, such as log-scale, suggested in the guidance. If normality cannot be satisfied by both original-scale and log-scale, nonparametric methods should be employed.

Other issues concerning the routine use of the logarithmic transformation of exposure responses are the equivalence limits and presentation of the results on the original scale. The guidance recommends that the bioequivalence limits of (80.00 percent, 125.00 percent) on the original scale for assessment of average bioequivalence be used. On the log-scale, they are [log(0.8), log(1.25)] = $(-0.2331, 0.2331)$, where log denotes the natural logarithm. This set of limits is symmetrical about zero on the log scale, but it is not symmetrical on the original scale. It should be noted that the rejection region of Schuirmann's two one-sided tests procedure associated with the new limits of (80.00 percent, 125.00 percent) is larger than that with the limits of

Bioavailability and Bioequivalence

(80.00 percent, 120.00 percent). As a result, a 90 percent confidence interval of (82.00 percent, 122.00 percent), for the ratio of averages of AUC(0–∞) between the test and reference formulations, will pass the bioequivalence test by the new limits, but not by the old limits. The new bioequivalence limits are 12.5 percent wider and 25 percent more liberal in the upper limit than the old limits. A new, wider upper bioequivalence limit may have an influence on the safety of the test formulation, which should be carefully examined if the new bioequivalence limits are adopted.

The FDA guidance requires that the results of analyses be presented on the log scale as well as on the original scale, which can be obtained by taking the inverse transformation. Because the logarithmic transformation is not linear, the inverse transformation of the results to the original scale is not straightforward (Liu and Weng 1991). For example, the point estimator of the ratio of averages on the original scale obtained from the antilog of the estimator of difference in averages on the log scale is biased and is always overestimated. Furthermore, the antilog of the standard deviation of the difference in averages on the log scale is not the standard deviation for the point estimator of the ratio of the averages on the original scale. Further research is needed for the presentation of the results on the original scale, especially the estimation of variability after the analyses are performed on the log scale.

For the limitation of average bioequivalence, consideration of individual therapeutic windows, and the objective of interchangeability, Chen (1995) summarized the merits of individual bioequivalence as follows:

1. Comparison of both averages and variances
2. Considerations of subject-by-formulation interaction
3. Assurance of switchability
4. Provision of flexible bioequivalence criteria for different drugs based on their therapeutic windows
5. Provision of reasonable bioequivalence criteria for drugs with highly intrasubject variability
6. Encouragement or reward of pharmaceutical companies to manufacture a better formulation

To achieve the objective of exchangeability among bioequivalent pharmaceutical products, the criteria for assessment of bioequivalence must possess certain important properties. Chen (1995, 1997) outlined the desirable characteristics of bioequivalence criteria proposed by the FDA which are provided in Table 10.4. In addition, to address the issues of intrasubject variability and subject-by-formulation interaction and to ensure drug switchability, valid statistical procedures, both estimation and hypothesis testing should be developed from the criteria to control the consumer's risk at the pre-specified nominal level (e.g., 5 percent). In addition, the statistical methods developed from the criteria should be able to provide sample size determination; to

238   *Quantitative Methods for Traditional Chinese Medicine Development*

TABLE 10.4

Desirable Features of Bioequivalence Criteria

Comparison of both averages and variances
Assurance of switchability
Encouragement or reward of pharmaceutical companies to manufacture a better formulation
Control of type I error rate (consumer's risk) at 5%
Allowance for determination of sample size
Admission of the possibility of sequence and period effects as well as missing values
User-friendly software application for statistical methods
Provision of easy interpretation for scientists and clinicians
Minimization of increased cost for conducting bioequivalence studies

Source: Chen, M.L., *Journal Biopharmaceutical Statistics*, 7, 5–11, 1997.

take into consideration the nuisance design parameters, such as period or sequence effects; and to develop user-friendly computer software. The most critical characteristics for any proposed criteria will be their interpretation to scientists and clinicians and the cost of conducting bioequivalence studies to provide inference for the criteria.

10.6 Frequently Asked Questions

Although the concepts of PBE and IBE for addressing drug prescribability and drug switchability have been discussed extensively since the early 1990s, the current FDA's position regarding the assessment of bioequivalence is that

> Average bioequivalence is required and individual/population bio-equivalence might be considered.

However, the FDA encourages that medical/statistical reviewers should be consulted if individual/population bioequivalence is to be used. For assessment of bioequivalence, some questions are frequently asked during the regulatory submission and review. In what follows, frequently asked questions in bioequivalence assessment are briefly described.

10.6.1 What If We Pass Raw Data Model but Fail Log-Transformed Data Model?

Most regulatory agencies including FDA, EMA, and WHO recommend that a log transformation of PK parameters of $AUC(0-t)$, $AUC(0-\infty)$, and C_{max} be performed before analysis. No assumption checking or verification of the log-transformed data is encouraged. However, the sponsors often conduct

Bioavailability and Bioequivalence 239

analysis based on both raw data and log-transformed data and submit the one passing bioequivalence testing. If the sponsor passes BE testing under the log-transformed data model, then there is no problem because it meets regulatory requirement. In practice, however, the sponsor may fail BE testing under the log-transformed data model but pass under the raw data model. In this case, the sponsor often provides scientific/statistical justification for the use of the raw data model. One of the most commonly seen scientific/statistical justifications is that the raw data model is a more appropriate statistical model than that of the log-transformed data model because all of the assumptions for the raw data model are met. However, for the raw data model, the bioequivalence limit is often expressed in terms of the ratio of the population means between the test and reference formulations, then the equivalence limit is expressed as a percentage of the population reference average which has to be estimated from the data. Therefore, the variability of the estimated reference average is not considered in the equivalence limit. Hence, the false positive rate for claiming average bioequivalence for the two one-sided tests procedure can be inflated to 50 percent. As a result, one should apply the modified two one-sided tests procedure using the raw data proposed by Liu and Weng (1995) to control the size at the nominal level.

Many researchers have criticized the use of log-transformed data as not scientific/statistically justifiable. Liu and Weng (1991) studied the distribution of log-transformed PK data assuming that the hourly concentrations are normally distributed. The results indicated that the log-transformed data are not normally distributed. Their findings argue against the use of log-transformed data because the primary normality assumption is not met and consequently the assurance of the obtained statistical inference is questionable. In this case, it is suggested that either another transformation such as Box-Cox transformation or a nonparametric method be considered. However, the interpretation of such a transformation is challenging to both pharmacokinetist and biostatistician.

10.6.2 What If We Pass AUC but Fail C_{max}?

On the basis of log-transformed data, the FDA requires that both AUC and C_{max} meet the (80.00 percent, 125.00 percent) bioequivalence limit for establishment of average bioequivalence. In practice, however, it is not uncommon to pass AUC (the extent of absorption) but fail C_{max} (the rate of absorption). In this case, average bioequivalence cannot be claimed according to the FDA guidance on bioequivalence. However, for C_{max}, the EMEA and WHO guidelines use a more relaxed equivalence margin of (70.00 percent, 143.00 percent). Thus, the sponsors often argue with the FDA based on the EMEA and WHO guidelines.

In the case when we pass AUC but fail C_{max}, Endrenyi et al. (1991) suggested considering C_{max}/AUC as an alternative bioequivalence measure for the rate of absorption. However, C_{max}/AUC is not currently selected as the required pharmacokinetic responses for approval of generic drug products by any of the regulatory authorities in the world including the US FDA, EMEA, and WHO. On the other hand, it is very likely that we may pass C_{max} but fail AUC. In this case, it is suggested that we may look at partial AUC as an alternative measure of bioequivalence (see, e.g., Chen et al. 2001) if we fail to pass BE testing based on AUC from 0 to the last time point or AUC from 0 to infinity.

10.6.3 What If We Fail by a Relatively Small Margin?

In practice, it is very possible that we fail BE testing for either AUC or C_{max} by a relatively small margin. For example, suppose the 90 percent confidence interval for AUC is given by (79.50 percent, 120.00 percent), which is slightly outside the lower limit of (80.00 percent, 125.00 percent). In this case, the FDA's position is very clear that "The rule is the rule and you fail." With respect to regulatory review and approval, the FDA is very strict about this rule that the 90 percent confidence interval has to be totally within the bioequivalence limit of (80.00 percent, 125.00 percent) as described in the 2003 FDA guidance. However, the sponsor usually performs either an outlier detection analysis or a sensitivity analysis to resolve the issue. In other words, if a subject is found to be an outlier statistically, it may be excluded from the analysis with appropriate clinical justification. Once the identified outlier is excluded from the analysis, a 90 percent confidence interval is recalculated. If the 90 percent confidence interval after excluding the identified outlier is totally within the bioequivalence limit of (80.00 percent, 125.00 percent), the sponsor then argues to claim bioequivalence.

10.6.4 Can We Still Assess Bioequivalence If There Is a Significant Sequence Effect?

As indicated by Chow and Liu (2008), under a standard two-sequence, two-period (2×2) crossover design, significant sequence effect is an indication of possible (1) failure of randomization, (2) true sequence effect, (3) true carryover effect, and/or (4) true formulation-by-period effect. Under the standard 2×2 crossover design, the sequence effect is confounded with the carryover effect. Therefore, if a significant sequence effect is found, the treatment effect and its corresponding 90 percent confidence interval cannot be estimated without bias owing to possible unequal carryover effects. However, in the 2001 FDA draft guidance, the following list of conditions is provided to rule out the possibility of unequal carryover effects:

1. It is a single-dose study.
2. The drug is not an endogenous entity.

Bioavailability and Bioequivalence 241

3. More than an adequate washout period has been allowed between periods of study and in the subsequent periods the pre-dose biological matrix samples do not exhibit a detectable drug level in any of the subjects.

4. The study meets all scientific criteria (e.g., it is based on an acceptable study protocol, and it contains a validated assay methodology).

The 2001 FDA draft guidance also recommends that sponsors conduct a bioequivalence study with parallel designs if unequal carryover effects become an issue.

10.6.5 What Should We Do When We Have Almost Identical Means but Still Fail to Meet the Bioequivalence Criterion?

It is not uncommon to run into the situation that we have almost identical means but still fail to meet bioequivalence criterion. This may indicate that (1) the variation of the reference product is too large to establish bioequivalence between the test product and the reference product, (2) the bioequivalence study was poorly conducted, and (3) the analytical assay methodology is inadequate and not fully validated. The concept of individual bioequivalence and/or population bioequivalence is an attempt to overcome this problem. As a result, it is suggested that either PBE or IBE be considered to establish bioequivalence. However, in our experience, unless the variability of the test formulation is much smaller than that of the reference formulation, it is still unlikely to pass either PBE or IBE. In addition to avoid masking effect of PBE or IBE, the 2001 FDA draft guidance requires that the geometric test/reference averages be within 80.00 to 125.00 percent, too.

10.6.6 Power and Sample Size Calculation based on Raw Data Model and Log-Transformed Model Are Different

The power analysis calculation and sample size based on the raw data model are different from those under the log-transformed model owing to the fact that they are different models. Under different models, means, standard deviations, and coefficients of variation are different. As mentioned before, for assessment of bioequivalence, all regulatory authorities including the FDA, EMEA, WHO, and Japan require log-transformation of $AUC(0-t)$, $AUC(0-\infty)$, and C_{max} be done before analysis and evaluation of bioequivalence. As a result, one should use differences in mean and standard deviation or coefficient of variation for power analysis and sample size calculation based on the method for the log-transformed model (see, e.g., Chapter 5 of Chow and Liu 2008).

Note that sponsors should make the decision as to which model (the raw data model or the log-transformed data model) will be used for bioequivalence

242   *Quantitative Methods for Traditional Chinese Medicine Development*

assessment. Once the model is chosen, appropriate formulas can be used to determine the sample size. Fishing around to obtain the smallest sample size is not good clinical practice.

10.6.7 Adjustment for Multiplicity

The 2003 FDA guidance for general considerations requires that for $AUC(0-t)$, $AUC(0-\infty)$ and C_{max}, the following information be provided: (1) geometric means, (2) arithmetic means, (3) ratio of means, and (4) 90 percent confidence interval.

In addition, the 2003 FDA guidance recommends that logarithmic transformation be provided for measures for bioequivalence demonstration using a bioequivalence limit of 80.00 to 125.00 percent. Therefore, to pass the average bioequivalence, each 90 percent confidence interval of $AUC(0-t)$, $AUC(0-\infty)$, and C_{max} must fall within 80 and 125 percent. It follows that according to the intersection-union principle (Berger 1982), the type I error rate of average bioequivalence is still controlled under the nominal level of 5 percent. Therefore, there is no need for adjustment due to multiple pharmacokinetic measures.

10.7 Other Applications

In pharmaceutical development, the concept of equivalence should not be limited to bioequivalence for approval of generic drug products. The concept of equivalence can be applied to substantial equivalence for medical devices and biosimilarity for follow-on biologics.

10.7.1 Medical Devices

For medical devices, on the basis of the risk of medical devices posed to the patient and/or user, the FDA categorized medical devices into three classes, Regulations for Class I devices require general controls while the Class II devices require both general controls and special controls. On the other hand, because of higher risks, in addition to general controls and special controls, the US FDA requests that Class III devices require a Premarket Approval (PMA) to obtain marketing clearance. However, for Class I and II devices, the sponsor can make a premarket notification through a 510 (k) submission to the FDA. Under 510 (k), the new device must demonstrate that it is at least safe and effective as a legally US market device or a predicate device. This concept of equivalence for approval of medical devices under 510 (k) is referred to as substantial equivalence. According to the FDA, a device is considered substantially equivalent if either it has (1) the same intended use as

Bioavailability and Bioequivalence

the predicate and (2) the same technological characteristics as the predicate, or it has (1) the same intended use as the predicate and (2) different technological characteristics and the information submitted to FDA. Therefore, in submissions under 510 (k), as compared to the predicate, a device must demonstrate two-sided equivalence in technological characteristics or a one-sided equivalence or noninferiority in safety and effectiveness.

10.7.2 Follow-On Biologics

Unlike small-molecule drug products, a generic version of a biologic product is only a similar biological drug product (SBDP) in comparison with the originator biological product. It should be noted that the SBDP are not like the small-molecule generic drug products, which are usually referred to as containing identical active ingredient(s) as the innovative drug product. The concept for the development of SBDP, which are made of living cells or organisms, is very different from that of the (small-molecule) generic drug products. The SBDP are usually referred to as biosimilars by the European Medicines Agency (EMA) of European Union (EU), follow-on biologics (FOB or FoB) by the US FDA, and subsequent entered biologics (SEB) by Health Canada.

10.7.2.1 Fundamental Differences

Biosimilars are fundamentally different from small-molecule generic drugs. Some of the fundamental differences between biosimilars and generic drugs are summarized in Table 10.5. As can be seen from the table, for example, small-molecule drug products are made by chemical synthesis, while large-molecule biologics are made of living cells or organisms. Small-molecule drug products have well-defined structures that are easy to characterize, while biosimilars have heterogeneous structures with mixtures of related molecules that are difficult to characterize. Small-molecule drug products

TABLE 10.5

Fundamental Differences between Generic Drugs and Biosimilars

Generic Drugs	Biosimilars
Made by chemical synthesis	Made by living cells or organisms
Defined structure	Heterogeneous structure
	Mixtures of related molecules
Easy to characterize	Difficult to characterize
Relatively stable	Variable
No issue of immunogenicity	Sensitive to environmental conditions such as light and temperature
	Issue of immunogenicity
Usually taken orally	Usually injected
Often prescribed by a general practitioner	Usually prescribed by specialists

244   *Quantitative Methods for Traditional Chinese Medicine Development*

are usually relatively stable, while biosimilars are known to be variable and very sensitive to environmental conditions such as light and temperature. A small change or variation during the manufacturing process may translate to a drastic change in clinical outcomes (e.g., safety and effectiveness). Small-molecule drug products that are often taken orally are generally prescribed by general practitioners, while biosimilars that are usually injected are often prescribed by specialists. In addition, unlike small-molecule drug products, biosimilars may induce unwanted immune responses that may cause a loss of efficacy or change in their safety profile. Moreover, with differences in the size and complexity of the active substance, important differences also include the nature of the manufacturing process.

10.7.2.2 Approval Pathway of Biosimilars

For approval of biosimilars in the European Union (EU), the EMA has issued guidelines describing general principles for the approval of similar biological medicinal products or biosimilars (EMA 2010). The guideline is accompanied by several concept papers that outline areas in which the agency intends to provide more targeted guidance. Specifically, the concept papers discuss approval requirements for four classes of human recombinant products containing erythropoietin, human growth hormone, granulocyte-colony stimulating factor, and insulin. The guideline consists of a checklist of documents published to date relevant to data requirements for biological pharmaceuticals. It is not clear what specific scientific requirements will be applied to biosimilar applications. In addition, it is not clear how the agency will treat innovator data contained in the reference product dossiers. The guideline provide a useful summary of the biosimilar legislation and previous EU publications, it provides few answers to the issues. On the other hand, for approval of follow-on biologics in the United States, it depends whether the biologic product is approved under the US Food, Drug, and Cosmetic Act (FD&C) or it is licensed under the US Public Health Service Act (PHS). As indicated, some proteins are licensed under the PHS Act, while some are approved under the FD&C Act. For products approved under an NDA (US FD&C Act), generic version of the products can be approved under an ANDA, e.g., under Section 505(b)(2) of FD&C Act. For products that are licensed under a BLA (US PHS Act), there exists no abbreviated BLA at present time.

As pointed out by Woodcock et al. (2007), for assessment of similarity of follow-on biologics, the FDA would consider the following factors regarding (1) the robustness of the manufacturing process, (2) the degree to which structural similarity could be assessed, (3) the extent to which the mechanism of action was understood, (4) the existence of valid, mechanistically related pharmacodynamic assays, (5) comparative pharmacokinetics, (6) comparative immunogenicity, (7) the amount of clinical data available, and (8) the extent of experience with the original product.

Bioavailability and Bioequivalence

In practice, there is a strong industrial interest and desire for the regulatory agencies to develop review standards and an approval process for biosimilars rather than an ad hoc case-by-case review of individual biosimilar applications. Under these considerations, the FDA published several draft guidances on assessment of biosimilar products on February 9, 2012. However, little or no information regarding criteria for biosimilarity was mentioned. More research on methodology development for assessing biosimilarity and interchangeability is urgently needed.

10.7.2.3 Biosimilarity

On March 23, 2010, the *Biologics Price Competition and Innovation* (BPCI) Act (as part of the Affordable Care Act) was enacted, which has given the FDA the authority to approve similar biological drug products. As indicated in the BPCI Act, a biosimilar product is defined as a product that is highly similar to the reference product notwithstanding minor differences in clinically inactive components and there are no clinically meaningful differences in terms of safety, purity, and potency. There are no clinically meaningful differences between a biosimilar and an originator biological product in terms of safety, purity, and potency. On the basis of this definition, we would interpret that a biological medicine is biosimilar to a reference biological medicine if it is highly similar to the reference in safety, purity, and potency. Here purity may be related to some important quality attributes at critical stages of the manufacturing process and potency has something to do with the stability and efficacy of the biosimilar product. However, little or no discussion regarding how similar is considered highly similar (or how close is considered sufficiently close) was mentioned in the BPCI Act.

10.7.2.4 Interchangeability

As indicated in the BPCI Act, a biological product is considered to be interchangeable with the reference product if (1) the biological product is biosimilar to the reference product; and (2) it can be expected to produce the same clinical result in any given patient. In addition, for a biological product that is administered more than once to an individual, the risk in terms of safety or diminished efficacy of alternating or switching between use of the biological product and the reference product is not greater than the risk of using the reference product without such alternation or switch. Thus, by definition, there is a clear distinction between biosimilarity and interchangeability. In other words, biosimilarity does not imply interchangeability, which is much more stringent. The BPCI Act states also that if a test product is judged to be interchangeable with the reference product then it may be substituted, even alternated, without a possible intervention, or even notification, of the health care provider.

246　Quantitative Methods for Traditional Chinese Medicine Development

10.7.2.5 Scientific Factors and Practical Issues

One of key scientific factors for assessing biosimilarity of follow-on biologics is "How similar is highly similar?" Neither the BPCI Act nor the FDA draft guidance on biosimilars provide definition of highly similar. In practice, one would think that the degree of similarity determine highly similar based on some given criteria for biosimilarity. However, there is little or no information regarding "What criteria are considered the most appropriate criteria for assessing biosimilarity and/or interchangeability?" Current practice is to adopt the (80.00 percent, 125.00 percent) criterion for assessment of bioequivalence for generic approval based on log-transformed pharmacokinetic responses such as AUC and C_{max} without any scientific justification. This criterion was found not appropriate due to the fundamental differences between generics and biosimilars (see, e.g., Chow et al. 2011). Another practical issue is related to the question "How many biosimilar studies are required for establishing biosimilarity of follow-on biologics?" As pointed out by BPCI Act, biosimilarity of biosimilars to the innovative biological product must be demonstrated in safety, purity, and potency. Thus, biosimilar studies could include clinical safety/tolerability and immunogenicity studies (safety), critical quality attributes at various stages of biological manufacturing process (purity), and efficacy study (potency). Furthermore, in the interest of drug interchangeability, "How to assess switching and/or interchangeability?" has become a debatable issue due to the definition of interchangeability as described in the BPCI Act. In practice, it is not possible to show that biosimilars can produce the same clinical result as compared to the reference product in any given patient. However, it is possible to demonstrate that they can produce the same clinical results in any given patient with certain assurances. On February 9, 2012, the FDA circulated draft guidance on scientific consideration for demonstration of biosimilarity of follow-on biologics. In the draft guidance, the FDA recommends a stepwise approach for providing the totality-of-the-evidence for assessing biosimilarity of follow-on biologics. However, no specific guidance was provided as to "How to implement stepwise approach and provide totality-of-the-evidence as suggested by the draft guidance of the FDA?" The guidance emphasizes the importance of reference standard. However, little or no information regarding "How to establish reference standards?" was mentioned in the draft guidance.

To address these scientific factors and practical issues, the FDA has hosted a couple of public hearings in November 2–3, 2010 and May 11, 2012. At the same time, many researchers have devoted to methodology development for assessing biosimilarity and/or interchangeability. In the past few years, despite several journals (e.g., *Statistics in Medicine, Journal of Biopharmaceutical Statistics, Generics and Biosimilar Initiatives,* and the *Chinese Journal of Pharmaceutical Analysis*) have published special issues on biosimilars attempting to address these scientific factors and practical issues, many scientific factors and practical issues still remain unsolved.

Bioavailability and Bioequivalence

10.8 Concluding Remarks

As indicated in Chapter 1, the FDA kicked off a critical path initiative to assist the sponsors in identifying the scientific challenges underlying the medical product pipeline problems. A critical path opportunities list was released in 2006 to bridge the gap between the quick pace of new biomedical discoveries and the slower pace at which those discoveries are currently developed into therapies. However, the assessment of bioequivalence for generic approval was not included until a year later. In May 2007, the FDA issued the critical path opportunities for generic drugs that lay out the opportunities as well as the challenges that are unique to the generic drug products. Note that the critical path opportunities for generic drugs were issued by the Office of Generic Drugs, Center for Drug Evaluation and Research. Consequently, the critical path opportunities for generic drugs are only confined to the traditional chemical drug products (it could include medical devices and biosimilars).

Although bioavailability for *in vivo* bioequivalence studies is usually assessed through the measures of the rate and extent to which the drug product is absorbed into the bloodstream of human subjects, for some locally acting drug products such as nasal aerosols (e.g., metered-dose inhalers) and nasal sprays (e.g., metered-dose spray pumps) that are not intended to be absorbed into the bloodstream, bioavailability may be assessed by measurements intended to reflect the rate and extent to which the active ingredient or active moiety becomes available at the site of action. For those local delivery drug products, the US FDA indicates that bioequivalence may be assessed, with suitable justification, by *in vitro* bioequivalence studies alone (see, e.g., Part 21 Codes of Federal Regulations Section 320.24). In practice, it is expected that *in vitro* bioequivalence testing has less variability (say, <10 percent) due to analytical testing results, while *in vivo* bioequivalence testing has larger variability (say, between 20 and 30 percent). Unlike small molecule drug products, biosimilars are expected to have much larger variability (say, 40 to 50 percent). The magnitude of variability has an impact on the corresponding criteria for assessment of bioequivalence or biosimilarity. To provide a better understanding, Table 10.6 provides a comparison of *in vitro* bioequivalence testing, *in vivo* bioequivalence testing and testing for biosimilarity of follow-on biologics.

Unlike most small molecule drug products that contain one single active ingredient, TCM usually contain several components. For assessment of bioequivalence, it is not clear whether bioequivalence assessment should be done on each components or in total. One of the major challenges is that the pharmacological activity of each component is usually unknown and cannot be characterized based on current technology. In practice, it is suggested that TCM be treated as a combinational drug product with multiple components. The problem is that the relative ratios (proportions) of these components are

248 *Quantitative Methods for Traditional Chinese Medicine Development*

TABLE 10.6

Comparison among *in vitro* BE Testing, *in vivo* BE Testing, and Biosimilarity Testing

	In vitro **BE Testing**	*In vivo* **BE Testing**	**Biosimilarity Testing**
Characteristic	Drug release/delivery	Drug absorption	Drug absorption
Experimental unit	Bottles	Healthy volunteers	Healthy volunteers or patients
Sample size	3 lots per treatment and 10 units from each lot	24 to 36 subjects	48 subjects or more
Variability	Controllable	Not controllable	Not controllable
Variability range	<10%	20%–30%	40%–50%
Criterion	(90.00%, 111.00%)	(80.00%, 125.00%)	SABE, e.g., (70.00%, 143.00%)
Assumption	IVIVC	Fundamental Bioequivalence Assumption	Totality-of-the-evidence

Note: IVIVC, *in vitro* and *in vivo* correlation; SABE, scaled average bioequivalence criterion.

usually unknown. A slightly change or variation of these relative ratios may result in a major change in clinical outcomes. In other words, it is an interesting question to the investigators whether the Fundamental Bioequivalence Assumption can be applied to drug products with multiple components if there is evidence of (1) possible drug-to-drug (component-to-component) interaction, (2) different dose response curves for different components, and (3) different ratios of the components may result in different clinical outcomes. In this case, pilot studies for determining the best combination (relative ratio) for achieving the optimal therapeutic effect and possible component-to-component interactions must be conducted. Once these have been established, regulatory guidance (for criteria, design, and methods for data analysis) for assessment of bioequivalence and/or biosimilarity for drug product with multiple components (e.g., TCMs) are necessarily developed so that standard methods that are similar to the assessment of bioequivalence described in this chapter can be established accordingly.

11

Population Pharmacokinetics

11.1 Introduction

For a drug product under development, it is of interest to study how the drug moves through the body and the processes of movement such as absorption (A), distribution (D), metabolism (M), and excretion (E) after drug administration. This leads to the study of pharmacokinetics (PK). The key concept of a PK study is to study what the body does to the drug, which is usually characterized by ADME of a drug product after administration. In practice, however, we cannot measure concentrations at the site of action directly. Instead, we can measure concentrations in blood, plasma, or serum that reflect ADME at the site of action. The site of action is defined as the site at which the drug will have its effect. Concentrations have valuable information regarding ADME that allows manipulation of concentrations in early drug development so that the concentrations will remain within the therapeutic window (or index) of safety and efficacy. The bioequivalence testing described in Chapter 10 is to show that the primary PK parameters such as AUC and C_{max}, which reflect the extent and rate of drug absorption of the test product are not too high to avoid toxicity (safety) on one hand and are not too low to produce response (efficacy) on the other hand as compared to those of the reference product (innovative or brand name drug product).

Population pharmacokinetics (population PK) is the study of the sources and correlates of variability in drug concentrations among individuals who are the target patient population receiving clinically relevant doses of a drug of interest (Aarons 1991). Thus, population PK is to study the relationship between dose and concentration for both individuals and the population of individuals. The study of individual PK parameters has become very popular because it is a representative sample of a population of such individuals. Individual PK parameters are usually estimated by fitting a PK model. The analysis of PK responses has emerged as a useful approach to ascertaining the nature of drug disposition in patient populations. Although such an analysis permits the evaluation of associations between patient characteristics and variation in drug disposition, it usually involves a nonlinear mixed effects model, which presents certain statistical and PK modeling difficulties. Such an analysis is usually performed after a considerably large database of concentrations, doses, and patient characteristics is established. For estimation of population PK parameters, a traditional approach is to employ a so-called standard two-stage (STS) method. At the first stage, we estimate individual parameters. Then, we treat the estimates as samples to obtain a confidence interval for the population parameters. This method, however, does not account for the variability of the estimates obtained from the first stage. To avoid individual estimates, Sheiner et al. (1972, 1977) proposed an alternative first-order (FO) method for estimation of the mean and variance of the population parameters by minimizing an extended least squares criterion. This method, which uses a nonlinear mixed effect model, is available in the software NONMEM (Beal and Sheiner 1980). Several other methods, including parametric and nonparametric, have been developed. These methods include the use of the EM algorithm (Dempster et al. 1977) and the Bayesian approach (Racine-Poon 1985). In addition, Prevost, in an unpublished report, proposed an iterative two-stage (ITS) method that uses a linearization of the model around the estimated parameters, under the assumption of a normal distribution of parameters (Steimer et al. 1984). The ITS method has been investigated by Lindstrom and Bates (1990) under different approximations. For nonparametric methods, Mallet (1986) developed a method based on maximum likelihood of the whole set of individual measurements. Schumitzky (1990) also proposed a nonparametric algorithm to estimate the distribution using an EM estimation approach. For a one-compartment model, these methods are available on the software NPEM (Jelliffe et al. 1990). For application of a recent development in linear and nonlinear mixed effects model to population PK, see Davidian and Giltinan (1995), Vonesh and Chinchilli (1997), and Davidian (2003).

As one of the primary objectives of a population PK study is to estimate accurately and precisely the kinetic parameters in a population and the population parameters quantify the mean kinetics in the population, the interindividual kinetic variability, and the intraindividual variability of measured kinetic responses, it is suggested that a valid and efficient design should be used in order to produce accurate and reliable estimates of population parameters. For this purpose, some design factors such as the number of subjects, the number of concentrations measured in each individual, and the sampling times of the biologic fluid (e.g., blood) in which the drug concentration is determined are necessarily considered for achieving the desired degree of accuracy and precision of the estimates of the population parameters. These design factors can be controlled to a certain extent by conducting a prospective population kinetic study. The most widely accepted theoretical approach of determining optimal sampling times for PK studies is based on the Fisher information matrix. A commonly used criterion for determining optimal sampling times is to maximize the determinant of the Fisher information matrix (or equivalently minimize the inverse of the determinant),

Population Pharmacokinetics 251

which is known as the D-optimality criterion. Following the concept of D-optimality, two approaches are commonly considered in designing a population PK study. These two approaches are the population Fisher information matrix approach (Wang and Endrenyi 1992) and the informative block randomized (IBR) approach (Ette et al. 1994).

The chapter is organized as follows. In Section 11.2, regulatory requirements for the use of population PK in pharmaceutical development are given. Approaches for population PK modeling are described in Section 11.3. Approaches to the design of population pharmacokinetic studies are discussed in Section 11.4. Section 11.5 gives an example to illustrate statistical methods described in this chapter. Section 11.6 provides some concluding remarks including study protocol, concerns/challenges of the population approach in population PK, the relationship between PK and pharmacodynamics (PD), the use of computer simulation, and software applications.

11.2 Regulatory Requirements

In 1999, the FDA issued guidance on Population Pharmacokinetics (FDA 1999). In this guidance, the FDA provides some recommendations on design and analysis of a population pharmacokinetic study. Also, included in this guidance are data handling such as missing data and outliers, population PK model development, and validation. These requirements are briefly summarized below.

11.2.1 Population PK Analysis

As indicated in the 1999 FDA guidance on Population PK, the population model defines at least two levels of hierarchy. At the first level, pharmacokinetic observations in an individual such as concentrations are viewed as arising from an individual probability model, whose mean is given by a pharmacokinetic model quantified by individual-specific parameters. At the second level, the individual parameters are regarded as random variables. Because the focus of a population PK study is on population of individual PK parameters, the FDA suggests the two commonly used methods, namely, the two-stage approach and the nonlinear mixed effects modeling approach are considered in population PK analysis. As pointed out by the FDA, although the traditional two-stage approach (when applicable) can yield adequate estimates of population characteristics, it may not be applicable in sparse data situations because individual parameters may be hard to estimate. The standard two-stage approach and the nonlinear mixed effects modeling approach will be discussed in detail in the next section.

11.2.2 Study Design

At the planning of a population PK study, it is suggested that certain preliminary pharmacokinetic information and the drug's major elimination pathways in humans should be available. In addition, a sensitive and specific assay capable of measuring the drug and all metabolites of clinical relevance should be available. When designing a population PK study, FDA suggests that some design considerations such as sampling times, number of samples per subject, and number of subjects be considered for an accurate and reliable assessment of population characteristics. Optimizing the sampling design is of particular importance when severe limitations exist on the number of subjects and/or samples per subject (e.g., in pediatric patients or the elderly). FDA recommends some informative designs proposed in the literature (e.g., Hashimoto and Sheiner 1991; Johnson et al. 1996; Sun et al. 1996) be used to ensure that there are enough patients not only for an accurate and precise estimation of the population parameters but also for detection of any subgroup differences with a desired power.

11.2.3 Population PK Model Development/Validation

For development of a population PK model, the FDA suggests that the objectives and hypotheses be stated clearly. It is recommended that all assumptions inherent in the population analysis be explicitly expressed. The criteria and rationale for model building procedures dealing with confounding, covariate, and parameter redundancy should be stated clearly. The steps taken for model building should be outlined clearly to permit the reproducibility of the analysis. For a developed population PK model, the FDA recommends that the reliability of the analysis results be examined through diagnostic plots, including predicted versus observed concentration, predicted concentration superimposed on the data, and posterior estimates of parameters versus covariate values. Whenever possible, evaluation for robustness using sensitivity analysis should be conducted.

For validation of a population PK model, because there is no consensus on an appropriate statistical approach to validation of population PK models, the FDA suggests focusing on the predictive performance aspect of validation either through an external validation or an internal validation. External validation is the application of the developed model to a new data set (validation data set) from another study, while internal validation refers to the use of data splitting (e.g., cross validation) and resampling techniques (e.g., bootstrapping). The predictive performance aspect of validation is defined as the evaluation of the predictability of the model developed using a learning or index data set when applied to a validation data set not used for model building and parameter estimation.

Note that the FDA indicated that not all population PK models need to be validated. If the population PK analysis results will be incorporated in

Population Pharmacokinetics 253

the drug label, model validation is encouraged and model validation procedures should be an integral part of the protocol. If population PK models are developed to explain variability with no dosage adjustment recommendation envisaged and to provide descriptive information for labeling, models can be tested for stability only.

11.2.4 Missing Data and Outlier

In population PK studies, missing values commonly occur at either PK response or covariates. Missing data are potential sources of bias. Excluding all subjects with any missing data will decrease the sample size. Thus, in certain situations, it may be better to impute missing values rather than to delete those subjects with missing values from analysis. As indicated in the 1999 FDA guidance, although many methods for imputation are available in the literature, the performance of imputation techniques in this context is not well studied. Thus, the FDA suggests that the imputation procedure should be described and a detailed explanation of how such imputations were done and the underlying assumptions made should be provided.

For outliers, either outlying individuals (intersubject variability) or outlying data points (intrasubject variability), the FDA requires that the reasons for declaring an outlying data point should be statistically convincing and if possible be pre-specified in the study protocol.

11.2.5 Timing for Application

The use of the population PK approach can help increase understanding of the quantitative relationship among drug input patterns, patient characteristics, and drug disposition. It is helpful in situations when the investigator wishes to identify factors that affect drug behavior or to explain variability in a target population. The population PK approach is especially helpful in certain adaptive study designs such as dose finding studies in early stages of drug development.

As indicated in the 1999 FDA guidance, the FDA advises that in certain circumstances such as (1) when the population for which the drug is intended is quite heterogeneous and (2) when the target concentration window is believed to be relatively narrow, the population PK approach is most likely to add value when a reasonable *a priori* expectation exists that intersubject kinetic variation may warrant altered dosing for some subgroups in the target population. The FDA also pointed out that the population PK approach is most likely used in phase I and late phase IIb of clinical development for estimation of population parameters of a response surface model where information is gathered on how the drug will be used in subsequent stages of drug development (see also Sheiner 1997). However, the FDA also noted that in phase I and much of phase IIb studies where patients are usually sampled extensively, complex methods of data analysis may not be needed.

The population PK approach can also be used in early phase IIa and phase III of drug development to gain information on drug safety (efficacy) and to gather additional information on drug pharmacokinetics in special populations. The population PK approach can also be useful in phase IV studies such as post-marketing surveillance or labeling change.

11.3 Population PK Modeling

As indicated earlier, the movement of a drug administered to a patient is studied via some population characteristics that describe absorption, distribution, metabolism, and elimination of the drug. These population characteristics are measured by some pharmacokinetic parameters such as the fraction of each dose that is absorbed when the drug is given by the oral route (absorption), volume of distribution of the drug with respect to its concentration (distribution) and the clearance of the drug with respect to its concentration in plasma (elimination). In practice, it is of interest to learn about the variation of PK parameters in a target patient population. This leads to the study of population pharmacokinetic modeling. In what follows, several approaches for estimation of population characteristics of pharmacokinetic parameters are described.

11.3.1 Traditional Two-Stage Method

The traditional approach for estimation of population characteristics of PK parameters consists of two stages, which are described below. At the first stage, for each of a number of patients, enough dosages are administered and enough plasma concentrations are drawn to allow the PK parameters to be estimated for each individual. Estimates of these PK parameters are often obtained based on a deterministic pharmacokinetic model (e.g., a one-compartment model or a multiple-compartment model). Then, at the second stage, based on estimates of the PK parameters obtained from each individual, an analysis of covariance model is considered to avoid effects due to possible confounding and/or interaction among covariates (e.g., demographics or patient characteristics) and to study the treatment effects (e.g., dosage and route of administration) and between-individual variation.

In practice, there are obvious obstacles to this traditional approach including the ethical issue and cost. From a statistical point of view, the traditional approach suffers the following disadvantages. First, the use of estimates based on a deterministic model from each individual does not take into consideration the variability of each individual (i.e., intraindividual variability). Second, sparse and/or haphazard sampling of each subject

Population Pharmacokinetics

may not provide accurate and reliable estimates of the PK parameters for each subject. To overcome this problem, the frequency of sampling for blood drawn is necessary, which may lead to the ethical concern. Third, the traditional approach may not be useful in describing population characteristics when there are a lot of demographic, physiological, and/or behavioral characteristics recorded for each subject such as weight, age, renal function, race, ethnicity, disease status, and so on which are often of interest to the investigator.

11.3.2 Nonlinear Mixed Effects Modeling Approach

As an alternative to the traditional two-stage method, the FDA suggests the use of a nonlinear mixed effects modeling approach. The approach of nonlinear mixed effects modeling is a nonlinear regression model that accounts for both fixed and random effects. It provides estimates of population characteristics that define the population distribution of the PK and/or PD parameters.

In the 1970s, Sheiner et al. (1972, 1977) laid the foundations of population pharmacokinetic modeling. They showed how, with data collected as part of routine patient care, such modeling can estimate the average values of PK parameters and the interindividual variances of those parameters in a patient population. With such sparsely sampled data from patients, their methodology produced estimates that were similar to published values derived with traditional methods.

11.3.2.1 First-Order Method

Let y_{ij} be the jth (plasma or serum) concentration obtained from the ith subject, where $j = 1,...,n_i$ and $i = 1,...,m$ and $N = \sum_{i=1}^{m} n_i$ is the total number of observations. Also, let x_{ij} be conditions of jth measurement (e.g., times, doses) from the ith subject. As discussed earlier, our focus is not on population mean concentration, but on population of individual PK parameters. This leads to the use of a nonlinear mixed effects model. Following the concept of the two-stage approach, for the first stage, we consider so-called intrasubject PK model. Consider the following model:

$$y_{ij} = f(x_{ij}, \beta_i) \cdot e_{ij}, \tag{11.1}$$

where

$$E(y_{ij}|\beta_i) = f(x_{ij}, \beta_i),$$
$$\mathrm{Var}(y_{ij}|\beta_i) = \upsilon\{f(x_{ij}, \beta_i), \xi\},$$

in which f dictated by compartment model, superposition of past doses, β_i is a $p \times 1$ vector of PK parameters, as an example

$$\beta_i = (F_i, Cl_i, V_{di})' \tag{11.2}$$

as considered by Sheiner et al. (1977). For the second stage, we consider the intersubject population model as follows:

$$\beta_i = d(a_i, \beta, b_i),$$

where a_i is the subject characteristic (covariate) of the ith subject and b_i is a $k \times 1$ vector of random effects which follows a k-variate distribution with mean 0 and variance-covariance matrices D. As a result, the two-stage hierarchy leads to the following intrasubject PK model (stage 1):

$$\begin{aligned} y_i &= f_i(\beta_i) \cdot e_i \\ &= f_i(\beta_i) \cdot R_i^{1/2}(\beta_i, \xi) \cdot \varepsilon_i \end{aligned} \tag{11.3}$$

where

$$\begin{aligned} E(y_i|b_i) &= f_i(\beta_i), \\ \mathrm{Var}(y_i|b_i) &= R_i(\beta_i \xi). \end{aligned}$$

Note that

$$P_{y|b}\left(y_i|x_{i1}, \dots, x_{in_i}, a_i, \beta, b_i, \xi\right) = P_{y|b}\left(y_i|\beta, b_i, \xi\right).$$

For the intersubject population model (stage 2), we have

$$\beta_i = d(a_i, \beta, b_i),$$

where

$$b_i \sim H = N_k(0, D).$$

Under this two-stage hierarchical model, the objectives are to (1) determine d (i.e., the relationship between PK and covariates), (2) estimate β (i.e., the relationship between PK and covariates), (3) estimate H (i.e., the variation in population), and (4) estimate β_i (i.e., characterize individuals and consequently optimize or individualized dosing). For achieving these objectives,

Population Pharmacokinetics 257

we consider maximizing the following likelihood function for obtaining the maximum likelihood estimates:

$$l(\beta,\xi,H) = \sum_{i=1}^{m} l_i(\beta,\xi,H)$$
$$= \sum_{i=1}^{m} P_{y|b}(y_i|\beta,b_i,\xi)dH(b_i). \tag{11.4}$$

Because of the complexity of the likelihood function (i.e., nonlinear in b_i), there exist no closed forms for the maximum likelihood estimates if they are not intractable. Beal and Sheiner (1982) considered first-order approximation about $b_i = 0$ assuming that $P_{y|b}$ is normal and $H = N_k(0, D)$. In other words, they considered

$$y_i = f_i\{d(a_i,\beta,b_i)\} + R_i^{1/2}(d(a_i,\beta,b_i),\xi)\cdot\varepsilon_i$$
$$\approx f_i\{d(a_i,\beta,0)\} + Z_i(\beta,0)b_i + R_i^{1/2}\{d(a_i,\beta,0)\}\cdot\varepsilon_i. \tag{11.5}$$

Then, approximate l_i by the n_i-variate normal with

$$E(y_i) \approx f_i\{d(a_i, \beta, 0)\},$$

and

$$\mathrm{Var}(y_i) \approx R_i\{d(a_i,\beta,0)\} + Z_i(\beta,0)DZ_i'(\beta,0).$$

This was implemented in the FORTRAN program in NONMEM (it was referred to as the FO method).

11.3.2.2 An Example

As an example, consider the specific case of digoxin as described by Sheiner et al. (1977). Suppose the population characteristics describing absorption, distribution, and elimination of the drug are of particular interest to the investigator. For absorption, the pharmacokinetic parameter considered is F_{oral}, which is the fraction of each dose that is absorbed when the drug is given by oral route. For distribution, the volume of distribution, denoted by V_d, of the drug with respect to its concentration in plasma is examined. For elimination, the clearance of the drug (Cl) with respect to its concentration in plasma is assessed. Suppose we wish to model the kinetics of a drug using the one-compartment open model. Without loss of generality, we will only consider the single-dose case. Let C_{ij} be the ith measured plasma concentration in the jth individual at time t_{ij}. Thus, the one-compartment open model leads to

$$C_{ij} = \left(\frac{F_j \cdot D_j}{V_{dj}} \right) \exp(-Cl_j / V_{dt} \cdot t_{ij}) \qquad (11.6)$$

where F_j is the fraction of drug absorbed by the jth individual when receiving a dose by the chosen route, D_j is the dose received by the jth individual, V_{dj} is the volume of distribution for the drug in the jth individual, Cl_j is the drug clearance for the jth individual, and t_{ij} is the time of drawing the ith sample in the jth individual ($t_{ij} = 0$ at the time of administration of the dose D_j). Note that although there are three unknown parameters: F_j, V_{dj}, and Cl_j, only two constants, F_j/V_{dj} and Cl_j/V_{dj} could be estimated for any individual from one single study. Now, suppose that drug clearance can be described by the following relation:

$$Cl_j = A + B \cdot Cl_j^{Cr}, \qquad (11.7)$$

where Cl_j^{Cr} is the creatinine clearance for the jth individual, a quantity that can be directly measured or can be estimated from other data such as serum creatinine value, A and B are some fixed constants which relate drug clearance to creatinine clearance. Further, suppose that the volume of distribution depends on renal function and has the following relationship:

$$V_{dj} = D + E \cdot Cl_j^{Cr}, \qquad (11.8)$$

where D and E are some fixed constants, which must be estimated from data. As it can be seen that Equations 11.1 through 11.3 are deterministic models. To have accurate and reliable assessment of population characteristics, we should take into consideration the variabilities associated with each deterministic model. This leads to

$$C_{ij} = \left(\frac{F_j \cdot D_j}{V_{dj}} \right) \exp(-Cl_j / V_{dj} \cdot t_{ij}) \cdot \varepsilon_{ij},$$

$$Cl_j = A + B \cdot Cl_j^{Cr} + \eta_j^{Cr}, \qquad (11.9)$$

$$V_{dj} = D + E \cdot Cl_j^{Cr} + \eta_j^{V},$$

where $\varepsilon_{ij}, \eta_j^{Cr}$, and η_j^{Cr} follow normal distribution with mean 0 and variances $\sigma_\varepsilon^2, \sigma_{Cl}^2$, and σ_V^2, respectively. Sheiner et al. (1977) suggested linearizing

Population Pharmacokinetics

model 11.4 first and then considering an approximation based on the first-term Taylor series expansion. After some algebra, model 11.4 becomes

$$C_{ij} = M_{ij} \left[1 + \left(\frac{Cl_j}{V_{dj}^2} t_{ij} - \frac{1}{V_{dj}} \right) \eta_j^V - \frac{t_{ij}}{V_{dj}} \eta_j^{Cr} \right] + \left(\alpha^2 M_{ij}^2 + 1 \right)^{1/2} \varepsilon_{ij}, \qquad (11.10)$$

where

$$M_{ij} = \left(\frac{F \cdot D_j}{V_{dj}} \right) \exp(-Cl_j / V_{dj} \cdot t_{ij}),$$

and F is the assumed constant bioavailability. Thus, we have

$$\begin{aligned} \text{Var}(C_{ij}) = &\, M_{ij}^2 \left(\frac{Cl_j}{V_{dj}^2} t_{ij} - \frac{1}{V_{dj}} \right)^2 \sigma_V^2 + M_{ij}^2 \left(\frac{t_{ij}}{V_{dj}} \right)^2 \sigma_{Cl}^2 \\ &- 2 \left(\frac{Cl_j}{V_{dj}^2} t_{ij} - \frac{1}{V_{dj}} \right) \left(\frac{t_{ij}}{V_{dj}} \right) M_{ij}^2 \sigma_{V,Cl}^2 + \left(\alpha^2 M_{ij}^2 + 1 \right) \sigma_\varepsilon^2, \end{aligned}$$

where $\sigma_{V,Cl}^2$ is the population covariance between Cl_j and V_{dj}.

11.3.2.3 Other Approximations

The first-order approximation is obvious biased and there is a room for improvement. A better approximation based on Laplace's approximation has been proposed in the literature (see, e.g., Wolfinger 1993; Vonesh 1996).

Assume that H is $N_k(0, D)$, $P_{y|b}$ is normal with $R_i(\xi)$. Then, we have

$$l_i = (2\pi)^{-(n_i + k)/2} \int |D|^{-1/2} \exp\{-q(y_i, b_i)/2\} db_i,$$

where

$$q(y_i, b_i) = \{y_i - f_i(\beta_i)'\} R_i^{-1}(\xi) \{y_i - f_i(\beta_i)\} + b_i' D^{-1} b_i.$$

Thus, we can solve $q'(y_i, b_i) = 0$ for $\hat{b}_i$. It can be verified that for large n_i

$$l_i \approx (2\pi)^{-n_i/2} |D|^{-1/2} |q''(y_i, \hat{b}_i)/2|^{-1/2} \exp\{-q(y_i, \hat{b}_i)/2\}.$$

260 *Quantitative Methods for Traditional Chinese Medicine Development*

Thus, $l_i \approx n_i$-variate normal with

$$E(y_i) \approx f_i\{d(a_i,\beta,\hat{b}_i)\} - Z_i\{\beta,\hat{b}_i\}\hat{b}_i,$$

and

$$\text{Var}(y_i) \approx Z_i\{\beta,\hat{b}_i\}DZ_i'\{\beta,\hat{b}_i\} + R_i(\xi).$$

As indicated by Davidian (2003), this approximation works remarkably well for sparse (i.e., small n_i) population PK data as long as intrasubject variation is small. This approximation has been implemented in many software packages. For example, nlme of S-plus, %nlinmix of SAS, and NONMEM.

Note that Mallet (1986) proposed the use of completely nonparametric approach for estimation of H. On the other hand, Davidian and Gallant (1993) assumed H has a nice density and estimate H along with other model components.

11.3.2.4 Bayesian Approach

Wakefield (1996) and Müller and Rosner (1997) proposed a three-stage hierarchy Bayesian approach by the following stages. For the first stage (stage 1), consider

$$\begin{aligned}
y_i &= f_i(\beta_i) \cdot e_i \\
&= f_i(\beta_i) \cdot R_i^{1/2}(\beta_i,\xi) \cdot \varepsilon_i,
\end{aligned}$$

where

$$\begin{aligned}
E(y_i|b_i) &= f_i(\beta_i), \\
\text{Var}(y_i|b_i) &= R_i(\beta_i,\xi),
\end{aligned}$$

and

$$P_{y|b}(y_i|x_{i1},\ldots,x_{in_i},a_i,\beta,b_i,\xi) = P_{y|b}(y_i|\beta,b_i,\xi)$$

At the second stage (stage 2), consider

$$\beta_i = d(a_i,\beta,b_i),$$

where

$$b_i \sim P_b|D(b_i|D) \text{ of } b_i \sim H.$$

Population Pharmacokinetics 261

At the third stage (stage 3), assume the following hyperprior

$$(\beta, \xi, D) \sim p_{\beta, \xi, D}(\beta, \xi, D).$$

Note that this approach has been implemented in PKBugs, which is a WinBUGS interface with built-in PK models.

11.4 Design of Population PK

As discussed in the previous section, the analysis of population PK parameters usually involves a nonlinear mixed effects model, the estimates of intersubject (or interindividual), intrasubject (or intraindividual) variability, and measurement error are extremely important. A relatively large intersubject variability may indicate that more patients are needed to have sound statistical inference for the parameters. On the other hand, if the intrasubject variability is much larger than the intersubject variability, more plasma samples may be needed to characterize the plasma concentration–time curve. An appropriate nonlinear mixed effects model should be able to account for these variations. For a PK model, it is of interest to estimate the population parameters and the difference in parameters between groups such as treatment group, sex, age, and race. The estimation of population parameters can be obtained based on plasma concentrations over time. Statistical inference for the difference in parameters between groups may be considered for assessing bioequivalence based on a pre-selected decision rule. The interpretation of these parameters, however, is important in evaluation of drug performance within and between groups.

When planning a population PK study, the design factors such as the number of subjects, the number of concentrations measured in each individual, and the sampling times of the biologic fluid (e.g., blood) in which the drug concentration is determined are necessarily considered for achieving optimal accuracy and precision of the estimates of the population parameters. In practice, the most widely accepted theoretical approach of determining optimal sampling times for PK studies is based on the Fisher information matrix. A commonly used criterion for determining optimal sampling times is to maximize the determinant of the Fisher information matrix (or equivalently minimize the inverse of the determinant), i.e., the D-optimality criterion. In other words, the design factors should be selected in order to reach D-optimality.

Sheiner and Beal (1983) and Al-Banna et al. (1990) studied the effect of these design factors in terms of the bias and precision of population kinetic parameters estimated obtained by the first-order method via computer simulation. Hashimoto and Sheiner (1991), on the other hand, explored the design

262 *Quantitative Methods for Traditional Chinese Medicine Development*

of experiments in pharmacokinetic/pharmacodynamic (PK/PD) investigations. Wang and Endrenyi (1992) considered a large sample approach for evaluation of the variances of parameter estimates for a population pharmacokinetic study. Their method was referred to as the population Fisher information matrix (PFIM) approach. Sun et al. (1996) proposed using an informative block (profile) randomized (IBR) approach to investigate the effect of sample times recording error (both systematic and random) on the estimates of the population PK parameters. When designing a population PK study, the FDA encourages that these informative designs be considered. Such designs should include enough patients in important subgroups to ensure accurate and precise parameter estimation and the detection of any subgroup differences. In what follows, the PFIM design and IBR design of population PK studies are described.

11.4.1 Population Fisher's Information Matrix Approach

Wang and Endrenyi (1992) proposed a large sample approach to evaluate the approximate asymptotic variances (or coefficients of variation) of the maximum likelihood estimators. The information is used to facilitate the selection of favorable experimental designs that lead to the precise estimation of population kinetic parameters by the first-order method. Wang and Endrenyi (1992) noted that the first-order method is identical to the maximum likelihood approach (applied to the first-order model) under the assumption of normally distributed errors. Thus, estimated variances might be normally distributed after suitable transformation.

Let β and $\hat{\beta}$ denote, respectively, a vector of k parameters and the corresponding vector of the maximum likelihood estimators. Let V represent the variance-covariance matrix of $\hat{\beta}$. Thus, the diagonal elements of V are the variances and the off-diagonal elements are the pairwise covariances of the elements of $\hat{\beta}$ Further, let J denote the inverse of V, i.e.,

$$J = V^{-1},$$

where each element of J, j_{rs} is given by

$$j_{rs} = E\left(\frac{\partial_l}{\partial\beta_r} \cdot \frac{\partial_l}{\partial\beta_r}\right) = -E\left(\frac{\partial^2 l}{\partial\beta_r \partial\beta_s}\right), r = 1, \ldots, k; s = 1, \ldots, k, \qquad (11.11)$$

where l is the log-likelihood function, E is the expectation of the random variable in the equation, and J is the Fisher's information matrix. Wang and Endrenyi (1992) proposed to estimate the information matrix J from the data using the following approximation:

Population Pharmacokinetics

$$j_{rs} \approx \left(\frac{\partial_l}{\partial \beta_r} \cdot \frac{\partial_l}{\partial \beta_r} \right) \approx - \left(\frac{\partial^2 l}{\partial \beta_r \partial \beta_s} \right), r = 1, \ldots, k; s = 1, \ldots, k, \qquad (11.12)$$

In practice, it is very tedious, if not impossible, to calculate the expected variances based on Equation 11.11, even for a simple kinetic model and a simple design. On the other hand, the computation of the observed variances by Equation 11.12 is quite feasible with the use of computers. The observed variances obtained from Equation 11.12 approach their true values as the sample size (i.e., the number of individuals) in the sample becomes larger.

It should be noted that in the context of population pharmacokinetics, the population kinetic parameters constitute β, the kinetic responses (e.g., drug concentrations) form the observations, and the dose and sampling times are examples of independent variables. Statistically, the set of kinetic responses from a given individual is regarded as a single observation in the multivariate sense. Moreover, the observations from different individuals are assumed to be independent. Thus, the sample size in a population kinetic study is the number of subjects.

The large sample approach, which is referred to as the PFIM approach, in conjunction with computer simulation is applied to facilitate the design of experiments that aim at the estimation of population pharmacokinetic parameters. PFIM approach proposed by Wang and Endrenyi (1992) is a numerical procedure that evaluates the efficiency of the different sampling designs, from which the most favorable one is selected. In addition, Wang and Endrenyi (1992) indicated that owing to its efficiency and effectiveness in assessing the variability of parameter estimates, the PFIM approach can serve as a tool for studying the relationship between experimental design and the precision of population parameter estimates. After selecting a suitable design for a prospective population pharmacokinetic study, the biases of the parameter estimates may be evaluated and the variability of the estimates confirmed by applying the simulation method for that design. If the calculated biases turn out to be substantial, the estimates obtained following data collection and analysis can be adjusted accordingly.

11.4.2 Informative Block Randomized Approach

Ette et al. (1994) proposed a method that combines the efficiency of D-optimality criteria and the robustness afforded by random sampling. This method was referred to as the informative block randomized (IBR) design. Based on the D-optimality criteria, Ette et al. (1994) considered three alternative sampling procedures with respect to the average PK parameter estimates. These sampling schemes include (1) the informative sampling scheme, (2) the randomized sampling scheme, and (3) the IBR sampling scheme, which are described below.

In the informative sampling scheme, each subject has an identical sampling scheme with sampling times specified according to the D-optimality criteria with all of the samples constrained to be within a specified sampling interval. In the randomized sampling scheme, samples are chosen at random from within the sampling intervals, while in the IBR sampling scheme, the sampling interval is divided into contiguous intervals and equal numbers of samples are chosen at random from each interval.

Ette et al. (1994) compared the efficiency of these informative sampling schemes with that of a conventional sampling scheme, in which sampling times are approximately equal spaced on a log-scale. The population PK parameter estimates obtained with the conventional sampling scheme are found to be inferior to those obtained from the informative, randomized, and IBR schemes. The performance of the three sampling schemes is similar in terms of the accuracy and precision of population PK parameter estimates. Sun et al. (1996) investigated the effect of sample times recording error (both systematic and random) on the estimation of population PK parameters under an IBR design for a drug with two compartment PKs for both single-dose and multiple-dose administrations. The PK profile was divided into three blocks and each subject was sampled across the blocks providing two samples per block. Sun et al. (1996) observed that negative systematic error in the recording of sample times resulted in efficient estimation of volume terms, whereas positive systematic error favored the efficient estimation of the clearance terms. These errors resulted in sufficient samples being located in critical regions for the estimation of volume terms (negative systematic error) and clearance terms (positive systematic error). Sun et al. (1996) concluded that the efficiency in the estimation of clearance was not severely compromised for moderate sampling time recording errors.

Roy and Ette (2005) compared the PFIM D-optimal and IBR designs and indicated that the IBR design is preferred for pragmatic reasons. Pragmatism would detect the use of designs that are easy to implement without loss of efficiency, and clinical trial simulations should be used to choose the appropriate design to meet study objectives.

11.4.3 Remarks

As indicated in the 1999 FDA guidance for Population Pharmacokinetics, three broad approaches (with increasing information content) exist for obtaining information about pharmacokinetic variability. These approaches include (1) single-trough sampling design, (2) multiple-trough sampling design, (3) full population PK sampling design. For the single-trough sampling design, a single blood sample is obtained from each patient at, or close to, the trough of the drug concentrations, shortly before the next dose, and a frequency distribution of plasma or serum levels in the sample of patients is calculated. The FDA pointed out that this approach will give a fairly accurate picture of the variability in trough concentrations in the target population

Population Pharmacokinetics 265

under the assumptions that (1) the sample size is large, (2) the assay and sampling errors are small, and (3) the dosing regimen and sampling times are identical for all patients. In practice, however, these assumptions are usually not met. Thus, the use of the single-trough sampling design is not encouraged except in situations where it is absolutely necessary.

For the multiple-trough sampling design, two or more blood samples are obtained near the trough of steady state concentrations from most or all patients. In addition to relating blood concentration to patient characteristics, it is possible to separate interindividual and residual variabilities. A multiple-trough sampling design requires fewer subjects than that of the single-trough sampling design. In addition, the relationship of trough levels to patient characteristics can be evaluated with greater precision.

The full population PK sampling design refers to a sampling design where blood samples are drawn from subjects at various times (typically one to six time points) following drug administration. The full population PK sampling design is also known as the experimental population pharmacokinetic design or full pharmacokinetic screen. The objective of the full population PK sampling design is to obtain, where feasible, multiple drug levels per patient at different times to describe the population PK profile. This design permits an estimation of pharmacokinetic parameters of the drug in the study population and an explanation of variability using the nonlinear mixed effects modeling approach. As indicated in the 1999 FDA guidance, the full population PK sampling design should be planned to explore the relationship between the pharmacokinetics of a drug and demographic and pathophysiological features of the target population (with its subgroups) for which the drug is being developed.

11.5 An Example

To illustrate statistical methods described in the previous sections, consider the theophylline data from Pinheiro and Bates (1995). Serum concentrations of the drug theophylline were collected in 12 subjects over a 25-hour period after oral administration of the drug. The concentration data are given in Table 11.1. Pinheiro and Bates (1995) considered the following first-order compartment model:

$$C_{it} = \frac{Dk_{ei}k_{ai}}{Cl_i(k_{ai} - k_{ei})}\left[e^{-k_{ei}t} - e^{-k_{ai}t}\right] + e_{it},$$

where C_{it} is the observed concentration of the ith subject at time t, D is the dose of theophylline, k_{ei} is the elimination rate constant for subject i, k_{ai} is

TABLE 11.1

Theophylline Concentration Data in 12 Subjects

Subject	Time	Conc	Dose	Wt
1	0.00	0.74	4.02	79.6
1	0.25	2.84	4.02	79.6
1	0.57	6.57	4.02	79.6
1	1.12	10.50	4.02	79.6
1	2.02	9.66	4.02	79.6
1	3.82	8.58	4.02	79.6
1	5.10	8.36	4.02	79.6
1	7.03	7.47	4.02	79.6
1	9.05	6.89	4.02	79.6
1	12.12	5.94	4.02	79.6
1	24.37	3.28	4.02	79.6
2	0.00	0.00	4.40	72.4
2	0.27	1.72	4.40	72.4
2	0.52	7.91	4.40	72.4
2	1.00	8.31	4.40	72.4
2	1.92	8.33	4.40	72.4
2	3.50	6.85	4.40	72.4
2	5.02	6.08	4.40	72.4
2	7.03	5.40	4.40	72.4
2	9.00	4.55	4.40	72.4
2	12.00	3.01	4.40	72.4
2	24.30	0.90	4.40	72.4
3	0.00	0.00	4.53	70.5
3	0.27	4.40	4.53	70.5
3	0.58	6.90	4.53	70.5
3	1.02	8.20	4.53	70.5
3	2.02	7.80	4.53	70.5
3	3.62	7.50	4.53	70.5
3	5.08	6.20	4.53	70.5
3	7.07	5.30	4.53	70.5
3	9.00	4.90	4.53	70.5
3	12.15	3.70	4.53	70.5
3	24.17	1.05	4.53	70.5
4	0.00	0.00	4.40	72.7
4	0.35	1.89	4.40	72.7
4	0.60	4.60	4.40	72.7
4	1.07	8.60	4.40	72.7
4	2.13	8.38	4.40	72.7
4	3.50	7.54	4.40	72.7
4	5.02	6.88	4.40	72.7

(*Continued*)

Population Pharmacokinetics

TABLE 11.1 (CONTINUED)

Theophylline Concentration Data in 12 Subjects

Subject	Time	Conc	Dose	Wt
4	7.02	5.78	4.40	72.7
4	9.02	5.33	4.40	72.7
4	11.98	4.19	4.40	72.7
4	24.65	1.15	4.40	72.7
5	0.00	0.00	5.86	54.6
5	0.30	2.02	5.86	54.6
5	0.52	5.63	5.86	54.6
5	1.00	11.40	5.86	54.6
5	2.02	9.33	5.86	54.6
5	3.50	8.74	5.86	54.6
5	5.02	7.56	5.86	54.6
5	7.02	7.09	5.86	54.6
5	9.10	5.90	5.86	54.6
5	12.00	4.37	5.86	54.6
5	24.35	1.57	5.86	54.6
6	0.00	0.00	4.00	80.0
6	0.27	1.29	4.00	80.0
6	0.58	3.08	4.00	80.0
6	1.15	6.44	4.00	80.0
6	2.03	6.32	4.00	80.0
6	3.57	5.53	4.00	80.0
6	5.00	4.94	4.00	80.0
6	7.00	4.02	4.00	80.0
6	9.22	3.46	4.00	80.0
6	12.10	2.78	4.00	80.0
6	23.85	0.92	4.00	80.0
7	0.00	0.15	4.95	64.6
7	0.25	0.85	4.95	64.6
7	0.50	2.35	4.95	64.6
7	1.02	5.02	4.95	64.6
7	2.02	6.58	4.95	64.6
7	3.48	7.09	4.95	64.6
7	5.00	6.66	4.95	64.6
7	6.98	5.25	4.95	64.6
7	9.00	4.39	4.95	64.6
7	12.05	3.53	4.95	64.6
7	24.22	1.15	4.95	64.6
8	0.00	0.00	4.53	70.5
8	0.25	3.05	4.53	70.5
8	0.52	3.05	4.53	70.5

(Continued)

TABLE 11.1 (CONTINUED)

Theophylline Concentration Data in 12 Subjects

Subject	Time	Conc	Dose	Wt
8	0.98	7.31	4.53	70.5
8	2.02	7.56	4.53	70.5
8	3.53	6.59	4.53	70.5
8	5.05	5.88	4.53	70.5
8	7.15	4.73	4.53	70.5
8	9.07	4.57	4.53	70.5
8	12.10	3.00	4.53	70.5
8	24.12	1.25	4.53	70.5
9	0.00	0.00	3.10	86.4
9	0.30	7.37	3.10	86.4
9	0.63	9.03	3.10	86.4
9	1.05	7.14	3.10	86.4
9	2.02	6.33	3.10	86.4
9	3.53	5.66	3.10	86.4
9	5.02	5.67	3.10	86.4
9	7.17	4.24	3.10	86.4
9	8.80	4.11	3.10	86.4
9	11.60	3.16	3.10	86.4
9	24.43	1.12	3.10	86.4
10	0.00	0.24	5.50	58.2
10	0.37	2.89	5.50	58.2
10	0.77	5.22	5.50	58.2
10	1.02	6.41	5.50	58.2
10	2.05	7.83	5.50	58.2
10	3.55	10.21	5.50	58.2
10	5.05	9.18	5.50	58.2
10	7.08	8.02	5.50	58.2
10	9.38	7.14	5.50	58.2
10	12.10	5.68	5.50	58.2
10	23.70	2.42	5.50	58.2
11	0.00	0.00	4.92	65.0
11	0.25	4.86	4.92	65.0
11	0.50	7.24	4.92	65.0
11	0.98	8.00	4.92	65.0
11	1.98	6.81	4.92	65.0
11	3.60	5.87	4.92	65.0
11	5.02	5.22	4.92	65.0
11	7.03	4.45	4.92	65.0
11	9.03	3.62	4.92	65.0
11	12.12	2.69	4.92	65.0

(*Continued*)

Population Pharmacokinetics

TABLE 11.1 (CONTINUED)

Theophylline Concentration Data in 12 Subjects

Subject	Time	Conc	Dose	Wt
11	24.08	0.86	4.92	65.0
12	0.00	0.00	5.30	60.5
12	0.25	1.25	5.30	60.5
12	0.50	3.96	5.30	60.5
12	1.00	7.82	5.30	60.5
12	2.00	9.72	5.30	60.5
12	3.52	9.75	5.30	60.5
12	5.07	8.57	5.30	60.5
12	7.07	6.59	5.30	60.5
12	9.03	6.11	5.30	60.5
12	12.05	4.57	5.30	60.5
12	24.15	1.17	5.30	60.5

the absorption rate constant for subject i, Cl_i is the clearance for subject i, and e_{it} are normal errors. To allow for random variability between subjects, Pinheiro and Bates (1995) further assumed that

$$Cl_i = e^{\beta_1 + b_{i1}},$$
$$k_{ai} = e^{\beta_2 + b_{i2}},$$
$$k_{ei} = e^{\beta_3},$$

where the β's denotes fixed-effect parameters and the b's denote random-effect parameters with an unknown covariance matrix. Under the above setting, the PROC NLMIXED procedure of SAS is given in Table 11.2. In Table 11.2,

TABLE 11.2

PROC NLMIXED Procedure of SAS

```
proc nlmixed data = theoph;
parms beta1 = -3.22 beta2 = 0.47 beta3 = -2.45
s2b1 = 0.03 cb12 = 0 s2b2 = 0.4 s2 = 0.5;
cl = exp(beta1 + b1);
ka = exp(beta2 + b2);
ke = exp(beta3);
pred = dose*ke*ka*(exp(-ke*time) - exp(-ka*time))/cl/(ka - ke);
model conc ~ normal(pred,s2);
random b1 b2 ~ normal([0,0], [s2b1,cb12,s2b2]) subject = subject;
run;
```

PARMS statement specifies starting values for the three β's and the four variance-covariance parameters. The clearance and rate constants are defined using SAS programming statements, and the conditional model for the data is defined to be normal with mean PRED and variance S2. The two random effects are b1 and b2, and their joint distribution is defined in the RANDOM statement. Note that brackets are used to define their mean vector (two zeros) and the lower triangle of their variance-covariance matrix (a general 2×2 matrix). A summary of the above PROC NLMIXED is given in Table 11.3, where Specifications lists the setup of the model and Dimensions indicates that there are 132 observations, 12 subjects, and 7 parameters.

PROC NLMIXED of SAS selects five quadrate points for each random effect, which produces a total grid of 25 points over which quadrate is performed. The PROC NLMIXED of SAS begins with a set of initial values (see, e.g., Table 11.4) and then provides iteration history (see, e.g., Table 11.5). Table 11.5 indicates that 10 iterations are required for the dual quasi-Newton algorithm to achieve convergence. The fitting information are summarized in Table 11.6, which lists the final optimized values of the log likelihood function and two information criteria in two different forms. Table 11.7 contains the maximum likelihood estimates of the parameters. Both s2b1 and s2b2 are marginally significant, indicating between-subject variability in the clearances and absorption rate constants, respectively. Note that there does not appear

TABLE 11.3

Summary of PROC NLMIXED of SAS

NLMIXED Procedure	
Specifications	
Data set	WORK.THEOPH
Dependent variable	Conc
Distribution for dependent variable	Normal
Random effects	b1 b2
Distribution for random effects	Normal
Subject variable	Subject
Optimization technique	Dual quasi-Newton
Integration method	Adaptive Gaussian Quadrature
Dimensions	
Observations used	132
Observations not used	0
Total observations	132
Subjects	12
Max obs per subject	11
Parameter	7
Quadrature points	5

Population Pharmacokinetics 271

TABLE 11.4

Initial Values of PROC NLMIXED of SAS

			Parameter				
beta1	beta2	beta3	s2b1	cb12	s2b2	s2	NegLogLike
−3.22	0.47	−2.45	0.03	0	0.4	0.5	177.789945

TABLE 11.5

History of Iterations

Iter	Calls	NegLogLike	Diff	MaxGrad	Slope
1	5	177.776248	0.013697	2.873367	−63.0744
2	8	177.7643	0.011948	1.698144	−4.75239
3	10	177.757264	0.007036	1.297439	−1.97311
4	12	177.755688	0.001576	1.441408	−0.49772
5	14	177.7467	0.008988	1.132279	−0.8223
6	17	177.746401	0.000299	0.831293	−0.00244
7	19	177.746318	0.000083	0.724198	−0.00789
8	21	177.74574	0.000578	0.180018	−0.00583
9	23	177.745736	3.88E-6	0.017958	−8.25E-6
10	25	177.745736	3.222E-8	0.000143	−6.51E-8

Note: GCONV convergence criterion satisfied.

TABLE 11.6

Fitting Information

Fit Statistics	Value
−2 log likelihood	355.5
AIC (smaller is better)	369.5
BIC (smaller is better)	372.9
Log likelihood	−177.7
AIC (smaller is better)	−184.7
BIC (smaller is better)	−186.4

to be a significant covariance between them, as seen by the estimate of cb12. The estimates of β_1, β_2, and β_3 are close to the adaptive quadrature estimates listed in the Table 3 of Pinheiro and Bates (1995). However, Pinheiro and Bates (1995) used a Cholesky-root parameterization for the random-effect variance matrix and a logarithmic parameterization for the residual variance. The PROC NLMIXED of SAS, on the other hand, uses the parameterization as given in Table 11.8, which yields similar results.

TABLE 11.7

Summary of Parameter Estimates

Parameter	Estimate	Standard Error	DF	t Value	Pr > |t|	Alpha	Lower	Upper	Gradient
beta1	-3.2268	0.05950	10	-54.23	<0.0001	0.05	-3.3594	-3.0942	-0.00009
beta2	0.4806	0.1989	10	2.42	0.0363	0.05	0.03745	0.9238	3.645E-7
beta3	-2.4592	0.05126	10	-47.97	<0.0001	0.05	-2.5734	-2.3449	0.000039
s2b1	0.02803	0.01221	10	2.30	0.0445	0.05	0.000833	0.05523	-0.00014
cb12	-0.00127	0.03404	10	-0.04	0.9710	0.05	-0.07712	0.07458	-0.00007
s2b2	0.4331	0.2005	10	2.16	0.0560	0.05	-0.01353	0.8798	-6.98E-6
s2	0.5016	0.06837	10	7.34	<0.0001	0.05	0.3493	0.6540	6.133E-6

Population Pharmacokinetics 273

TABLE 11.8

Alternative Parameterization in SAS

proc nlmixed data = theoph;
parms l11 = –1.5 l2 = 0 l13 = –0.1 beta1 = –3 beta2 = 0.5 beta3 = –2.5
ls2 = –0.7;
s2 = exp(ls2);
l1 = exp(l11)
l3 = exp(l13);
s2b1 = l1*l1*s2;
cb12 = l2*l1*s2;
s2b2 = (l2*l2 + l3*l3)*s2;
cl = exp(beta1 + b1);
ka = exp(beta2 + b2);
ke = exp(beta3);
pred = dose*ke*ka*(exp(–ke*time) – exp(–ka*time))/cl/(ka – ke);
model conc ~ normal (pred, s2);
random b1 b2 ~ normal ([0, 0], [s2b1, cb12, s2b2]) subject = subject;
run;

11.6 Discussion

11.6.1 Study Protocol

A population PK study is either considered as an add-on to a clinical trial or a stand-alone study. It should be noted that the objectives of the add-on population PK study should not compromise the objectives of the primary clinical study. In practice, a stand-alone population PK study is more comprehensive. As indicated in the 1999 FDA guidance on Population Pharmacokinetics, a study design protocol should include (1) a clear statement of the objectives of the population PK analysis, (2) sampling design, (3) data collection procedures, (4) data checking procedures, (5) procedures for handling missing data, (6) specific PK parameters to be estimated, (7) covariates to be estimated, (8) model assumptions and model selection criteria, (9) sensitivity analysis and validation procedure (if planned), and (10) special user-friendly case report forms for PK evaluation.

11.6.2 Concerns and Challenges

In population modeling, statistical methods for assessment of means and variances of pharmacokinetic parameters for a patient population are well-established based on sparse data collected under conditions of routine patient care. However, Nedelman (2005) indicated that there are the following potential concerns: (1) unobserved confounding variables may bias the statistical inferences, (2) conditions under which data are collected may lead to inaccuracies of reporting or recording, (3) correlations among important predictor variables may reduce statistical efficiency, and (4) costs cannot be controlled by principles of study design. To overcome these problems, Nedelman (2005) proposed a method for diagnosing the possible presence of confounding. In addition, Nedelman (2005) also proposed a model to capture the influence of data inaccuracies.

In practice, there are many issues/challenges when implementing a population PK as an add-on to clinical trial. These issues/challenges include, but are not limited to (1) the maintenance of blinding (2) data management and/or data merging in multicenter trials, (3) modifying inclusion/exclusion criteria without compromising primary objectives of the clinical trial, (4) complexity of PK procedures, and (5) monitoring PK aspects of study such as dosing history, demographics, sampling times, and sample processing and handling.

11.6.3 PK/PD

As indicated earlier, the key concept of a PK study is to study what the body does to the drug, while the key concept of a pharmacodynamic (PD) study is to study what the drug does to the body. Figure 11.1 illustrates the relationship between PK and PD and among dose, concentration and response. As a result, a PK/PD study is to study the relationship between dose and response, which provides insight information regarding (1) how best to choose doses at which to evaluate a drug, (2) how best to use a drug in a population, and (3) how best to use a drug to treat individual patients or subpopulations of patients. As can be seen from Figure 11.1, PK is to study the relationship between dose and concentration.

PK is only part of the full story. Population PK/PD study collects PK/PD data on same subjects. Suppose PD responses y_{ij}^* at times t_{ij}^*. Consider the plasma concentration C_{ij} taken at t_{ij}^*. Then, the intrasubject PD model could be described as follows:

$$y_{ij}^* = g(C_{ij}, a_i) + e_{ij}^*.$$

As a result, the intrasubject joint PK/PD model can be described as follows:

$$y_{ij} = f(x_{ij}, \beta_i) + e_{ij}, y_{ij}^* = g\left(f(x_{ij}^*, \beta_i)a_i\right) + e_{iju}^*,$$

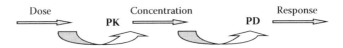

FIGURE 11.1
Relationship between PK and PD.

Population Pharmacokinetics

where

$$\beta_i = d(a_i, \beta, b_i), a_i = d^*(a_i, a, b_i^*),$$

and

$$\left(\beta_i', a_i'\right) \sim H.$$

11.6.4 Computer Simulation

Because of the complexity of a population PK study, it is suggested that a trial simulation be conducted to evaluate the performance of various designs for population PK studies for design selection. Trial simulation is a process that uses computers to mimic the conduct of a population PK study by creating virtual patients and extrapolating (or predicting) PK responses for each virtual patient based on pre-specified PK models. In practice, trial simulation of often considered to predict potential PK responses under different assumptions and various design scenarios at the planning stage of a population PK study for better planning (i.e., for achieving optimal accuracy and precision for estimation of population characteristics of the target patient population under study) of the actual study.

11.6.5 Software Applications

For population PK studies, many software packages are available. Most of them were developed based on maximum likelihood approach. To name of few, these software packages include (1) NONMEN (Beal and Sheiner 1989), which was the first software package developed for population pharmacokinetic/pharmacodynamic analyses, (2) NLME (Pinheiro and Bates 2000), which is a generic function of S-Plus (3) NLINMIX (Wolfinger 1993) and PROC NLMIXED, which are a macro and a generic function of SAS, and (4) WinNonlin or WinNonlinMix (Pharsight). These approaches also allow the evaluation of the influence of individual covariates on the parameters through the addition of fixed effects parameters or the incorporation of interoccasions variability, which quantifies the variability of the parameters of one individual during different occasions of sampling through the addition of random effects with variances to be estimated (Karlsson and Sheiner 1993). Software packages for analysis based on other approaches are also available. For example, NPLM (Mallet 1986) is developed for nonparametric maximum likelihood approach. On the other hand, SAS macros for Bayesian EM algorithm (Racine-Poon and Smith 1990) are also available. Edler (1998) provided a list of PK/PD software packages that were available up to 1998. This list included 72 software packages. This list, however, has not yet been updated.

12

Experience of Generic Drug Products with Multiple Components

12.1 Introduction

When an innovative drug product is going off patent protection, as indicated in Chapter 10, pharmaceutical or generic companies may file an Abbreviated New Drug Application (ANDA) for generic approval. As indicated in 21 CFR 320.24, bioavailability and bioequivalence may be established by *in vivo* and *in vitro* studies or with suitable justification by *in vitro* studies alone. *In vivo* studies include pharmacokinetic/pharmacodynamic (PK/PD) studies, bioavailability/bioequivalence (BA/BE) studies, and clinical studies, while *in vitro* studies are referred to as dissolution test/dissolution profile comparison and *in vitro* tests for content uniformity, prime/re-prime, spray pattern, plume geometry, and droplet distribution. For *in vivo* bioequivalence testing, the FDA requires that bioavailability and bioequivalence studies be conducted to provide substantial evidence of similar drug absorption of the proposed generic drug product to the innovative (brand name) drug product (FDA 2003a). *In vivo* bioequivalence testing is based on the Fundamental Bioequivalence Assumption that drug absorption is predictive of clinical outcomes. Similarly, *in vitro* bioequivalence testing for drug release or delivery is mainly based on *in vivo* and *in vitro* correlation (IVIVC). IVIVC indicates that there is well-established correlation between *in vivo* test results and *in vitro* test results. In other words, drug release/delivery is predictive of drug absorption. In this chapter, unlike most Western medicines that contain a single active ingredient, experience of generic drug products with multiple components is discussed. A typical example of Western medicines with multiple components is Premarin (conjugated estrogen) that was approved by the FDA intended for treating moderate to severe post-menopausal dyspareunia.

Conjugated estrogen tablets are an important medication for post-menopausal women. They are intended not only for treatment of moderate to severe vasomotor symptoms associated with menopause but also to prevent estrogen deficiency-induced osteoporosis and a variety of other conditions associated with estrogen deficiency. Other indications include palliative

278   *Quantitative Methods for Traditional Chinese Medicine Development*

therapy for breast and prostate cancers. The conjugated estrogen tablets contain four primary active ingredients: unconjugated estrone, estrone sulfate, unconjugated equilin, and equilin sulfate. The innovator products are exclusively derived from natural sources. Multiple strengths at 0.3, 0.625, 0.9, 1.25, and 2.5 mg are currently available in the marketplace. Thus, conjugated estrogen tablets are considered drug products similar to TCM because they contain multiple active ingredients (components).

On August 21, 1991, the FDA issued guidance on *Guidance for Conjugated Estrogen Tablets*—In vivo *Bioequivalence and* In vitro *Drug Release* (FDA 1991). As indicated in the FDA guidance, to obtain approval for all five strengths, the sponsors are required to conclude the average bioequivalence (ABE) based on two fasting studies conducted at the strengths of 0.625 and 1.25 mg, respectively, and a nonfasting study at the strength of 1.25 mg. For each study, the evidence of bioequivalence for *all* active ingredients needs to be established in order to claim bioequivalence. For other strengths, if dose proportionality and dissolution profiles are acceptable, then the study at the strength of 2.5 mg could be waived through the evidence of bioequivalence for fasting and nonfasting studies at the strength of 1.25 mg tablets. Similarly, the studies at the strengths of 0.3 and 0.9 mg could be waived if dose proportionality and dissolution profiles are acceptable and the fasting exhibits bioequivalence.

One of the primary objectives of the 1991 FDA guidance is to recommend the statistical design and analysis to establish the average bioequivalence of generic copies of conjugated estrogen tablets over all five strengths. There are, however, many important statistical issues embedded in the guidance. These issues include the study design, the multiplicity of studies and active ingredients, sample size determination, the use of baseline measurements, logarithmic transformation versus the presence of a significant first-order carryover effects, and others. Furthermore, if bioequivalence is conducted for nonfasting and fasting studies at the strength of 1.25 mg and the fasting study on the 0.625 mg tablets, then approval for the strengths of 0.3, 0.9, and 2.5 mg can be granted solely based on the data of dissolution profiles between the reference and test formulations under the assumption of proportionality. The 1991 FDA guidance, however, only requires that descriptive statistics for percent release be provided and does not require any statistical evidence for the similarity of dissolution profiles of drug products.

In the next couple of sections, *in vivo* single fasting bioequivalence study and *in vitro* drug release testing for conjugated estrogen tablets are briefly outlined and discussed. A review on FDA conjugated estrogen bioequivalence guidance is provided in Section 12.4 followed by some concluding remarks.

12.2 *In Vivo* Single Fasting Bioequivalence Study

12.2.1 Study Design

For assessment of bioequivalence between a test and a reference product of conjugated estrogen tablets, the 1991 FDA guidance recommends that a rather sophisticated four-sequence, three-period crossover design for two treatments be used. The design is illustrated in Table 12.1.

This four-sequence, three-period crossover design is made of two dual two-sequence, three-period crossover designs. It consists of the pairs of (TRT, RTR) and (RTT, TTR). The first-order residuals or residual effect stated repeatedly in the guidance are, in fact, the first-order carryover effect. There are 11 degrees of freedom (df) associated with a total 12 sequence-by-period means. Three df's are designated for sequence effects, which can be tested based on intersubject variability. The remaining eight df's are associated with the effects whose statistical inferences are based on intrasubject variability. Among them, two df's are for the period effects and one df is for each of the treatment effects, the first-order carryover effect, the interaction between the treatment and the first-order carryover effect, and second-order carryover effect. The remaining two df's are for two particular sequence-by-period interaction contrasts which are of little interest in real application. The analysis of variance (ANOVA) table for this four-sequence, three-period design given in Table 12.2 summarizes the source of variation and degrees of freedom under the assumption of an equal number of subjects in each sequence.

From the ANOVA table in Table 12.2, it can be seen that the four-sequence, three-period design provides estimates for the treatment effect in the presence of the first-order carryover effect. Moreover, under this design, the second-order carryover effect and treatment-by-first-order carryover interaction can

TABLE 12.1

Four-Sequence, Three-Period Crossover Design for Two Treatments

	Period		
Sequence	I	II	III
1	T	R	T
2	R	T	R
3	R	T	T
4	T	R	R

Note: R, reference product; T, test product.

TABLE 12.2

Analysis of Variance Table for the Design in Table 12.1

Source of Variation	Degrees of Freedom
Intersubject	$4n - 1$
Sequence	3
Residual	$4n - 4$
Intrasubject	$8n$
Treatment	1
Period	2
First-order carryover	1
Treatment × first-order carryover	1
Second-order carryover	1
Sequence × period contrasts	2
Residual	$8(n - 1)$
Total	$12n - 1$

Note: n = number of subjects per sequence.

also be tested. In practice, however, if washout periods of sufficient length are provided between periods of, for example, at least seven days, it is reasonable to assume that there are no second-order carryover effects and treatment-by-first-order interaction. Because the four-sequence, three-period design is more complicated than the standard 2 × 2 crossover design, it suffers from the following drawbacks:

1. It might be very time-consuming to complete the study;
2. It might increase the number of dropouts;
3. It might increase the chance of making errors in the randomization schedules.

To overcome these difficulties, as an alternative, a simpler design—the two-sequence, three-period design—is proposed. This design consists of (RTT, TRR). Under this design, the treatment effect can also be estimated in the presence of the first-order carryover effect provided that there are no second-order carryover effects. For this design, there are a total of five degrees of freedom associated with a total of six sequence-by-period means. The ANOVA table for this dual design is given in Table 12.3.

For this two-sequence dual design, the treatment effect can be estimated in the presence of the first-order carryover effect. In addition, the treatment effect and the first-order carryover effect are not correlated to each other. These two effects, however, are correlated in the four-sequence, three-period design that is recommended by the FDA guidance. Furthermore, for this two-sequence dual design, as indicated in the ANOVA table, both inference of treatment and first-order effects, are based on the unpaired t-test. Although the robust analysis is also available for the design given in Table 12.1, the

Experience of Generic Drug Products with Multiple Components

TABLE 12.3

Analysis of Variance Table for the Dual
Design

Source of Variation	Degrees of Freedom
Intersubject	$2n - 1$
Sequence	1
Residual	$2(n - 1)$
Intrasubject	$4n$
Treatment	1
Period	2
First-order carryover	1
Residual	$4(n - 1)$
Total	$6n - 1$

Note: n = number of subjects per sequence.

analysis is based on the weighted means with the inverse of variances of treatment effects from each dual pair as the weights. Hence, one has to estimate the variance to apply Satterwaite's method to approximate degrees of freedom. Both designs can be used to estimate intrasubject variability. Both designs, however, only use half of the data for estimation of intrasubject variability for each formulation. From these comparisons, the dual design (RTT, TRR) is preferred for evaluation of bioequivalence for conjugated estrogen tablets.

12.2.2 Sample Size

The FDA guidance states that statistical power considerations suggest that the study may require at least 36 subjects to meet the confidence interval criteria. The sample size, however, should be determined based on the following: (1) the study design, (2) the intrasubject variability, (3) the required power, and (4) the mean ratio between the test and the reference formulation.

For the four-sequence, four-period design as recommended by the FDA guidance, the variance for the estimated treatment effect in the presence of the first-order carryover effect is given as

$$V(F|C) = \left(\frac{6}{13n} \right) \sigma^2,$$

where sigma is the intrasubject variability. On the other hand, the variance for the estimated treatment effect for the two-sequence dual design (RTR, TRR) is given as

$$V(F|C) = V(F) = \left(\frac{3}{4n} \right) \sigma^2.$$

The ratio of these two variances is about 1.625. Hence, the four-sequence, three-period design is 62.5 percent more efficient than the proposed two-sequence dual design. The sample size sequence for an equivalence limit d and a nominal significance level of alpha and a power of beta can be obtained from direct application of the formula given by Chow and Liu (2008) to these two designs. For assessment of average bioequivalence, under a crossover design, sample size required for establishment of bioequivalence can be obtained through the evaluation of the power function for testing the following interval hypotheses:

$$H_0: \mu_T - \mu_R \leq \theta_L \quad \text{or} \quad \mu_T - \mu_R \geq \theta_L \quad \text{vs.} \quad H_a: \theta_L < \mu_T - \mu_R < \theta_U, \quad (12.1)$$

where θ_L and θ_U are some clinically meaningful limits for equivalence. The concept of interval hypotheses is to show equivalence by rejecting the null hypothesis of inequivalence. The above hypotheses can be decomposed into two sets of one-sided hypotheses:

$$H_{01}: \mu_T - \mu_R \leq \theta_L, \quad \text{vs.} \quad H_{a1}: \mu_T - \mu_R > \theta_L.$$

and

$$H_{02}: \mu_T - \mu_R \geq \theta_U, \quad \text{vs.} \quad H_{a2}: \mu_T - \mu_R > \theta_U.$$

Schuirmann (1987) proposes two one-sided test procedures for the above two one-sided hypotheses. We can reject the null hypothesis of bioinequivalence if

$$T_L = \frac{\bar{Y}_T - \bar{Y}_P - \theta_L}{\hat{\sigma}_d \sqrt{(1/n_1) + (1/n_2)}} > t(\alpha, n_1 + n_2 - 2)$$

and

$$T_U = \frac{\bar{Y}_T - \bar{Y}_P - \theta_U}{\hat{\sigma}_d \sqrt{(1/n_1) + (1/n_2)}} < -t(\alpha, n_1 + n_2 - 2)$$

Let $\theta = \mu_T - \mu_P$ and $\phi_s(\theta)$ be the power of Schuirmann's two one-sided tests at θ. Assuming that $n_1 = n_2 = n$, the power at $\theta = 0$ is given by

$$1 - \beta = \phi_s(0)$$
$$= P\left\{ \frac{-\Delta}{\hat{\sigma}_d \sqrt{2/n}} + t(\alpha, 2n - 2) < \frac{Y}{\hat{\sigma}_d \sqrt{2/n}} < \frac{\Delta}{\hat{\sigma}_d \sqrt{2/n}} - t(\alpha, 2n - 2) \right\},$$
$$(12.2)$$

Experience of Generic Drug Products with Multiple Components

where $Y = \bar{Y}_T - \bar{Y}_P$. Because a central t distribution is symmetric about 0, the lower and upper endpoints are also symmetric about 0:

$$\frac{-\Delta}{\hat{\sigma}_d\sqrt{2/n}} + t(\alpha, 2n-2) = -\left\{\frac{\Delta}{\hat{\sigma}_d\sqrt{2/n}} - t(\alpha, 2n-2)\right\}.$$

Therefore, $\phi_S(0) \geq 1 - \beta$ implies that

$$\left|\frac{\Delta}{\hat{\sigma}_d\sqrt{2/n}} - t(\alpha, 2n-2)\right| \geq t(\beta/2, 2n-2)$$

or that

$$n(\theta = 0) \geq 2[t(\alpha, 2n-2) + t(\beta/2, 2n-2)]^2\left[\frac{\hat{\sigma}_d}{\Delta}\right]^2. \tag{12.3}$$

If we must have an 80 percent power for detection of a 20 percent difference of placebo mean, then Equation 12.3 becomes

$$n(\theta = 0) \geq 2[t(\alpha, 2n-2) + t(\beta/2, 2n-2)]^2\left[\frac{CV}{20}\right]^2. \tag{12.4}$$

We will now consider the case where $\theta \neq 0$. Because the power curves of Schuirmann's two one-sided test procedures are symmetric about zero (Phillips 1990), we will only consider the case where $0 < \theta = \theta_0 < \Delta$. In this case, the statistic

$$\frac{Y - \theta_0}{\hat{\sigma}_d\sqrt{2/n}}$$

has a central t distribution with $2n - 2$ degrees of freedom. The power of Schuirmann's two one-sided test procedures can be evaluated at θ_0, which is given by

$$1 - \beta = \phi_S(\theta_0)$$
$$= P\left\{\frac{-\Delta - \theta_0}{\hat{\sigma}_d\sqrt{2/n}} - t(\alpha, 2n-2) < \frac{Y - \theta_0}{\hat{\sigma}_d\sqrt{2/n}} < \frac{\Delta - \theta_0}{\hat{\sigma}_d\sqrt{2/n}} - t(\alpha, 2n-2)\right\}. \tag{12.5}$$

284 *Quantitative Methods for Traditional Chinese Medicine Development*

Note that unlike the case where $\theta = 0$, the lower and upper endpoints are not symmetric about 0. Therefore, if we choose

$$\frac{\Delta - \theta_0}{\hat{\sigma}_d \sqrt{2/n}} - t(\alpha, 2n - 2) = t(\beta/2, 2n - 2),$$

then the resultant sample size may be too large to be of practical interest, and the power may be more than we need. As an alternative, Chow and Liu (2008) consider the inequality for obtaining an approximate formula for n

$$\phi_S(\theta_0) \le P \left\{ \frac{Y - \theta_0}{\hat{\sigma}_d \sqrt{2/n}} < \frac{\Delta - \theta_0}{\hat{\sigma}_d \sqrt{2/n}} - t(\alpha, 2n - 2) \right\}.$$

As a result, $\phi_S(\theta_0) \ge 1 - \beta$ gives

$$\frac{\Delta - \theta_0}{\hat{\sigma}_d \sqrt{2/n}} - t(\alpha, 2n - 2) = t(\beta, 2n - 2)$$

or

$$n(\theta_0) \ge 2[t(\alpha, 2n - 2) + t(\beta, 2n - 2)]^2 \left[\frac{\hat{\sigma}_d}{\Delta - \theta_0} \right]^2. \tag{12.6}$$

Similarly, if we must have an 80 percent power for detection of a 20 percent difference of placebo mean, then Equation 12.6 becomes

$$n(\theta_0) \ge [t(\alpha, 2n - 2) + t(\beta, 2n - 2)]^2 \left[\frac{CV}{\Delta - \theta_0'} \right]^2, \tag{12.7}$$

where

$$\theta_0' = 100 \times \frac{\theta_0'}{\mu_P}$$

For high-order crossover designs (Table 12.4), sample size required for achieving an 80 percent establishment of average bioequivalence can be similarity obtained. Let $m = 1$ (Balaam design), 2 (two-sequence dual design), 3 (four-period design with two sequences), and 4 (four-period design with four sequences) and denote the following:

$$v_1 = 4n - 3, \quad v_2 = 4n - 4, \quad v_3 = 6n - 5, \quad v_4 = 12n - 5;$$

Experience of Generic Drug Products with Multiple Components

TABLE 12.4

Commonly Used Higher-Order Crossover Designs

Design	Sequence	Period	Design
1	4	2	Balaam design
2	2	3	Two-sequence dual design
3	2	4	Four-period design with two sequences
4	4	4	Four-period design with four sequences

$$b_1 = 2, \quad b_2 = \frac{3}{4}, \quad b_3 = \frac{11}{20}, \quad b_4 = \frac{1}{4}.$$

Hence the formula of n required to achieve a $1 - \beta$ power at the α level of significance for the mth design when $\theta = 0$ is given by

$$n \geq b_m[t(\alpha, v_m) + t(\beta/2, v_m)^2]\left[\frac{CV}{\Delta}\right]^2, \tag{12.8}$$

and if $\theta = \theta_0 > 0$, the approximate formula for n is given

$$n(\theta_0) \geq b_m[t(\alpha, v_m) + t(\beta, v_m)^2]\left[\frac{CV}{\Delta - \theta}\right]^2, \tag{12.9}$$

For $m = 1, 2, 3,$ and 4.

For bioequivalence assessment under a parallel group design, the sample size required for establishment of bioequivalence can be similarly obtained as follows:

If we assume that $n = n_1 = n_2$, then

$$\begin{aligned}
n &= \frac{\left(\sigma_1^2 + \sigma_2^2\right)[Z(\alpha) + Z(\beta)]^2}{\Delta^2}, \\
&= \frac{2\sigma^2[Z(\alpha/2) + Z(\beta)]^2}{\Delta^2}, \quad \text{if } \sigma_1^2 = \sigma_2^2
\end{aligned} \tag{12.10}$$

For the one-sided test, the above expression for the required sample size becomes

$$n = \frac{\left(\sigma_1^2 + \sigma_2^2\right)[Z(\alpha) + Z(\beta)]^2}{\Delta^2}. \tag{12.11}$$

Note that when the population variance is unknown, the choice of sample size is not straightforward. For example, when the true value is $\mu = \mu_0 + \Delta$, the statistic

$$\frac{\bar{Y} - (\mu_0 + \Delta)}{s/\sqrt{n}}$$

follows a noncentral t distribution and noncentrality parameter $\delta = \Delta/\sigma$.

12.2.3 Remarks

It should be noted that the four-sequence, three-period design contains four sequences while the proposed two-sequence dual design only involves two sequences. Assume that the intra-subject variability and the equivalence limits are the same, the total number of subjects required by the FDA guidance design is 23 percent more than the proposed two-sequence dual design. Hence, there is another reason to use the dual design. It should be noted, however, that comparison of relative efficiency among different designs take into account the (1) total exposures to drug, (2) total number of subject-days, (3) total number of assays, and (4) relative costs of the above factors.

Because only a single dose is administered to the subject within each period, the total exposures, the total number of subject-days, and assays can, therefore, be measured by the period as the unit. Hence, the discussion of relative efficiency based on the number of subjects implicitly takes these factors partially into consideration. Liu (1995) discussed relative efficiency of replicated crossover designs in assessment of average bioequivalence.

12.2.4 Multiplicity of Studies and Ingredients

The FDA guidance requires that the sponsor establish evidence of bioequivalence in one fasting study at the strength of 1.25 mg and another fasting study at the strength of 0.625 mg to obtain approval for all strengths. To claim bioequivalence for one study, however, one has to show equivalence for all four active ingredients, that is, unconjugated estrone and equilin as well as conjugated estrone and equilin. Hence, the probability for concluding bioequivalence may be low. For example, if the probability that each ingredient of the generic version is, in fact, bioequivalent to its corresponding ingredient of the innovator product is 90 percent (i.e., power), then the probability of concluding bioequivalence for one study is $(0.9)^4 = 0.6561$ under the assumption of no dependence among four active ingredients and the probability of concluding bioequivalence for two fasting studies is only about 0.43. If conclusion of bioequivalence is based solely on the 90 percent confidence interval for all ingredients and all studies, then the probability for the generic product to meet the FDA requirement for at least one ingredient can also

Experience of Generic Drug Products with Multiple Components 287

be calculated. Because the approach of the 90 percent confidence interval is operationally equivalent to the two one-sided tests procedure at a nominal significance level of 5 percent, the probabilities of claiming bioequivalence for at least one active ingredient for one study given that they are, in fact, not bioequivalent, are 0.1855 for one study and 0.3366 for two studies.

As a result, there is a dilemma regarding the requirements for concluding bioequivalence in the FDA guidance. On the one hand, if the generic product is truly bioequivalent for each component, owing to the multiplicity of testing, the probability to claim bioequivalence for all four ingredients for two studies is only 43 percent. Hence, the requirement seems somewhat restricted and unfair to sponsors. On the other hand, if the probability of falsely claiming bioequivalence between the test and reference formulation is 5 percent for an individual ingredient, then the probability of claiming at least one active ingredient is 34 percent. Therefore, the rules stated in the FDA guidance cannot minimize the high risk of committing a type I error. In this case, techniques of multiple comparisons might be applied. The dependence among active ingredients which always exists, however, must be taken into consideration. More research is needed in this area.

12.2.5 Baseline Adjustment

The FDA guidance requires that for each active ingredient, the −48 hours and −24 hours blood samples be collected. The measurements at these two time points and the one immediately prior to dosing (i.e., time 0) serve as the baseline measurements for each of the four ingredients. The FDA guidance suggests taking the average of these three measurements as a single baseline value. The FDA guidance requires the sponsors to provide the pharmacokinetic data of concentrations, area under the plasma concentration-time curve (AUC) and the peak concentration (C_{max}) with and without baseline corrections. If there is a huge fluctuation among the three baseline measurements, however, then the average might not be robust enough to represent the true underlying baseline values. In this case, performing an analysis of variance based on these three repeated measurements without dosing is suggested to quantify the measurement error variability for the assay. If the measurement error is relatively small, the average of the three measurements is a reliable estimate for the baseline value of each subject. On the other hand, if the measurement error variability appears to be large, then caution should be exercised in using the average baseline value for correction of observed pharmacokinetic responses.

As suggested by the FDA guidance, an analysis of covariance with the single mean baseline value obtained from the first period is the covariate. If one assumes that each mean baseline value from the first period is different from subject to subject, however, then the covariate is confounded with the subject effect. In addition, because the treatment effect is estimated from the intrasubject contrast from each subject and, for the same subject, the mean baseline obtained from the first period is the same for the entire design and

288   *Quantitative Methods for Traditional Chinese Medicine Development*

the influence of the covariate will be cancelled out due to the contrasts. As a result, the estimate of the treatment effect will not be affected by this covariate. In other words, use of the mean baseline from the first period fails to determine whether or not the model has adequately adjusted for the differences in subjects' underlying estrogen level. Furthermore, because the covariate is a continuous variable and the subject is a class variable when performing PROC GLM of SAS, the least squares means given by the SAS statement LSMEANS for the treatment effect will be declared impossible to estimate if the number of subjects is different among sequences. One way to use the mean baseline of the first period as a covariate is to perform analysis of covariance for the intrasubject contrasts computed from each subject. In addition, it is suggested that an analysis of variance with the baseline values be performed to check whether the baseline values are the same at the beginning of each period. This is an alternative method to check the possible carryout effect.

12.2.6 Logarithmic Transformation versus the Presence of a Significant First-Order Carryover Effect

The FDA guidance suggests that a logarithmic transformation be performed if a significant first-order carryover effect is found ($p < 0.05$). In addition, the FDA guidance states that the reason for this is the inability to estimate the treatment effect if the term of first-order carryover effect is included in the model. Furthermore, in the absence of a significance first-order carryover effect, the analysis should be based on the untransformed data. From the ANOVA table given in Table 12.2, for the four-sequence, three-period crossover design, unlike the standard 2×2 crossover design, it is well known that the treatment effect can be estimated even in the presence of a significant first-order carryover effect. Thus, whether or not to take logarithmic transformation has no impact on the statistical significance of the first-order carryover effect. It has an impact, however, upon the distribution of the data. To be consistent with the *Guidance on Statistical Procedures for Bioequivalence Using a Standard Twotreatment Crossover Design* issued in 1992, it is recommended that a logarithmic transformation be performed for corrected and uncorrected AUC and peak concentration. As a result, the bioequivalence limits should also be changed to (80 percent, 125 percent) accordingly.

12.3 *In Vivo* Drug Release Testing

The FDA guidance only requires that for each time interval, the percent drug release for each dosage unit, the mean percent drug released, the range of percent drug released for the 12 dosage units, and the percent

Experience of Generic Drug Products with Multiple Components   289

coefficient of variation about the mean be provided. The guidance, however, does not specify how to compare the two dissolution profiles between the test and reference formulations. Because for each dosage unit the percent drug release at different time intervals are correlated, the traditional one-way and two-way analysis of variance and analysis of covariance are not appropriate (Gill 1988). Hence, the technique for repeated measurements should be used for consideration of correlated responses (Lindsey 1993). One simple way is to assume the compound symmetry for the covariance matrix because one only has to estimate two variance components. There are only 12 dosage units, however, this estimation of variance components might not be precise and this assumption might also be difficult to verify. This method, however, is more statistically sound than the one- or two-way ANOVA or ANCOVA.

Most analyses for dissolution data are conducted to test whether two profiles are different. This approach is based on the null hypothesis that two profiles are the same and the alternative that two profiles are not the same. Hence, failure to reject the null hypothesis can only result in the conclusion that there is insufficient evidence that the two profiles are not equal and cannot imply that the two profiles are the same. In addition, the rejection of the null hypothesis is not due to a truly meaningful difference but a very small variability. This is particularly true for dissolution testing. *In vitro* release testing is usually conducted under much more tightly controlled conditions than *in vivo* bioequivalence testing. The variability is small enough to declare a trivial difference as statistically significant. As a result, the concept of bioequivalence should be applied to *in vitro* dissolution testing. The null and alternative hypotheses should be reformulated as follows:

Null hypothesis: Two dissolution curves are not similar

Alternative hypothesis: Two dissolution curves are similar (equivalent)

If one rejects the above null hypothesis, one claims that the dissolution profiles are similar. The equivalence limits should be determined by researchers in this area and preferably by some fixed numbers that are independent of the results of reference formulations. Similar to the bioequivalence problem, the approach of confidence interval should be used because it can provide a measure for the closeness of the difference between the two curves with a probability statement and it can be used as a tool to judge whether the two curves are equivalent. One might suggest computing a 90 percent confidence interval for each time interval. The problem of multiplicity mentioned above, however, still remains.

Tsong (1995) defined similarity in two ways. Two dissolution profiles are said to be globally similar if the difference in average dissolution rates is less than 10 percent at all time points. For some specific time points, if the differences in average dissolution rates are less than 15 percent, then the two dissolution profiles are said to be locally similar at these time points. The problem of multiplicity, however, still remains with his definition of similarity. In order to avoid this problem, constructing a 90 percent confidence interval based on the combined difference from all time integrals is suggested. The combined difference can be weighted averages of all differences from different time points. The weights can be chosen depending upon the relative importance of each time point.

In order to take the USP specifications into consideration when comparing the two dissolution profiles, Chow and Ki (1997) proposed a time series approach which accounts for correlation between dissolution at different time points. In addition, the following procedure may be considered.

Step 1: Individual curve – each individual curve must meet all USP specifications at each of the specified time intervals. Otherwise, reject that the two curves are similar.

Step 2: Comparison of the dissolution curves of drug products – conduct the comparison of the dissolution curves between the test and reference formulations only if step 1 is skipped. Two dissolution curves are declared similar if the 90 percent confidence interval based on the combined difference is within the pre-specified limits. Otherwise, reject.

12.4 Issues on FDA Conjugated Estrogen Bioequivalence Guidance

For the *in vivo* single dose fasting bioequivalence study, the study design, sample size determination, multiplicity of studies and ingredients, use of baseline measurements, and logarithmic transformation have been discussed. The four-sequence, three-period design suggested by the FDA guidance is very sophisticated yet unnecessarily complicated. It does, however, provide estimates of the treatment, first-order carryover effects, and second-order carryover effects in the presence of each other. The inference can be obtained based on the intrasubject variability. Hence, the statement: "This requirement results from the inability to estimate the least squares means for treatment effects when a term for residual effects is included in the statistical model:" made in footnote five at the bottom of the page nine of the FDA guidance is not valid for the four-sequence, three-period crossover design. In addition, contrary to the statement on the page nine of the FDA guidance, taking logarithmic transformation of observed pharmacokinetic responses has no impact on the statistical significance of the first-order carryover effect. On the other hand, the description of the use of the mean baseline value from the first period as a covariate in the FDA guidance will not be able to

Experience of Generic Drug Products with Multiple Components 291

evaluate whether or not the model has adequately adjusted for the differences of the estrogen levels among subjects.

As an alternative, the use of the dual design (RTT, TRR) to investigate the bioequivalence in conjugated estrogen tablets is suggested. This two-sequence dual design can also provide an unbiased estimation of the treatment effect in the presence of the first-order carryover effect and its inference is also based on the intrasubject variability. Formulas for sample size determination for the two designs are also provided. It appears that the total number of subjects required for the four-sequence, three-period crossover design is more than that for the two-sequence dual design.

The multiplicity of studies and active ingredients is a much more complicated statistical issue. To control an overall study-wise type I error, a 90 percent confidence interval can be constructed, on log scale, based on the observed maximum difference among the four active ingredients and the upper quantile of the studentized range distribution. If the resulting 90 percent confidence interval, after inverse antilog transformation, is within (80.00 percent, 125.00 percent), then bioequivalence is concluded for the study.

With respect to *in vitro* drug release (dissolution) testing, the sampling times are 2.0, 5.0, and 8.0 hours for 0.3, 0.625, and 0.9 mg tablets and 2.0, 5.0, 8.0, and 10.0 hours for 1.25 and 2.5 mg tablets. It appears that a dissolution profile might not satisfactorily be characterized by three or four time points. Choosing at least five time points is recommended for an adequate description of a dissolution curve. On the other hand, the FDA guidance only requires 12 dosage units. The sampling plan stated in USP, however, might test up to 24 dosage units. It is not known whether 12 dosage units are enough to pass the USP test. Note that it is extremely important to consider the USP dissolution test with the USP sampling plan (Chow and Liu 1995) as a component of the criteria for determination of similarity between the two dissolution curves.

Recently, The FDA published *Guidance for Industry—Immediate Release Solid Oral Dosage Forms Scale-up and Postapproval Changes (SUPAC): Chemistry, Manufacturing, and Controls, In Vitro Dissolution Testing and In Vivo Bioequivalence Documentation*. This guidance adopted the concept of similarity for comparison between two dissolution profiles. In addition, it requests the sponsor to use the following similarity factor f2 to compare dissolution profiles based on at least 12 individual dosage units:

$$f_2 = 50 \log_{10} \left\{ \left[1 + \frac{1}{n} \Sigma (R_i - T_i)^2 \right]^{-0.5} \times 100 \right\},$$

where R_i and T_i are percent dissolved at time point i.

This similarity factor is a logarithmic reciprocal square root transformation of one plus the mean squared (the average sum of squares) differences in percent dissolved between the test and reference products over all time points. The FDA suggests that two dissolution profiles are declared similar if f_2 is between 50 and 100. First, it is not clear from the guidance whether the percent dissolved is referred to as the cumulative percent dissolved up to time point t or as the incremental percent dissolved observed from the previous time point $t - 1$ to the current time point t. Second, it is not known if R_i and T_i are the average of percent dissolved of all dosage units at the time point t or refer to the percent dissolved of individual dosage units, respectively, for the test and reference drug products. Third, the range of f_2 is from $-\infty$ to 100, and it is not symmetric about zero.

It is understandable, therefore, that a value of 100 for f_2 corresponds to a value of zero for the mean squared differences in percent dissolved over all time points. On the other hand, the selection of 50 for f_2 as the lower limit for claiming similarity requires explanation and clarification because it indicates that the mean squared difference is 99, which seems very arbitrary and presents no meaningful explanation. Finally, the guidance does not provide any references regarding the statistical justification for the use of f_2 in assessment of similarity between two dissolution profiles. Consequently, thorough research in both theoretical and applied statistics is required before any regulations in assessment of similarity between dissolution profiles can be put into practice.

12.5 Concluding Remarks

Following the publication of the 1991 FDA guidance on conjugated estrogen tablets, Liu and Chow (1996) provided a comprehensive review of the guidance with recommendations for future bioequivalence studies for drug products with multiple components. It should be noted that although regulatory guidance on *in vivo* bioequivalence testing for drug product and on *in vitro* bioequivalence testing for nasal aerosols and nasal sprays drug products for local action are well established (FDA 2003a,b), they focus on drug products with a single active ingredient rather than drug products with multiple active ingredients or components. For drug products with multiple components (e.g., TCMs), many scientific factors and/or statistical issues as described in Chapter 12 of this book still remain unsolved.

Unlike traditional Western medicines that usually contain single active ingredient, conjugated estrogen tablets contain several primary active ingredients (components) such as unconjugated estrone, estrone sulfate, unconjugated equilin, and equilin sulfate, which are considered drug products with multiple components. Regulatory requirements for assessment of drug products with multiple components in terms of good drug characteristics

Experience of Generic Drug Products with Multiple Components 293

such as purity, quality, safety, potency, and stability are similar but slightly different owing to possible component-to-component interaction and their relative relationships in mechanism of action and pharmacological activity. In practice, because TCMs usually contain a number of active and inactive components, they can be treated as drug products with multiple components like conjugated estrogen tablets. Thus, the FDA experience on study design, sample size determination, and multiplicity of components for evaluation of conjugated estrogen tablets is helpful for development of TCMs.

13

Stability Analysis for Drug Products with Multiple Components

13.1 Introduction

For every drug product in the marketplace, the US FDA requires that an expiration dating period (or shelf life) must be indicated on the immediate container label. The shelf life is defined as the time interval at which the characteristics of a drug product (e.g., strength) will remain within the approved specifications after manufacture. Along this line, Shao and Chow (2001b) studied several statistical procedures for estimation of drug shelf life. Before a shelf life of a drug product can be granted by the FDA, the manufacturers (drug companies) need to demonstrate that the average drug characteristics can meet the approved specifications during the claimed shelf-life period through a stability study.

For determination of the shelf life of a drug product, both the FDA stability guidelines and the stability guidelines issued by the International Conference on Harmonization (ICH) requires that a long-term stability study be conducted to characterize the degradation of the drug product over a time period under appropriate storage conditions. Both the FDA and ICH stability guidelines suggest that stability testing be performed at 3-month intervals during the first year, 6-month intervals during the second year, and annually thereafter. The degradation curve can then be used to establish an expiration dating period or shelf life applicable to all future batches of the drug product.

For a single batch, the FDA stability guidelines indicate that an acceptable approach for drug products that are expected to decrease with time is to determine the time at which the 95 percent one-sided lower confidence bound for the mean degradation curve intersects the acceptable lower product specification limit, e.g., as specified in the USP/NF (FDA 2000). More details regarding design and analysis of stability studies can be found in the work of Chow (2007).

295

296 *Quantitative Methods for Traditional Chinese Medicine Development*

13.2 Regulatory Requirements

As indicated earlier, the US FDA issued the first stability guidelines. However, specific requirements on statistical design and analysis of stability studies were not available until 1987 (FDA 1987). These guidelines were subsequently revised to reflect changes in the regulatory environment for international harmonization (FDA 1998). In the interest of having international harmonization of stability testing requirements for a registration application within the three areas of the European Union (EU), Japan, and the United States, a tripartite guideline for the stability testing of new drug substances and products was developed by the Expert Working Group (EWG) of the ICH and released in 1993. In what follows, regulatory requirements for stability testing as described in the FDA stability guidelines and ICH guidelines for stability will be briefly described.

13.2.1 FDA Stability Guidelines

The purpose of the 1987 FDA stability guidelines is twofold. One objective is to provide recommendations for the design and analysis of stability studies to establish an appropriate expiration dating period and product requirements. The other objective is to provide recommendations for the submission of stability information and data to the FDA for investigational and new drug applications and product license applications. The 1987 FDA stability guidelines indicate that a stability protocol must describe not only how the stability is to be designed and carried out but also the statistical methods to be used for analysis of the data. As pointed out by the 1987 FDA stability guidelines, the design of a stability protocol is intended to establish an expiration dating period applicable to all future batches of the drug product manufactured under similar circumstances. Therefore, as indicated in the 1987 FDA stability guidelines, the design of a stability study should be able to take into consideration the following variabilities: (1) individual dosage units, (2) containers within a batch, and (3) batches.

The purpose is to ensure that the resulting data for each batch are truly representative of the batch as a whole and to quantify the variability from batch to batch. In addition, the 1987 FDA stability guidelines provide a number of requirements for conducting a stability study for determination of an expiration dating period for drug products. Some of these requirements are summarized below.

13.2.1.1 Batch Sampling Consideration

The 1987 FDA guidelines indicate that at least three batches and preferably more should be tested to allow for some estimate of batch-to-batch variability and to test the hypothesis that a single expiration dating period for all

Stability Analysis for Drug Products with Multiple Components 297

batches is justifiable. It is a concern that testing a single batch does not permit assessment of batch-to-batch variability and that testing of two batches may not provide a reliable estimate. It should be noted that the specification of at least three batches being tested is a minimum requirement. In general, more precise estimates can be obtained from more batches.

13.2.1.2 Container (Closure) and Drug Product Sampling

To ensure that the samples chosen for stability study can represent the batch as a whole, the 1987 FDA stability guidelines suggest that selection of such containers as bottles, packages, and vials from the batches be included in the stability study. Therefore, it is recommended that at least as many containers be sampled as the number of sampling times in the stability study. In any case, sampling of at least two containers for each sampling time is encouraged.

13.2.1.3 Sampling Time Considerations

The 1987 FDA stability guidelines suggest that stability testing be done at 3-month intervals during the first year, 6-month intervals during the second year, and annually thereafter. In other words, it is suggested that stability testing be performed at 0, 3, 6, 9, 12, 18, 24, 36, and 48 months for a 4-year duration of a stability study. However, if the drug product is expected to degrade rapidly, more frequent sampling is necessary.

13.2.2 ICH Guidelines for Stability

The ICH Q1A guidelines for stability are usually referred to as the parent guidelines for stability because (1) they have been revised a couple of times and (2) they are the foundation of subsequent guidelines for stability developed by the ICH EWG since it was issued in 1993 (ICH Q1A 1993; ICH Q1A [R2] 2003). The ICH Q1A (R2) guidelines for stability, provide a general indication of the requirements for stability testing but leave sufficient flexibility to encompass the variety of practical situations required for specific scientific situations and characteristics for the materials being evaluated. The ICH guidelines for stability establish the principle that information on stability generated in any of the three areas of the EU, Japan, and the United States would be mutually acceptable in both of the other two areas provided that it meets the appropriate requirements of the guidelines and the labeling is in accordance with national and regional requirements. Table 13.1 lists ICH guidelines related to stability testing issued in the past decade. It should be noted that the choice of test conditions defined in the ICH guidelines is based on an analysis of the effects of climatic conditions in the three areas of the EU, Japan, and the United States. Therefore, the main kinetic temperature in any region of the world can be derived from climatic data (ICH

298   *Quantitative Methods for Traditional Chinese Medicine Development*

TABLE 13.1

ICH Guidelines Related to Stability Testing

ICH Guideline	Date Issued	Description
Q1A	1993	Stability testing of new drug substances and products
Q1A (R2)	2003	Stability testing of new drug substances and products
Q1B	1996	Photostability testing of new drug substance and products
Q1C	1997	Stability testing of new dosage forms
Q1D	2003	Bracketing and matrixing designs for stability testing of new drug substances and products
Q1E	2004	Evaluation of stability data
Q1	2004	Stability data package for registration applications in climatic zones III and IV
Q3A	2003	Impurities in new drug substances
Q3B (R)	2003	Impurities in new drug products
Q5C	1995	Stability testing of biotechnological/biological products
Q6A	1999	Specifications: test procedures and acceptance criteria for new drug substances and new drug products: chemical substances
Q6B	1999	Specifications: test procedures and acceptance criteria for new drug substances and new drug products: biotechnological/biological products

Q1F 2004). Basically, the ICH Q1A (R2) guidelines for stability are similar to the 1987 FDA stability guidelines and the current FDA draft guidelines for stability (FDA 1998). For example, the ICH guidelines suggest that testing under the defined long-term conditions normally be done every 3 months over the first year, every 6 months over the second year, and annually thereafter. It requires that the container to be used in the long-term real-time stability evaluation be the same as or simulate the actual packaging used for storage and distribution. For the selection of batches, it requires that stability information from accelerated and long-term testing be provided on at least three batches and the long-term testing should cover a minimum of 12 months' duration on at least three batches at the time of submission. For the drug product, it is required that the three batches be of the same formulation and dosage form in the containers and closure proposed for marketing. Two of the three batches should be at least pilot scale. The third batch may be smaller (e.g., 25,000 to 50,000 tablets or capsules for solid oral dosage forms). However, the ICH Q1A (R2) guidelines for stability also requires that the first three production batches of the drug substances or drug product manufactured post approval, if not submitted in the original registration application, be placed on the long-term stability studies using the same stability protocol as in the approved drug application. For storage conditions, the ICH Q1A (R2) guidelines require that accelerated testing be carried out

Stability Analysis for Drug Products with Multiple Components 299

at a temperature at least 15°C above the designated long-term storage temperature in conjunction with the appropriate relative humidity conditions for that temperature. The designated long-term testing conditions will be reflected in the labeling and retest date. The retest date is the date when samples of the drug substance should be reexamined to ensure that material is still suitable for use. The ICH Q1A (R2) guidelines for stability also indicate that where significant change occurs during 6 months of storage under conditions of accelerated testing at $40 \pm 2°C/75 \pm 5\%$ relative humidity, additional testing at an intermediate condition (such as $30 \pm 2°C/60 \pm 5\%$ relative humidity) should be conducted for drug substances to be used in the manufacture of dosage forms tested long term at 25°C/60% relative humidity in considered failure to meet the specification.

For the evaluation of stability data, the ICH Q1A (R2) guidelines for stability indicate that statistical methods should be employed to test goodness of fit of the data on all batches and combined batches (where appropriate) to the assumed degradation line or curve. If it is inappropriate to combine data from several batches, the overall retest period may depend on the minimum time a batch may be expected to remain within acceptable and justified limits. A retest period is defined as the period of time during which the drug substance or drug product can be considered to remain within specifications and therefore acceptable for use in the manufacture of a given drug product, provided that it has been stored under the defined conditions.

13.2.3 Remarks

As indicated earlier, the EU, Japan, and the United States have different but similar stability requirements (see, e.g., Mazzo 1998). On the basis of the different requirements, pharmaceutical companies may have to conduct stability tests repeatedly for different markets. The ICH guidelines for stability are an attempt to harmonize these requirements so that information generated in any of the three areas of the EU, Japan, and the United States would be acceptable to the other two areas. In what follows, we briefly summarize the differences in requirements regarding stability aspects among the EU, Japan, and the United States, which were discussed in a workshop on stability testing held in Brussels, Belgium, November 5–7, 1991.

13.2.3.1 Minimum Duration of Stability Testing

In the EU it is required to file an application based on the results of stability tests performed after at least 6 months of storage. In the United States, however, the FDA requires that a minimum of 12 months of stability data be provided. The Ministry of Health, Labor, and Welfare (MHLW) of Japan requires 12 months. Statistically, it is undesirable to extrapolate a drug shelf life too far beyond the sampling intervals under study. Therefore, as a rule

300   *Quantitative Methods for Traditional Chinese Medicine Development*

of thumb, it is suggested that stability extrapolation not extend beyond 6 months. Stability data should be obtained to cover up to 6 months prior to the desired expiration dating period. In other words, if a desired shelf life is 18 months, stability testing should cover at least a 1-year period. However, as indicated in the 1987 FDA stability guidelines, although a tentative shelf life may be granted based on a short-term stability study, the pharmaceutical companies are expected to have commitment to obtain complete data that cover the full expiration dating period.

13.2.3.2 Minimum Number of Batches Required for Stability Testing

Under the current stability guidelines, the FDA requires at least three batches, and preferably more should be tested to allow a reasonable estimation of batch-to-batch variability and to test the hypothesis that a single expiration dating period for all future batches is justifiable. However, the EU requires only that stability data on two batches of the active drug substances be submitted for the evaluation of a drug expiration period. For the number of batches required in stability testing, the MHLW's requirement is consistent with the FDA's. The 1987 FDA stability guidelines provide some justification for the use of a minimum number of three batches for stability testing. The 1987 FDA stability guidelines indicate that a single batch does not permit assessment of batch-to-batch variability, and testing two batches provides an unreliable estimate. To provide a more precise estimate of drug shelf life, it is preferred to have stability testing on more batches. However, practical considerations such as cost, resources, and capacity may prevent the collection of data from more batches. As a result, the specification that at least three batches be tested has become a minimum requirement representing a compromise between statistical and regulatory considerations and actual practice.

13.2.3.3 Definition of Room Temperature

According to the USP/NF, the definition of room temperature is between 15° and 30°C in the United States. However, in the EU, the room temperature is defined as being 15° to 25°C, while in Japan, it is defined being 1° to 30°C. If the drug product is sensitive to the temperature range 0 to 30°C, degradation of the drug product may vary from one temperature to another within the range. Therefore, it is important to investigate the stability of the drug product at different ranges of temperatures if the drug product is to be marketed in different regions. In this case harmonization of the definition of room temperature may not be useful. However, if the drug product is not sensitive to this range of temperatures, harmonization of the definition of room temperatures may be needed so that similar stability testing need not be conducted repeatedly to fulfill different requirements.

Stability Analysis for Drug Products with Multiple Components — 301

13.2.3.4 Extension of Shelf Life

In practice, when a New Drug Application (NDA) submission is filed, there are usually limited data available on the stability of the drug product. In the United States it is a common practice for the FDA to tentatively grant marketing authorization of the drug product based on limited stability data. However, it is required by the FDA that a pharmaceutical company submit the results of stability studies obtained up to the expiration date granted. However, the EU does not accept an extension of shelf life beyond real-time data submitted.

13.2.3.5 Least Stable Batch

When there is a batch-to-batch variation, or the batches are not equivalent, the European Health Authorities expect the pharmaceutical industry to consider the least stable batch for the determination of shelf life and to refrain from averaging the values statistically. When there is batch-to-batch variation, the 1987 FDA stability guidelines suggest considering the minimum of individual shelf lives. It should be noted that the use of the least stable batch for determination of shelf life is conservative.

13.2.3.6 Least Protective Packaging

The MHLW of Japan prefers to determine the drug shelf life based on the results of stability testing using the least stable packaging material instead of testing the product in all packages. The 1987 FDA stability guidelines, however, encourage sampling of at least two containers of each packaging material for each sampling time in all cases. The idea of testing the least stable packaging material is well taken. However, how to identify the least stable packaging material is an interesting statistical question. To identify the least stable packaging material, a pilot study may be required. As a result, a fractional factorial design may be applied. However, it should be noted that the selected pilot design should be able to avoid any possible confounding and interaction effects.

13.2.3.7 Replicates

In Japan each test must be repeated three times without provision for scientific and statistical justification. The 1987 FDA stability guidelines, however, encourage testing an increasing number of replicates at later sampling times, particularly the latest sampling time. The reason for doing this is that it will increase the precision of the estimation of the expiration dating period because the degradation is most likely to occur at later sampling time points than at earlier time points for long-term stability studies. Although the accuracy and precision of the estimated shelf life based on replicates of test results will be improved, it is not clear how much improvement the test

302   *Quantitative Methods for Traditional Chinese Medicine Development*

replicates will achieve. Replications at each sampling time point not only increase the precision of the estimation for shelf life but also provide data on the lack-of-fit test for fitting individual simple linear regressions to each batch. In practice, it is of interest to investigate the impact of replicates at each sampling time point on the accuracy and precision of shelf-life estimation.

13.2.3.8 General Principles

The ICH stability guideline suggests the following general principles for the evaluation of stability of biosimilar products. These general principles indicate that the applicant should

1. Develop data to support the claimed shelf life.
2. Consider any external conditions affecting potency, purity and quality.
3. Primary data to support the requested shelf life should be based on long–term, real-time, real-condition stability studies. The design of the long-term stability program is critical.
4. Retest periods are not appropriate for biotech/biological.

13.3 Statistical Model and Methods

13.3.1 Statistical Model

Consider the case where the drug characteristic is expected to decrease with time. The other case can be treated similarly. Assume that drug characteristic decreases over time linearly (i.e., the degradation curve is a straight line). In this case, the slope of the straight line is considered as the rate of stability loss of the product. Let X_j be the jth sampling (testing) time point (i.e., 0 months, 3 months, etc.) and Y_{ij} be the corresponding testing result of the ith batch ($j = 1,...,n; i = 1,...,k$). Then

$$Y_{ij} = \alpha_i + \beta_i X_j + e_{ij}, \tag{13.1}$$

where e_{ij} are assumed to be independent and identically distributed (i.i.d.) random errors with mean 0 and variance σ_e^2. The total number of observations is $N = kn$. The α_i (intercepts) and β_i (slopes) vary randomly from batch to batch. It is assumed that α_i ($i = 1,...,k$) are independent, identically, distributed (i.i.d.) with mean a and variance σ_a^2, and that β_i ($i = 1,...,k$) are i.i.d. with mean b and variance σ_b^2. The $e_{ij}, \alpha_i,$ and β_i are mutually independent.

If $\sigma_a^2 = 0$ (i.e., α_i are equal), then the above model has a common intercept. Similarly, if $\sigma_b^2 = 0$ (i.e., β_i are equal), then the above model has a common slope. If both $\sigma_a^2 = 0$ and $\sigma_b^2 = 0$, then there is no batch-to-batch variation

Stability Analysis for Drug Products with Multiple Components

and the above model reduces to a simple linear regression. Under the above model, Chow and Shao (1989) proposed several statistical tests for batch-to-batch variation.

13.3.2 Statistical Methods

13.3.2.1 Fixed Batches Approach

If there is no batch-to-batch variation, a commonly used method for fitting the above model is the ordinary least squares (OLS) and a 95% lower confidence bound for $E(Y) = a + b\xi$, the expected drug characteristic at time ξ, can be obtained as

$$\hat{a} + \hat{b}\xi - t_{0.95}S(\xi),$$

where $\hat{a}$ and $\hat{b}$ are the OLS estimators of a and b, respectively, $t_{0.95}$ is the one-sided 95th percentile of the t distribution with $N - 2$ degrees of freedom, and

$$S^2(\xi) = \text{MSE}\left\{\frac{1}{N} + \frac{(\xi - \bar{X})^2}{k\sum_{j=1}^{n}(X_j - \bar{X})^2}\right\},$$

where

$$\bar{X} = \frac{1}{n}\sum_{j=1}^{n}X_j$$

and

$$\text{MSE} = \frac{1}{N-2}\sum_{i=1}^{k}\sum_{j=1}^{n}(Y_{ij} - \hat{a} - \hat{b}X_j)^2.$$

The estimated shelf life can be obtained by solving the following equation:

$$\eta = \hat{a} + \hat{b}\xi - t_{0.95}S(\xi),$$

where η is a given approved lower specification limit.

When there is a batch-to-batch variation (i.e., there are different intercepts and different slopes), the FDA recommends the minimum approach be used for estimation of the shelf life of a drug product. The minimum

304   *Quantitative Methods for Traditional Chinese Medicine Development*

approach considers the minimum of the estimated shelf lives of the individual batches. The minimum approach, however, has received considerable criticism because it lacks of statistical justification. As an alternative, Ruberg and Hsu (1990) proposed an approach using the concept of multiple comparisons to derive some criteria for pooling batches with the worst batch. The idea is to pool the batches that have slopes similar to the worst degradation rate with respect to a predetermined similarity (equivalence) limit.

13.3.2.2 Random Batches Approach

As indicated in the FDA guideline, the batches used in long-term stability studies for establishment of drug shelf life should constitute a random sample from the population of future production batches. In addition, all estimated shelf lives should be applicable to all future batches. As a result, statistical methods based on a random effects model seem more appropriate. In recent years, several methods for determination of drug shelf life with random batches have been considered. See, for example, Chow and Shao (1989, 1991), Murphy and Weisman (1990), Chow (1992), and Shao and Chow (1994). Under the assumption that batch is a random variable, stability data can be described by a linear regression model with random coefficients. Consider the following model:

$$Y_{ij} = X'_{ij}\beta_i + e_{ij},$$

where Y_{ij} is the jth assay result (percent of label claim) for the ith batch, X_{ij} is a $p\times l$ vector of the jth value of the regressor for the ith batch and X'_{ij} is its transpose, β_i is a $p\times l$ vector of random effects for the ith batch, and e_{ij} is the random error in observing Y_{ij}. Note that $X'_{ij}\beta_i$ is the mean drug characteristic for the ith batch at X_{ij} (conditional on β_i). The primary assumptions for the model are similar to those for Model 4.1. Because X_{ij} is usually chosen to be x_j for all i, where x_j is a $p\times l$ vector of nonrandom covariate which could be of the form $(1, t_j, t_j w_j)'$ or $(1, t_j, w_j, t_j w_j)'$, where t_j is the jth time point and w_j is the jth value of $q\times l$ vector of nonrandom covariate (e.g., package type and dosage strength). Denote $x_j = x(t_j, w_j)$, where $x(t, w)$ is a known function of t and w. If there is no batch-to-batch variation, the average drug characteristic at time t is $x(t)'\beta$ and the true shelf life is equal to

$$\bar{t}_{true} = \inf\{t : x(t)'\beta \le \eta\},$$

which is an unknown but nonrandom quantity. The shelf life is then given by

$$\hat{t} = \inf\{t : L(t) \le \eta\},$$

Stability Analysis for Drug Products with Multiple Components

where

$$L(t) = x(t)'\bar{b} - t_{\alpha,nk-p} \left[\frac{x(t)'(X'X)^{-1}x(t)}{k(nk-p)} \text{SSR} \right]^{1/2}$$

where SSR is the usual sum of squared residuals from the ordinary least squares regression.

When there is batch-to-batch variation, t_{true} is random since β_i is random. Chow and Shao (1991) and Shao and Chow (1994) proposed considering an $(1 - \alpha) \times 100\%$ lower confidence bound of the εth quantile of t_{true} as the labeled shelf life, where ε is a given small positive constant. That is,

$$P\{t_{\text{label}} \le t_\varepsilon\} \ge 1 - \alpha,$$

where t_ε satisfies

$$P\{t_{\text{true}} \le t_\varepsilon\} = \varepsilon.$$

It follows that

$$t_\varepsilon = \inf\{t : x(t)'\beta - \eta = z_\varepsilon \sigma(t)\}$$

where $z_\varepsilon = \Phi^{-1}(1 - \varepsilon)$ and $\sigma(t)$ is the standard deviation of $x(t)'\beta_i$. As a result, the shelf life is given by

$$\hat{t} = \inf\{t : x(t)'\bar{b} \le \bar{\eta}(t)\},$$

where

$$\bar{\eta}(t) = \eta + c_\kappa(\varepsilon, \alpha) z_\varepsilon \sqrt{v(t)},$$

$$c_\kappa(\varepsilon, \alpha) = \frac{1}{\sqrt{k} z_\varepsilon} t_{\alpha,K-1,\sqrt{k} z_\varepsilon},$$

$$v(t) = \frac{1}{k-1} x(t)'(X'X')^{-1} X'SX(X'X')^{-1} x(t).$$

Note that $t_{\alpha,k-1,\sqrt{k} z_\varepsilon}$ is the αth upper quantile of the noncentral t distribution with $k - 1$ degrees of freedom and noncentrality parameter $\sqrt{k} z_\varepsilon$.

306   *Quantitative Methods for Traditional Chinese Medicine Development*

13.3.2.3 Remarks

As indicated in the FDA stability guidelines, the estimated shelf life of a drug can be obtained at the time point at which the 95 percent one-sided lower confidence limit for the mean degradation curve intersects the acceptable lower specification limit. In practice, it is of interest to study the bias of the estimated shelf life. If the bias is positive, the estimated shelf life overestimates the true shelf life. On the other hand, if there is a downward bias, the estimated shelf life is said to underestimate the true shelf life. In the interest of the safety of the drug product, the FDA might prefer a conservative approach, which is to underestimate rather than overestimate the true shelf life. Sun et al. (1999) studied distribution properties of the estimated shelf life proposed by Chow and Shao (1991) and Shao and Chow (1994) for both cases with and without batch-to-batch variation. The result indicate that when there is no batch-to-batch variation (i.e., $\sigma_a^2 = \sigma_b^2 = 0$), there is a downward bias which is given by

$$\frac{t_\alpha \sigma_e}{b^2} \left[\frac{b^2}{n} + \frac{(b\bar{X} + a - \eta)^2}{\sum_{j=1}^{n} (X_j - \bar{X})^2} \right]^{1/2},$$

where t_α, is the $(1 - \alpha)$th quantile of the t distribution with $k - 1$ degrees of freedom.

13.3.3 Two-Phase Shelf-Life Estimation

Unlike most drug products, some drug products are required to be stored at several temperatures such as $-20°$, $5°$, and $25°C$ (room temperature) in order to maintain stability until use (Mellon 1991). The drug products of this kind are usually referred to as frozen drug products. Unlike the usual drug products, a typical shelf-life statement for frozen drug products usually consists of multiple phases with different storage temperatures. For example, a commonly adopted shelf life statement for frozen products could be either (1) 24 months at $-20°C$ followed by 2 weeks at $5°C$ or two days at $25°C$ or (2) 24 months at $-20°C$ followed by 2 weeks at $5°C$ and one days at $25°C$. As a result, the drug shelf life is determined based on a two-phase stability study. The first-phase stability study is to determine drug shelf life under frozen storage condition such as $-20°C$, while the second-phase stability study is to estimate drug shelf life under refrigerated or ambient conditions. A first-phase stability study is usually referred to as a frozen study, and a second-phase stability study is known as a thawed study.

Because the stability study of a frozen drug product consists of frozen and thawed studies, the determination of the shelf life involves a two-phase linear regression. The frozen study is usually conducted similar to a regular

Stability Analysis for Drug Products with Multiple Components 307

long-term stability study except the drug is stored at frozen condition. In other words, stability testing will normally be conducted at 3-month intervals during the first year, 6-month intervals during the second year, and annually thereafter. Stability testing for the thawed study is conducted following the stability testing for the frozen study, which may be performed at 2-day intervals up to 2 weeks. It should be noted that the stability at the second phase (i.e., thawed study) might depend on the stability at the first phase (i.e., frozen study). In other words, an estimated shelf life from the thawed study following stability testing at 3 months of the frozen study may be longer than that obtained from the thawed study following the frozen study at 6 months. For simplicity, Mellon (1991) suggested that stability from the frozen study and the thawed study be analyzed separately to obtain a combined shelf life for the drug product. As an alternative, Shao and Chow (2001a) consider the following method for determination of drug shelf lives for the two phases based on a similar concept proposed by Chow and Shao (1991) and Shao and Chow (1994).

13.3.3.1 First-Phase Shelf Life

For the first-phase shelf life, we have stability data

$$Y_{ik} = \alpha + \beta t_i + \varepsilon_{ik},$$

where $i = 1,\ldots, I \geq 2$ (typically, $t_i = 0, 3, 6, 9, 12, 18$ months), $k = 1,\ldots, K_i \geq 1$, α and β are unknown parameters, and ε_{ik}'s are i.i.d. random errors with mean 0 and variance $\sigma_1^2 > 0$. The total number of data for the first phase is $n_1 = \Sigma_i K_i \, (= IK$ if $K_i = K$ for all i). At time t_i, $K_{ij} > I$ second-phase stability data are collected at time intervals $t_{ij}, j = 1,\ldots, J \geq 2$. The total number of data for the second phase is $n_2 = \Sigma_i \Sigma_j K_{ij} \, (= IJK$ if $K_{ij} = K$ for all i and j). Data from two phases are independent. Typically, $t_{ij} = t_i + s_j$, where $s_j = 1, 2, 3$ days, etc.

Let $\alpha(t)$ and $\beta(t)$ be the intercept and slope of the second-phase degradation line at time t. Because the degradation lines for the two phases intersect,

$$\alpha(t) = \alpha + \beta t.$$

Then, at time t_i, $i = 1,\ldots, I$, we have stability data

$$Y_{ijk} = \alpha + \beta t_i + \beta(t_i)s_j + e_{ijk},$$

where $\beta(t)$ is an unknown function of t and e_{ijk}'s are i.i.d. random errors with mean 0 and variance $\sigma_{2i}^2 > 0$. We assume that $\beta(t)$ is a polynomial in t. Typically,

$$\beta(t) = \beta_0 \quad \text{Common slope model,}$$

$$\beta(t) = \beta_0 + \beta_1 t \quad \text{Linear trend model,}$$

or

$$\beta(t) = \beta_0 + \beta_1 t + \beta_2 t^2 \quad \text{Quadratic trend model.}$$

In general,

$$\beta(t) = \sum_{h=0}^{H} \beta_h t^h,$$

where β_h's are unknown parameters and $H + 1 < \Sigma_j K_{ij}$ for all i and $H < I$.

The first-phase shelf life can be determined based on the first-phase data $\{Y_{ik}\}$ as the time point at which the lower product specification limit intersects the 95 percent lower confidence bound of the mean degradation curve (FDA 1987; ICH 1993). Let $\hat{\alpha}$ and $\hat{\beta}$ be the least squares estimators of α and β, based on the first phase data, and let

$$L(t) = \hat{\alpha} + \hat{\beta}t - t_{0.05;n_1-2}\sqrt{v(t)}$$

be the 95 percent lower confidence bound for $\alpha + \beta t$, where $t_{0.05;n_1-2}$ is the upper 0.05 quantile of the t distribution with $n_1 - 2$ degrees of freedom,

$$v(t) = \hat{\sigma}_1^2 \frac{nt^2 - \left(2\sum_{i,k} t_i\right)t + \sum_{i,k} t_i^2}{n\sum_{i,k} t_i^2 - \left(\sum_{i,k} t_i\right)^2},$$

and

$$\hat{\sigma}_1^2 = \frac{1}{n_1 - 2}\sum_{i,k}(Y_{ik} - \hat{\alpha} - \hat{\beta}t_i)^2$$

is the usual error variance estimator based on residuals. Suppose that the lower limit for the drug characteristic is η (we assume that $\alpha + \beta t$ decreases as t increases). Then the first-phase shelf life is the first solution of $L(t) = \eta$, i.e.,

$$\hat{t} = \inf\{t : L(t) \le \eta\}.$$

Note that the first-phase shelf life is constructed so that

$$P\{\hat{t} \le \text{the true first-phase shelf life}\} = 95\%$$

Stability Analysis for Drug Products with Multiple Components

assuming that e_{ik}'s are normally distributed. Without the normality assumption, result approximately holds for large n_1. We now consider the second-phase shelf life, which is described below.

13.3.3.2 Case of Equal Second Phase Slopes

To introduce the idea, we first consider the simple case where the slopes of the second-phase degradation lines are the same. When $\beta(t) \equiv \beta_0$, the common slope β_0 can be estimated by the least squares estimator based on the second-phase data:

$$\hat{\beta}_0 = \frac{\sum_{i,j,k}(s_j - \bar{s})Y_{ijk}}{\sum_{i,j,k}(s_j - \bar{s})^2},$$

where s_j is the second-phase time intervals and $\bar{s}$ is the average of s_j's. The variance of $\hat{\beta}_0$ is

$$V(\hat{\beta}_0) = \frac{\sigma_2^2}{\sum_{i,j,k}(s_j - \bar{s})^2},$$

which can be estimated by

$$\hat{V}(\hat{\beta}_0) = \frac{\hat{\sigma}_2^2}{\sum_{i,j,k}(s_j - \bar{s})^2},$$

where

$$\hat{\sigma}_2^2 = \frac{1}{n_2 - 2}\sum_{i,j,k}(Y_{ijk} - (\hat{\alpha} + \hat{\beta}t_i) - \hat{\beta}_0 s_j)^2.$$

For fixed t and s, let

$$v(t,s) = v(t) + \hat{V}(\hat{\beta}_0)s^2$$

and

$$L(t,s) = \hat{\alpha} + \hat{\beta}t + \hat{\beta}_0 s - t_{0.05;n_1+n_2-4}\sqrt{v(t,s)}.$$

310　　*Quantitative Methods for Traditional Chinese Medicine Development*

For any fixed t less than the first-phase true shelf life, i.e., t satisfying $\alpha + \beta t > \eta$, the second-phase shelf life can be estimated as

$$\hat{s}(t) = \inf\{s \geq 0 : L(t, s) \leq \eta\}$$

(if $L(t, s) < \eta$ for all s, then $\hat{s}(t) = 0$). That is, if the drug product is taken out of the first-phase storage condition at time t, then the estimated second-phase shelf life is $\hat{s}(t)$.

The justification for $\hat{s}(t)$ is that for any t satisfying $\alpha + \beta t > \eta$,

$$P\{\hat{s}(t) \leq \text{the true second-phase shelf life}\} = 95\%$$

assuming that e_{ik} and e_{ijk} are normally distributed. Without the normality assumption, the above result approximately holds for large n_1, and n_2.

In practice, the time at which the drug product is taken out of the first-phase storage condition is unknown. In such a case we may apply the following method to assess the second-phase shelf life. Select a set of time intervals $t_l < \hat{t}$, $l = 1,\ldots, L$, and construct a table (or a figure) for $(t_l, \hat{s}(t_l))$, $l = 1,\ldots, L$. If a drug product is taken out of the first-phase storage condition at time t_0, which is between t_l and t_{l+1}, then its second-phase shelf life is $\hat{s}(t_{l+1})$. However, a single shelf-life label may be required. We propose the following method.

13.3.3.3 Determination of a Single Two-Phase Shelf-Life Label

In most cases, $L(\hat{t}, s)$ is less than η for all s, i.e., $\hat{s}(\hat{t}) = 0$. Hence, we propose to select a $\hat{t}_1 < \hat{t}$ such that $\hat{s}(\hat{t}) > 0$ and use $\hat{t}_1 + \hat{s}(\hat{t}_1)$ as the two-phase shelf-life label. The justification for this two-phase shelf-life label is

1. If the drug product is stored under the first-phase storage condition until time $\hat{t}_1$, then

$$P\{\hat{t}_1 \leq \text{the true first-phase shelf life}\} \geq 95\%$$

because $\hat{t}_1 < \hat{t}$.

2. If the drug product is taken out of the first-phase storage condition at time $\hat{t}_1 < \hat{t}$, then its estimated second-phase shelf life is $\hat{s}(\hat{t})$, and

$$P\{\hat{s}(\hat{t}_1) \leq \text{the true second phase shelf life at time } t_0\}$$

$$\geq P\{\hat{s}(\hat{t}_0) \leq \text{the true second phase shelf life at time } t_0\}$$

$$\geq 95\%$$

However, this two-phase shelf-life label is very conservative if t_0 is much less than $\hat{t}_1$.

Stability Analysis for Drug Products with Multiple Components 311

A general rule of choosing $\hat{t}_1$ is that $\hat{t}_1$ should be close to $\hat{t}$, while $\hat{s}(\hat{t})$ is reasonably large. For example, if the units of the first- and second-phase shelf lives are month and day, respectively, and if $\hat{t} = 24.5$, then we can choose $\hat{t}_1 = 24$; if $\hat{t} = 24$, then we choose $\hat{t}_1 = 23$. A table of $(t_l, \hat{s}(t_i))$, $l = 1,\dots, L$, will be useful for the selection of $\hat{t}_1$.

13.3.3.4 General Case of Unequal Second-Phase Slopes

In general, the slope of the second-phase degradation line varies with time. Let $\overline{Y}_i$ be the average of Y_{ijk}'s with a fixed i, $Z_{ijk} = Y_{ijk} - \overline{Y}_i$, and $X_{hij} = (s_j - \overline{s})t_i^h$. Then the least squares estimator of $(\beta_0,\dots,\beta_H)$, denoted by $(\hat{\beta}_0,\dots,\hat{\beta}_H)$, is the least squares estimator of the following linear regression model:

$$Z_{ijk} = \sum_{h=0}^{H} \beta_h X_{hij} + \text{error}.$$

Let

$$\hat{\beta}(t) = \sum_{h=0}^{H} \hat{\beta}_h t^h$$

and

$$\hat{V}(\hat{\beta}(t)) = \hat{\sigma}_2^2 \mathbf{1}'(X'X)^{-1}\mathbf{1},$$

where $\mathbf{1}' = (1, t, t^2, \dots, t^H)$, X is the design matrix and

$$\hat{\sigma}_2^2 = \frac{1}{n_2 - (H+2)} \sum_{i,j,k} \left(Z_{ijk} - \sum_{h=0}^{H} \hat{\beta}_h X_{hij} \right)^2.$$

The second-phase shelf-life and the two-phase shelf-life label can be determined in the same way as described in the previous section with

$$L(t, s) = \hat{\alpha} + \hat{\beta}t + \hat{\beta}(t)s - t_{0.05;n_1+n_2-(H+4)}\sqrt{v(t, s)}$$

and

$$v(t, s) = v(t) + \hat{V}(\hat{\beta}(t))s^2.$$

312   *Quantitative Methods for Traditional Chinese Medicine Development*

For the proposed method for two-phase shelf-life estimation, assume that the assay variabilities are the same across different phases. Detailed information regarding two-phase shelf-life estimation can be found in the work of Shao and Chow (2001a) and Chow and Shao (2002). In practice, the assay variability may vary from phase to phase. In this case, the proposed method is necessarily modified for determination of the expiration dating period of the drug product.

In practice, it is of interest to determine the allocation of sample size at each phase. For a fixed total of sample size, it is of interest to examine the relative efficiency for estimation of shelf lives using either more sampling time points in the first phase or less sampling time points in the second phase or less sampling time points in the first phase and more sampling time points in the second phase. The allocation of sampling time points at each phase then becomes an interesting research topic for two-phase shelf-life estimation. In addition, because the degradation at the second phase is highly correlated with the degradation at the first phase, it may be of interest to examine such correlation for future design planning.

13.4 Stability Designs

Because stability data are analyzed using a linear regression, the selection of observations that will give the minimum variance for the slope is to take one half at the beginning of the study and one half at the end. The beginning of the stability study is usually called $t = 0$. Stability studies are typically done at several different times. In practice, there is no unique best design. Thus, the choice of design must use the fact that analyses will be done after additional data are collected. Nordbrock (1992) introduced several designs that are commonly considered in stability studies. These designs are briefly described below.

13.4.1 Basic Matrix 2/3 on Time Design

A complete long-term study for one strength of a dosage form in one package has three batches, with all three tested every 3 months in the first year, every 6 months in the second year, and annually thereafter. Thus, if a 36-month shelf life is desired and the complete study is used, each of the three batches is tested at 0, 3, 6, 9, 12, 18, 24, and 36 months. The basic matrix 2/3 on time design has only two of the three batches tested at intermediate time points (other than at times of 0 and 36), as presented in Table 13.2. If an analysis is to be done after 18 months (e.g., for a registration application), the basic matrix 2/3 on time design can be modified by testing all batches at 18 months.

Stability Analysis for Drug Products with Multiple Components

TABLE 13.2

Basic Matrix 2/3 on Time Design

Batch	Test Times		
A	0, 3,	9, 12,	24, 36
B	0, 3,	6, 12,	18, 36
C	0,	6, 9,	18, 24, 36

13.4.2 Matrix 2/3 on Time Design with Multiple Packages

The first extension of the basic design is when one strength is packaged into three packages (i.e., when each batch is packaged into each of three packages). The basic matrix 2/3 on time design is applied to each package in a balanced fashion, as presented in Tables 13.3 and 13.4. Balance is defined as each batch is tested twice at each intermediate time point, and each package is tested twice at each intermediate time point. If an analysis is done after 18 months (e.g., for a registration application), this design can be modified by testing all batch-by-package combinations at 18 months.

13.4.3 Matrix 2/3 on Time Design with Multiple Packages and Multiple Strengths

When three strengths (say, 10, 20, and 30) are manufactured using different weights of the same formulation, giving nine sub-batches, we further assume that there are three packages for each strength. In this case, the basic matrix 2/3 on time design can be applied to each of the nine sub-batches in a balanced fashion (see Table 13.5). In this design, each sub-batch is tested twice at

TABLE 13.3

Matrix 2/3 on Time Design
with Multiple Packages

Batch	Pkg 1	Pkg 2	Pkg 3
A	T1	T2	T3
B	T2	T3	T1
C	T3	T1	T2

Note: Pkg 1, package 1; etc.

TABLE 13.4

Test Code Definitions

Code	Test Times after Time 0		
T1	3,	9, 12,	24, 36
T2	3,	6, 12,	18, 36
T3		6, 9,	18, 24, 36

Note: Batches are tested at time 0.

TABLE 13.5

Matrix 2/3 on Time Design with Multiple Packages and Multiple Strengths

Batch	Strength	Pkg 1	Pkg 2	Pkg 3
A	10	T1	T2	T3
A	20	T2	T3	T1
A	30	T3	T1	T2
B	10	T2	T3	T1
B	20	T3	T1	T2
B	30	T1	T2	T3
C	10	T3	T1	T2
C	20	T1	T2	T3
C	30	T2	T3	T1

Note: Pkg 1, package 1; etc.

each intermediate time point, each package is tested twice at each intermediate time point for each batch, each batch is tested 6 times at each intermediate time point, and each package is tested 6 times at each intermediate time point. If an analysis is done after 18 months (e.g., for a registration application), this design can be modified by testing all batch-by-strength-by-package combinations at 18 months.

13.4.4 Matrix 1/3 on Time Design

A further reduction in the amount of testing is accomplished by reducing the testing in each of the preceding designs from 2/3 to 1/3. For example, the basic 1/3 on time design has one of the three batches tested at each intermediate time point, as presented in Table 13.6. If an analysis is done after 18 months (e.g., for a registration application), the basic matrix 1/3 on time design can be modified by testing all batches at 18 months.

13.4.5 Matrix on Batch-by-Strength-by-Package Combinations

If there are multiple strengths and multiple packages, one could also choose to test only a portion of the batch-by-strength-by-package combinations. An example of when this might be appropriate is when there are three batches, each made into two strengths, giving six sub-batches. Although

TABLE 13.6

Basic Matrix 1/3 on Time Design

Batch	Test Times			
A	0, 3,	12,		36
B	0,	6,	18,	36
C	0,	9,	24, 36	

Stability Analysis for Drug Products with Multiple Components 315

TABLE 13.7

Matrix 1/2 on Time and Matrix on Batch × Strength × Package

Batch	Strength	Pkg 1	Pkg 2	Pkg 3
A	10	T1	T2	–
A	20	T2	–	T1
B	10	T2	–	T1
B	20	–	T1	T2
C	10	–	T1	T2
C	20	T1	T2	–

three packages will be used, the batch size is small and only two packages can be manufactured in each strength sub-batch. A matrix design on batch-by-strength-by-package combinations is presented in Table 13.7, with two packages selected for each of the six sub-batches, and where time is also matrixed by the factor 1/2. This design is approximately balanced because two packages are tested per sub-batch, one or two strengths are tested for each selected package by batch, four sub-batches are tested for each package, etc. Similar statements for the balance on time can be made.

13.4.6 Uniform Matrix Design

Another approach to design is the uniform matrix design, for which the same time protocol is used for all combinations of the other design factors (Murphy 1996). The strategy is to delete certain times (e.g., the 3-, 6-, 9-, and 18-month time points); therefore, testing is done only at 12, 24, and 36 months. This design has the advantages of simplifying the data entry of the study design and eliminating time points that add little to reducing the variability of the slope of the regression line. The disadvantage is that if there are major problems with the stability, there is no early warning because early testing is not done. Further, it may not be possible to determine if the linear model is appropriate (e.g., it may not be possible to determine whether there is an immediate decrease followed by very little decrease). However, the major disadvantage is that this design is probably not acceptable to some regulatory agencies.

13.4.7 Comparison of Designs

Nordbrock (1992) compared designs based on the power approach. This approach computes the probability that a statistical test will be significant when there is a specified alternative slope configuration. Power can be computed easily in Statistical Analysis Software (SAS, SAS Institute Inc., Cary, North Carolina). The strategy is to compute power for several designs and then to choose the design that has acceptable power and the smallest sample size (or cost). Acceptable power is not well defined at this stage. Other methods of comparing designs are given by Ju and Chow (1995) and Pong and

316   *Quantitative Methods for Traditional Chinese Medicine Development*

Raghavarao (2000), where the criterion is the precision for estimating shelf life.

When evaluating designs, it is also important to answer the question "What is the probability of being able to defend the desired shelf life with the study?" (see, e.g., Nordbrock 1994). In other words (assuming that the parameter is expected to decrease over time), what is the probability that the 95 percent one-sided lower confidence bound for the slope will be acceptable for specified values of the slope(s) for particular subsets of data, which may include, for example, only one strength and/or only one package? It is important to know at the design stage what the statistical penalty (with respect to shelf life) might be if differences among packages and/or strengths are found. Similarly, Nordbrock (2000) compared matrix designs to full designs using the probability of achieving the desired shelf life.

Chow and Liu (1995) indicated that a matrixing design might be applicable to strength if there is no change in proportion of active ingredients, container size, and immediate sampling time points. The application of a matrixing design to situations such as closure systems, orientation of containers during storage, packaging form, manufacturing process, and batch size should be evaluated carefully. It is discouraged to apply a matrixing design to sampling times at two endpoints (i.e., the initial and the last) and at any time points beyond the desired expiration date. If the drug product is sensitive to temperature, humidity, and light, the matrixing design should be avoided.

13.5 Stability Analysis for Drug Products with Multiple Active Components

In the previous sections we only considered a drug product with a single active ingredient. In practice, some drug products may contain multiple active ingredients. For example, Premarin (conjugated estrogens, USP) is known to contain at least five active ingredients: estrone, equilin, 17α-dihydroequilin, 17α-estradiol, and 17β-dihydroequilin. Other examples include combinational drug products, such as the traditional Chinese medicines. For a drug product with multiple active ingredients (or components), an ingredient-by-ingredient (or component-by-component) stability analysis may not be appropriate, because these active ingredients may have some unknown interactions. In this section, the basic idea for obtaining an estimate of drug shelf life for drug products with multiple components (e.g., TCMs) is described.

13.5.1 Basic Idea

Let $y(t, k)$ be the potency of the kth ingredient at time t after the manufacture of a given drug product, $k = 1,..., p$. For ingredient k, its shelf life is the time

Stability Analysis for Drug Products with Multiple Components 317

interval at which $E[y(t, k)]$ (the expectation of $y[t, k]$) remains within a specified limit, whereas the shelf life for the drug product may be the time interval at which $E[f(y(t, 1),..., y(t, p))]$ remains within the specified limits, where f is a function (such as a linear combination of $y[t, 1],..., y[t, p]$) that characterizes the impact of all active ingredients. In general, f is a vector-valued function with a dimension $q \leq p$. If data are observed from $y(t, 1),..., y(t, p)$ and the function f in the previous discussion is a known function, then stability analysis can be made by using the transformed data $z(t) = f[y(t, 1),..., y(t, p)]$. If the dimension of f is 1, then $z(t)$ can be treated as a single ingredient. If the dimension of f is $q > 1$, then one may define the shelf life to be the minimum of the shelf lives $\tau_1,..., \tau_q$, where τ_h is the shelf life when the hth component of $z(t)$ is treated as a single ingredient. One special case is where f is the identity function so that the shelf life is the minimum of all shelf lives corresponding to different ingredients $y(t, k)$, $k = 1,..., p$. In practice, however, f is typically unknown. Although the best way to estimate f is to fit a model between the y and z variables, it requires data observed from both y and z, which is not a common practice in the pharmaceutical industry, because the variable z is not clearly defined in many problems, such as the traditional Chinese medicines (see, e.g., Chow et al. 2006). Chow and Shao (2006) assumed that the components of z are linear combinations of the components of y and proposed a method to establish the shelf life. Note that Chow and Shao's approach is basically an application of the factor model in multivariate analysis (see, e.g., Johnson and Wichern 1998).

13.5.2 Models and Assumptions

Let $y(t)$ denote the p dimensional vector whose kth component is the potency of the kth ingredient at time t after the manufacture of a given drug product, $k = 1,..., p$. We assume that the drug potency is expected to decrease with time. If $p = 1$, that is, $y(t)$ is univariate, the current established procedure to determine a shelf life is to use the time at which a 95 percent lower confidence bound for the mean degradation curve $E[y(t)]$ intersects the acceptable lower product specification limit as specified in the 1987 FDA stability guidelines (see also ICH Q1A [R2] 2003). Let η be the vector whose kth component is the lower product specification limit as specified in the USP/NF for the kth component of $y(t)$. Chow and Shao (2006) proposed a statistical method for determining the shelf life of a TCM following a similar idea suggested by the FDA, assuming that the components are linear combinations of some factors. Let $y(t)$ denote the p dimensional vector whose kth component is the potency of the kth ingredient at time t after the manufacture of a given TCM, $k = 1, ..., p$. Assume that, for any t,

$$y(t) - E[y(t)] = LF_t + \varepsilon_t, \qquad (13.2)$$

where L is a $p \times q$ nonrandom unknown matrix of full rank, F_t and ε_t are unobserved independent random vectors of dimensions q and p, respectively, $E(F_t) = 0$, $\text{Var}(F_t) = I_q$ (the identity matrix of order q), $E(\varepsilon_t) = 0$, $\text{Var}(\varepsilon_t) = \Psi$, and

Ψ is an unknown diagonal matrix of order p. Let $z(t) = (L'L)^{-1} L'y(t)$. It follows from Equation 13.2 that

$$z(t) - E[z(t)] = F_t + (L'L)^{-1} L'\varepsilon_t. \tag{13.3}$$

Now, let $x(t)$ be an s dimensional covariate vector associated with $y(t)$ at time t. Chow and Shao (2007) assume the following model at any time t:

$$E[y(t)] = Bx(t), \text{ Var}[y(t)] = \Sigma, i = 1,...,m, j = 1,...,n, \tag{13.4}$$

where B is a $p \times s$ matrix of unknown parameters and $\Sigma > 0$ is an unknown $p \times q$ positive definite covariate matrix. Because $z(t) = (L'L)^{-1}L'y(t)$, it follows from Equation 13.4 that

$$E[z(t)] = \gamma'x(t) = (L'L)^{-1}L'Bx(t), \quad i = 1,...,m, j = 1,...,n, \tag{13.5}$$

where $\gamma = B'L(L'L)^{-1}$.

13.5.3 Shelf-Life Determination

Suppose that we independently observe data y_{ij}, $i = 1,...,m$, $j = 1,...,n$, where y_{ij} is the jth replicate of $y(t_i)$ and $t_1,...,t_m$ are designed time points for the stability analysis. Define

$$x_i = x(t_i), \quad z_{ij} = (L'L)^{-1}L'y_{ij}, \quad i = 1, ..., m, j = 1, ..., n. \tag{13.6}$$

Consider the case where $q = 1$. If z_{ij}'s are observed, according to FDA (1987), the expiration dating period (or shelf life) is given by

$$\tau = \inf\{t : l(t) \le \eta\}, \tag{13.7}$$

where η is the lower product specification limit as specified in the USP/NF. However, z_{ij}'s are not observed but y_{ij}'s. Thus, the lower confidence bound $l(t)$ in Equation 13.7 needs to be modified as follows:

$$l(t) = \hat{\gamma}'x(t) - t_{0.95, mn-s}\sqrt{x(t)'Vx(t)}, \tag{13.8}$$

where

$$V = \frac{mn - 1}{mn} \sum_{i=1}^{m} \sum_{j=1}^{n} (\hat{\gamma}_{i,j} - \hat{\gamma})(\hat{\gamma}_{i,j} - \hat{\gamma})',$$

in which $\hat{\gamma}_{i,j}$ is the estimator of γ with the (i,j)th data point deleted. For the case where $1 < q \le p$, let $\hat{B}$ be least squares estimator of B, λ_k be the kth largest eigenvalue of the sample covariance matrix based on $y_{ij} - \hat{B}x_i$, $i = 1,...,m$, $j = 1,...,n$,

Stability Analysis for Drug Products with Multiple Components 319

and e_k be the normalized eigenvector corresponding to λ_k. Then, estimator $\hat{L}$ of L is the $p \times q$ matrix whose kth column is $\lambda_k e_k$, $k = 1,\ldots,q$. Let $\hat{\gamma}_k$ be the kth column of $\hat{\gamma} = \hat{B}'\hat{L}(\hat{L}'\hat{L})^{-1}$, which is an $s \times q$ matrix. Thus, we have

$$l_k(t) = \hat{\gamma}_k' x(t) - t_{0.95/q, mn-s} \sqrt{x(t)' V_k x(t)}, \tag{13.9}$$

where

$$V_k = \frac{mn-1}{mn} \sum_{i=1}^{m} \sum_{j=1}^{n} (\hat{\gamma}_{k,i,j} - \hat{\gamma}_k)(\hat{\gamma}_{k,i,j} - \hat{\gamma}_k)',$$

in which $\hat{\gamma}_{k,i,j}$ is the same as $\hat{\gamma}_k$ but calculated with the (i,j)th data point deleted. Then, $l_k(t)$, $k = 1,\ldots,q$ are approximate 95 percent simultaneous lower confidence bounds for $\varsigma(t)$, $k = 1,\ldots,q$, where $\varsigma_k(t)$ is the kth component of $E[z(t)] = \gamma' x(t)$. An estimated shelf life is then given by

$$\tau = \min_{k=1,\ldots,q} \tau_k,$$

where τ_k is defined by the right-hand side of Equation 13.8 with $l(t)$ replaced by $l_k(t)$ and is, in fact, an estimated shelf life for the kth component of z with confidence level $(1 - 0.05/q) \times 100\%$.

13.5.4 An Example

To illustrate the proposed method for determining the shelf life of a drug product with multiple active ingredients, consider a stability study conducted for a traditional Chinese herbal medicine, which is newly developed for treatment of patients with rheumatoid arthritis. This medicine contains three active botanical components, namely *Herba epimedii* (HE), B extract, and C extract. Each of the three components has been used as an herbal remedy since ancient times and is well documented in the Chinese Pharmacopoeia. The proportions of each components are summarized below:

Component	Formulation
HE	60 mg
B	25 mg
C	25 mg
Excipient	90 mg
Total	200 mg

To establish a shelf life for this product, a stability study was conducted for a time period of 18 months under a testing condition of 25°C/60% relative humidity. The lower product specification limit for each component is 90%.

320   *Quantitative Methods for Traditional Chinese Medicine Development*

TABLE 13.8

Stability Data of the Traditional Chinese Medicine

Component	Sampling Time Point (Month)					
	0	**3**	**6**	**9**	**12**	**18**
HE	99.6	97.5	96.8	96.2	94.8	95.3
	99.7	98.3	97.0	96.0	95.1	94.8
	100.2	99.0	98.2	97.1	95.3	94.6
B	99.5	98.4	96.3	95.4	93.2	91.0
	100.5	98.5	97.4	94.9	94.5	92.1
	99.3	99.0	97.3	95.0	93.1	91.5
C	100.0	99.5	98.9	98.2	97.9	97.5
	99.8	99.4	99.0	98.5	98.0	97.9
	101.2	99.9	100.3	99.5	98.9	98.0

TABLE 13.9

$l(t)$ Values for Various t

t	19	20	21	22	23	24	25	26	27	28
$l(t)$	4.97	4.36	3.75	3.14	2.52	1.90	1.28	0.66	0.03	−0.60

Stability data (percent of label claim) at each sampling time point for the three components are given in Table 13.8.

Since $p = 3$, we consider that $q = 1$. Using the proposed procedure described in the previous sections, we obtain $l(t)$ in Equation 9.8 for various t (month) as shown in Table 13.9. Hence, the estimated shelf life for this product is 27 months.

13.5.5 Discussion

This section introduces the method for determining the shelf life of a drug product with p active ingredients proposed by Chow and Shao (2006). Basically, Chow and Shao (2007) assume that these active ingredients are linear combinations of q factors. Because these factors are chosen using principal components, the first factor can be viewed as the primary active factor, and the second factor can be viewed as the secondary active factor. Chow and Shao (2007) assume that active ingredients decrease with time. If one or more ingredients increase with time, then a transformation such as $g(y) = -y$ or $g(y) = 1/y$ may be applied. If p is small or moderate, then $q = 1$ is recommended. If p is large, then adding a few more factors may be considered. Because the principal components are orthogonal, adding more factors will not affect the previous selected factors (except that $t_{0.95,mn-s}$ is changed to $t_{1-0.05/q,mn-s}$) so that one can compare the results in a sensitivity analysis. Finally, adding more factors always results in a more conservative procedure. Note that in their proposed approach, Chow and Shao (2007) assume

Stability Analysis for Drug Products with Multiple Components 321

that there is no significant toxic degradant in the test drug product with multiple components. This is a reasonable assumption for most traditional Chinese medicines because multiple ingredients are used to reduce toxicities when used in conjunction with primary therapy. However, when toxic degradation products are detected, special attention should be paid to (1) identity (chemical structure), (2) cross reference to information about biological effects and the significance of the concentration likely to be encountered, and (3) indications of pharmacological action or inaction as indicated in the FDA guidelines for stability analysis. Chow and Shao's approach is useful when different ingredients degrade not independently of each other, which is the case for most traditional Chinese medicines. If multiple ingredients degrade independently, then an ingredient-by-ingredient analysis may be appropriate. If Chow and Shao's approach is applied, it is suggested that q be selected as $q = 1$ or $q = 2$ factors that are ingredients having the most variability.

13.6 Stability Analysis with Discrete Responses

For solid oral dosage forms such as tablets and capsules, the FDA stability guideline indicates that following characteristics should be studied in stability studies: (1) tablets—appearance, friability, hardness, color, odor, moisture, strength, and dissolution, and (2) capsules—strength, moisture, color, appearance, shape brittleness, and dissolution. Some of these characteristics are measured using a discrete rating scale. As a result, the usual methods for stability analysis may not be appropriate. Chow and Shao (2003) proposed some statistical methods for estimation of drug shelf life based on discrete responses with and without batch-to-batch variation following the concept as described in the FDA stability guideline. For illustrative purposes, their method for the case of random batches is briefly described below.

Suppose that there are k batches of a drug product in a stability study and that from the ith batch, y_{ij}, $j = 1,\ldots,n_i$, binary responses are observed at some time points. Consider the following logistic regression model:

$$E(y_{ij}) = \psi(\beta'x_{ij}), \quad i = 1,\ldots,k, \quad \text{Var}(y_{ij}) = \tau(\beta'x_{ij}), \quad j = 1,\ldots,n_i, \quad (13.10)$$

where $\psi(z) = e^z/(1 + e^z)$, $\tau(z) = \psi(z)[1 - \psi(z)]$, x_{ij} is a p vector of covariates, β is a p vector of unknown parameters, and β' its transpose. Typically, $x'_{ij} = (1,t_{ij})$, $\left(1,t_{ij},t_{ij}^2\right)$, $(1, t_{ij}, w_{ij}t_{ij})$, or $(1, t_{ij}, w_{ij}, w_{ij}t_{ij})$, where t_{ij} is the jth time point for batch i and w_{ij} is a vector of covariates such as the bottle size or container type. Where there is a batch-to-batch variation, the parameter vector β in Equation 13.10 takes different values for different batches and, thus, should be denoted by β_i, $i = 1,\ldots,k$. Some researchers considered β_is as unknown fixed effects when estimating drug shelf life (see, e.g., Ruberg

322 *Quantitative Methods for Traditional Chinese Medicine Development*

and Hsu 1992). This fixed effect approach, however, may not provide a shelf life that is applicable to all future batches of the same drug product based on stability data from the k batches. Alternatively, Shao and Chow (1994) considered a random batch approach by considering the following mixed effects model:

$$E\left(y_{ij}|\beta_i\right) = \psi\left(\beta_i'x_{ij}\right), \quad i = 1,\ldots,k,$$

$$\mathrm{Var}\left(y_{ij}|\beta_i\right) = \tau\left(\beta_i'x_{ij}\right), \quad j = 1,\ldots,n_i, \qquad (13.11)$$

$$\beta_i's \text{ are independently distributed as } N(\beta, \Sigma),$$

where ψ and τ are the same as those in Model 13.10, $E(y_{ij}|\beta_i)$ and $\mathrm{Var}(y_{ij}|\beta_i)$ are the conditional expectation and variance of y_{ij} given that random effect β_i, $\beta = E(\beta_i)$ is an unknown vector, and $\Sigma = \mathrm{Var}(\beta_i)$ is an unknown covariance matrix. If $\Sigma = 0$, then there is no batch-to-batch variation and Model 13.11 reduces to Model 13.10.

Now let $\psi\left[\beta_{\text{future}}'x(t)\right]$ be the mean degradation at time t for a future batch of the drug product. The true shelf life for this batch is then given by

$$t_{\text{future}}^* = \inf\{t : \beta_{\text{future}}'x(t) \leq \psi^{-1}(\eta)\},$$

which is a random variable because β_{future} is random. Consequently, a shelf-life estimator should be a 95 percent lower prediction bound (instead of a lower confidence bound) for t_{future}^*. Because $\beta_i s$ are unobserved random effects, the prediction bound has to be obtained based on the marginal model specified by

$$E\left(y_{ij}\right) = E\left[E\left(y_{ij}|\beta_i\right)\right] = E\left[\psi\left(\beta_i'x_{ij}\right)\right]$$

and

$$\mathrm{Var}(y_{ij}) = \mathrm{Var}\left[E\left(y_{ij}|\beta_i\right)\right] + E\left[\mathrm{Var}\left(y_{ij}|\beta_i\right)\right] = \mathrm{Var}\left[\psi\left(\beta_i'x_{ij}\right)\right] + E\left[\tau\left(\beta_i'x_{ij}\right)\right].$$

However, either $E(y_{ij})$ nor $\mathrm{Var}(y_{ij})$ is an explicit function of $\beta_i'x_{ij}$ and, hence, an efficient estimator of β, such as the maximum likelihood estimator, is difficult to compute. Furthermore, when k is small, the computation of the maximum likelihood estimator requires an iteration process that may not converge. Alternatively, Chow and Shao (2003) proposed the following method for a small k (say $k = 3$).

Stability Analysis for Drug Products with Multiple Components 323

Assume that n_is are large so that Model 13.10 can be fitted within each fixed batch. For each fixed i, let $\hat{\beta}_i$ be a solution of

$$\sum_{j=1}^{n_i} x_{ij}\left[y_{ij} - \psi\left(\beta_i' x_{ij}\right)\right] = 0,$$

i.e., $\hat{\beta}_i$ is the maximum likelihood estimator of β_i based on the data observed from the ith batch, given β_i. For large n_i, $\hat{\beta}_i$ is approximately distributed as $N[\beta_i, V_i(\beta_i)]$, conditioning on β_i, where

$$V_i(\beta_i) = \left[\sum_{j=1}^{n_i} x_{ij} x_{ij}' \tau\left(\beta_j' x_{ij}\right)\right]^{-1}.$$

Unconditionally, $\hat{\beta}_i$ is approximately distributed as $N(\beta, D_i)$, where

$$D_i = E\left[\mathrm{Var}(\hat{\beta}_i | \beta_i)\right] + \mathrm{Var}\left[E(\hat{\beta}_i | \beta_i)\right] \approx E\left[V_i(\beta_i)\right] + \mathrm{Var}(\beta_i) = E\left[V_i(\beta_i)\right] + \sum.$$

Let

$$\hat{\beta} = \frac{1}{k}\sum_{i=1}^{k}\hat{\beta}_i.$$

Then $\hat{\beta}$ is approximately distributed as $N(\beta, k^{-1}D)$, where $D = k^{-1}\sum_{i=1}^{k} D_i$. Define

$$v(t) = x(t)'\left[\frac{1}{k-1}\sum_{i=1}^{k}(\hat{\beta}_i - \hat{\beta})(\hat{\beta}_i - \hat{\beta})'\right]x(t).$$

Then $\left[\hat{\beta}'x(t) - \psi^{-1}(\eta)\right]/\sqrt{v(t)/k}$ is approximately distributed as the non-central t distribution with $k - 1$ degrees of freedom and the noncentrality parameter of $\left[\beta'x(t) - \psi^{-1}(\eta)\right]/\sqrt{x(t)'\Sigma x(t)}$. Following the idea of Shao and Chen (1997), Chow and Shao (2003) proposed the following approximate 95 percent lower prediction bound for t^*_{future} as an estimated shelf life

$$\hat{t}^*_{\mathrm{future}} = \inf\left\{t : L(t) \le \psi^{-1}(\eta)\right\}, \tag{13.12}$$

324   *Quantitative Methods for Traditional Chinese Medicine Development*

where

$$L(t) = \hat{\beta}'x(t) - \rho_{0.95}(k)\sqrt{\frac{v(t)}{k}}, \tag{13.13}$$

$\rho_0(k)$ satisfies

$$\int_0^1 P\{T_k(u) \le \rho_a(k)\} du = a,$$

$T_k(u)$ denotes a random variable with the noncentral t distribution having $k - 1$ degrees of freedom and the noncentrality parameter of $\sqrt{k}\Phi^{-1}(1-u)$, and Φ is the standard normal distribution function. Values of $\rho_{0.95}(k)$ are given by Shao and Chen (1997).

13.6.1 Remarks

It can be shown that $\hat{t}^*_{\text{future}}$ in Equation 13.12 is an approximate 95 percent lower prediction bound for the true shelf life t^*_{future} (see, e.g., Chow and Shao 2003). Note that $\hat{t}^*_{\text{future}}$ in Equation 13.12 has the same form as the $\hat{t}^*$ except that $L(t)$ is replaced by a more conservative bound in Equation 13.13 that incorporates the batch-to-batch variability. Chow and Shao (2003) also proposed some tests for batch-to-batch variation to determine whether the method (i.e., random batch approach) described above is appropriate.

In practice, it may be of interest to consider a mixture of a continuous response variable (e.g., strength) and a discrete response variable including binary response or ordinal response with more than two categories (e.g., color or hardness) for estimation of drug shelf life. This requires further research.

13.7 Concluding Remarks

For the study of drug stability, the FDA guidelines require that all drug characteristics be evaluated. In most drug products, we obtain an estimated drug shelf life based primarily on the study of the stability of the strength of the active ingredient. However, some drug products may contain more than one active ingredient. For example, Premarin (conjugated estrogens, USP) is known to contain at least five active ingredients: estrone, equilin, 17α-dihydroequilin, 17α-estradiol, and 17β-dihydroequilin. The specification limits for each component are different. To ensure identity, strength, quality,

Stability Analysis for Drug Products with Multiple Components 325

and purity, it is suggested that each component be evaluated separately for determination of drug shelf life. In this case, although a similar concept can be applied, the method suggested in the FDA stability guidelines is necessarily modified. It should be noted that the assay values observed from each component might not add up to a fixed total, which is due to the possible assay variability for each component. The modified model should be able to account for these sources of variation. Pong and Raghavarao (2001) proposed a statistical method for estimation of drug shelf life for drug products with two components. The distributions of shelf life for two components were evaluated by Pong and Raghavarao (2002) under different designs.

14

Case Studies

14.1 Introduction

Traditional Chinese medicine (TCM) development the Western way involves nonclinical development and preclinical/clinical development. The purpose of nonclinical development is to ensure the quality of the TCM meets product specification and regulatory standards during the development process. Quality assurance can always be achieved by identifying, reducing/eliminating, and/or controling variabilities due to various sources of raw materials, in-process materials, and final finished products. As a result, raw materials, in-process materials, and final finished products are usually tested for consistency at various stages of the TCM development process. On the other hand, the purpose of preclinical/clinical development focuses on safety and efficacy of the TCM under development, although it is debatable whether a well-established Chinese herbal medicine should be tested in animals before it is tested in humans.

In recent years, much of the modern research on TCM has focused on integrating TCM with Western medicine (e.g., cancer research). This integrated approach makes use of Western medicine's strength in attacking the diseases under study with TCM's strength of supporting the patient. As an example, in a cancer trial treating 211 patients with lung cancer, Chen (2002) reported that 1-year survival rates of patients undergoing chemotherapy combined with herbal medicine was 85 percent compared to one year survival rate of 69 percent for patients treated by chemotherapy alone. In some cases, on the other hand, the principal investigator uses TCM treatment alone to treat patients with advanced cancer. While this approach is not preferred by many practitioners, de Lemos (2002) indicated that TCM treatment by itself could have an effect on cancer progression.

One of the major criticisms in TCM development is that the Chinese doctor only reports successful clinical cases, while those failed cases are not documented. This has led to a significant bias for a fair and reliable evaluation of the TCM under development. The purpose of this chapter is to examine the effectiveness of TCM development the Western way through a review of case studies both nonclinically and clinically across various therapeutic areas.

The remainder of this chapter is organized as follows. In Section 14.2, the concept of quality by design proposed by the FDA is introduced with an application in the manufacturing process of TCM. Section 14.3 provides a review of several (isolated) successful clinical cases that indicated TCM treatment work. Case studies for TCM development in cancer care, cardiovascular diseases (hypertension prescription), acupuncture in treating diabetes, and TCM treatment for multiple sclerosis are discussed in Section 14.4. Some concluding remarks are given in Section 14.5.

14.2 Nonclinical Quality by Design

14.2.1 Concept of Quality by Design

In the pharmaceutical industry, it is recognized that a reasonable high-quality product can only be achieved at a great effort and cost. In practice, pharmaceutical companies mainly focus on development rather than putting their emphasis on manufacturing. In many cases, the manufacturing process is not only unable to meet pre-specified quality standard but also to predict effects scale-up on final products. Quality by design (Qbd) is a concept that assumes quality could be planned and that most quality crises and problems relate to the way in which quality was planned. In recent years, the FDA has considered quality by design as a vehicle for the transformation of how drugs are discovered, developed, and commercially manufactured. In the past few years, the FDA has implemented the concepts of QbD into its premarket processes. The focus of this concept is that quality should be built into a product with an understanding of the product and process by which it is developed and manufactured along with a knowledge of the risks involved in manufacturing the product and how best to mitigate those risks. This is a successor to the "quality by QC" (or "quality after design") approach that the companies took up until the 1990s. Winkle (2007) provides a comprehensive comparison of the traditional approach with the systematic QbD approach (see Table 14.1).

Winkle (2007) pointed out that the implementation of quality by design is not only beneficial to industry but also to FDA. As an example, from the perspective of the pharmaceutical industry, quality by design ensures the production of better products with fewer problems in manufacturing. The use of quality by design not only reduces the number of manufacturing supplements required for postmarket changes at the same time it allows for implementation of new technology to improve manufacturing without regulatory scrutiny. In addition, it can also improve interaction with FDA reviewers and consequently speed up the review/approval process. On the other hand, from the perspective of FDA, the implementation of quality by design will,

Case Studies 329

TABLE 14.1

A Comparison between Traditional Approach and QbD Systematic Approach

Aspects	Traditional	Quality by Design
Pharmaceutical development	Empirical Univariate experiments	Systematic Multivariate experiments
Manufacturing process	Fixed	Adjustable
Process control	In-process testing for go/no-go Offline analysis with slow response	PAT utilized for feedback and feed forward at real time
Product specification	Primary means of quality control Based on batch data	Overall quality control strategy Based on desired product performance (safety and efficacy)
Control strategy	Based on intermediate and end product testing	Risk-based Controls shifted upstream Real-time release upstream
Lifecycle management	Reactive to problems Scale-up and post-approval changes	Continual improvement enabled within design space

Source: Modified from Winkle, 2007. PDA/FDA Joint Regulatory Conference, September 24, 2007.

Note: PAT, process analytical technology.

first, not only enhance scientific foundation for review but also provide better coordination across review, compliance, and inspection divisions within the FDA. Second, it not only improves information in regulatory submissions and quality of review but also provides for better consistency and for more flexibility in decision making. Moreover, it ensures decisions are made on science and not on empirical information. Quality by design not only involves various disciplines in decision making but also allows the FDA to use limited resources to address higher risks more efficiently.

14.2.2 Statistical Method for QbD

The concept of quality by design (QbD) has been widely accepted and applied in the pharmaceutical manufacturing industry. There are still two key issues to be addressed in the implementation of QbD for herbal drugs. The first issue is the quality variation of herbal raw materials, and the second issue is the difficulty in defining the acceptable ranges of critical quality attributes (CQAs). Most recently, Yan et al. (2014) proposed a feedforward control strategy and a method for defining the acceptable ranges of CQAs. To introduce the methodology of feedforward control strategy proposed by Yan et al. (2014), the following notations are helpful.

For simplicity, italic letters are used for scalars and lowercase letters denote vectors. Data matrices are denoted with capital letters. For a batch process, the data recorded in M batches of production are composed of three parts denoted by X, Z, and Y, i.e., matrix X (M × K) comprises K attributes measured on raw materials; matrix Z (M × J) consists of J process parameters; and matrix Y (M × I) comprises I attributes measured on the intermediates or products. x_{new} (1 × K) is the vector consisting of the attributes of the new input materials. $Lo_{x,k}$ and $Hi_{x,k}$ are the minimum and maximum of the kth material attributes in historical batches. z_{new} (1 × J) is the vector consisting of the process parameters that will be used in the new batch of production and $z_{new,j}$ is the jth process parameter. $Lo_{z,j}$ and $Hi_{z,j}$ are the lower limit and upper limit of the jth process parameter. $y_{des,i}$ is the desired value of the ith CQA, and $Lo_{des,i}$ and $Hi_{des,i}$ are the lower control limit and upper control limit of the ith CQA. The predicted value of the ith CQA of the intermediate produced with process parameters of z_{new} is denoted by $\hat{y}_i$. Vector $b_{i,x}$ (1 × K) comprises the regression coefficients that describe the effects of input material attributes on the ith CQA. Vector $b_{i,z}$ (1 × J) comprises the regression coefficients that describe the effects of process parameters on the ith CQA.

The feedforward control strategy for adjusting process parameters according to input material attributes and the method for defining the acceptable ranges of CQAs are described by the following steps.

Step 1: Modeling the effects of input material attributes and process parameters on the CQAs simultaneously. First, using the data (X, Z, Y) obtained from industrial production or design of experiments (DOE), the quantitative relationship that links input material attributes and process parameters to CQAs is established in the form of Y = f (X, Z). As the number of input variables is usually large compared with the number of batches and the input variables are usually intercorrelated, partial least squares (PLS) regression (Eriksson et al. 2001) is commonly used for this situation, instead of multivariable linear regression. With the established model, the CQAs can be predicted based on x_{new} and z_{new} before the process is conducted.

Step 2: Establishing the optimization model for calculating the best process parameters. On the basis of the regression models in step 1, an optimization model, see Equations 14.1 through 14.3 below, is built taking process parameters z_{new} as the decision variables. The input material attributes x_{new} are included in the coefficients of the objective function and the constraint functions. z_{new} can be optimized to make the predicted CQAs as close to the targeted values as possible and in the control limits of $Lo_{des,i}$ and $Hi_{des,i}$ In other words, minimize z_{new} with respect to the following objective function:

$$\sum_{i=1}^{I} w_i \cdot \left(\frac{\hat{y}_i - y_{des,i}}{y_{des,i}} \right)^2, \tag{14.1}$$

such that

$$Lo_{des,i} \leq \hat{y}_i \leq Hi_{des,i}, \quad 1 \leq i \leq I \tag{14.2}$$

Case Studies 331

and

$$Lo_{z,j} \leq z_{\text{new},j} \leq Hi_{z,j}, \quad 1 \leq j \leq J. \tag{14.3}$$

The objective function (Equation 14.1) is a weighted square of the error between the predicted values and the desired values of CQAs. The weight w_i represents the importance of the ith CQA. Other terms relating to process efficiency can be added into the objective function if needed, as in the research of Muteki and MacGregor (2008). Equation 14.2 is the constraint of the control range of each CQA, and Equation 14.3 is the constraint of the adjustment range of each process parameter. A constraint based on the inter-correlation of process parameters can be added. However, this constraint is not used in the case study of this work because the process parameters in the design of experiments are orthogonal.

Step 3: Defining the feasible material space. Some methods for defining the specifications of input materials have been proposed in the literature (Duchesne and Macgregor 2004; Garcia-Munoz 2009; Cui et al. 2012). A simple way for defining the specifications of input materials is based only on the quality of materials that produced products of acceptable quality in the historical batches. The adjustment effects of process parameters are not included in this way, however, which makes the acceptable ranges of input material attributes small and, consequently, some materials will be misclassified as unacceptable. Therefore, in this study the feasible material space (FMS) is determined under the feedforward control circumstance, and it is the ranges of material attributes that make the optimization model in step 2 produce feasible solutions. The method for calculating the FMS is described as follows. For simpler formula derivation, the ith CQA can be predicted using Equation 14.4 if the interaction terms between input material attributes and process parameters were not included in the regression models established in step 1.

$$\hat{y}_i = b_{i,x} \cdot x_{\text{new}}^T + b_{i,z} \cdot z_{\text{new}}^T \quad 1 \leq i \leq I. \tag{14.4}$$

If some terms, such as square terms, were included in the regression models established in step 1, then these terms are included in x_{new} and z_{new} of Equation 14.4 and the corresponding regression coefficients are included in $b_{i,x}$ and $b_{i,z}$. The expression $b_{i,x} \cdot x_{\text{new}}^T$ represents the effect of input materials on the CQAs, whereas $b_{i,z} \cdot z_{\text{new}}^T$ represents the effect of process parameters on the CQAs and its range is the adjustment capacity of process parameters. Each $\hat{y}_i$ should be in the range of $Lo_{des,i}$ and $Hi_{des,i}$ to make the intermediate acceptable. This leads to

$$Lo_{des,i} - \max\left(b_{i,z} \cdot z_{\text{new}}^T\right) \leq b_{i,x} \cdot x_{\text{new}}^T \leq Hi_{des,i} - \min\left(b_{i,z} \cdot z_{\text{new}}^T\right) \quad 1 \leq i \leq I. \tag{14.5}$$

Thus, the adjustment range of each process parameter in z_{new} is given by

$$Lo_{z,j} \le z_{new,j} \le Hi_{z,j} \quad 1 \le j \le J. \tag{14.6}$$

The knowledge space of the input material is limited; that is, the ranges of material attributes that have been studied are confined. Therefore, the material attributes should be in the knowledge space to make the prediction of CQAs reliable (Equation 14.7). A constraint based on the intercorrelation structure of the material attributes can be added as shown by Duchesne and Macgregor (2004); however, it is not used in this work for simplicity.

$$Lo_{x,k} \le x_{new,k} \le Hi_{x,k} \quad 1 \le k \le K \tag{14.7}$$

Then the feasible material space can be calculated from Equations 14.5 through 14.7. Moreover, if the interaction terms between input material attributes and process parameters were included in the regression models established in step 1, Equation 14.5 would be a little complicated. However, after substituting the variables by numeric values, the FMS can still be defined by numerical computation.

Step 4: Defining the acceptable ranges of CQAs for the previous process. As the intermediate produced by the previous process is taken as the input material for the current process being studied, the FMS for this current process places limits on the acceptable ranges of CQAs for the previous process. Therefore, the acceptable ranges of CQAs for the previous process can be defined based on the FMS, or simply, are the same as the FMS.

14.2.3 Case Study of QbD

In the case study of the ethanol precipitation process of Danshen (Radix Salvia miltiorrhiza) injection, regression models linking input material attributes, and process parameters to CQAs were built first and an optimization model for calculating the best process parameters according to the input materials was established. Then, the feasible material space was defined and the acceptable ranges of CQAs for the previous process were determined.

Ethanol precipitation is a commonly used purification process in the manufacturing of herbal drugs (Gong et al. 2010, 2011; Huang and Qu 2011; Zhang et al. 2013). The first three manufacturing processes of Danshen injection are shown in Figure 14.1, including extraction, concentration, and ethanol precipitation, which are the typical starting manufacturing processes for many herbal drugs. The herbal raw materials are first extracted by hot water, and then the extract is treated by a concentration process conducted under reduced pressure and heating to obtain the concentrate. Then, in the ethanol precipitation process, with the addition of ethanol into the concentrate, large amounts of impurities of poor solubility in ethanol are precipitated. The quality variation of herbal raw materials has led to the batch-to-batch

Case Studies

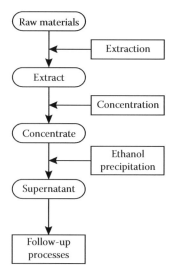

FIGURE 14.1
Flow chart of the first three manufacturing processes of *Danshen* injection. The manufacturing processes are shown in rectangles. The raw materials and intermediates are shown in ellipses.

quality fluctuation of the concentrates. Therefore, a process control strategy is needed that can adjust the process parameters to compensate for the impact of the quality fluctuation of the concentrates. On the other hand, the APIs are precipitated together with the impurities, and it is difficult to determine how many APIs should be retained in the supernatant. Therefore, for many herbal drug manufacturing processes such as ethanol precipitation, the acceptable ranges of CQAs are not well defined. The ethanol precipitation process of Danshen injection was taken as an application example for the methodology of the feedforward control strategy.

Ethanol precipitation experiments were conducted following Table 14.2 in random order. During the process, the ethanol solution of designed concentration was pumped the raw materials by the extraction and concentration processes (Figure 14.1). In the extraction process, the Danshen crude drug is extracted with boiling water at a temperature of about 100°C. Then in the concentration process, the extract is concentrated under reduced pressure at a temperature of about 80°C to obtain the concentrate. The analytical-grade ethanol was purchased from Lingfeng Chemical Reagent Co., Ltd. (Shanghai, China). Deionized water was produced using a Mili-Q academic water purification system (Milford, Massachusetts, USA). The ethanol solutions of different ethanol concentrations used in the experiments were prepared by ethanol and deionized water. The HPLC-grade acetonitrile and trifluoroacetic acid were purchased from Merck (Darmstadt, Germany). Standard substances of four phenolic acids, including danshensu (DSS), protocatechuic aldehyde (PA), rosmarinic acid (RA), and salvianolic acid B (SaB) were

334 *Quantitative Methods for Traditional Chinese Medicine Development*

TABLE 14.2

Box-Behnken Design for Ethanol Precipitation with Four Factors Including Two
Material Attributes and Two Process Parameters

Standard Order	Water Content in Concentrate (g/g)	Ethanol Concentration (v/v)	Ethanol Flow Rate (mL/min)	Ethanol Consumption (mL/g)
DOE 1	0.44	0.92	20	2.1
DOE 2	0.50	0.92	20	2.1
DOE 3	0.44	0.98	20	2.1
DOE 4	0.50	0.98	20	2.1
DOE 5	0.47	0.95	16	1.7
DOE 6	0.47	0.95	24	1.7
DOE 7	0.47	0.95	16	2.5
DOE 8	0.47	0.95	20	2.5
DOE 9	0.44	0.95	20	1.7
DOE 10	0.50	0.95	20	1.7
DOE 11	0.44	0.95	20	2.5
DOE 12	0.50	0.95	20	2.5
DOE 13	0.47	0.92	16	2.1
DOE 14	0.47	0.98	16	2.1
DOE 15	0.47	0.92	24	2.1
DOE 16	0.47	0.98	24	2.1
DOE 17	0.44	0.95	16	2.1
DOE 18	0.50	0.95	16	2.1
DOE 19	0.44	0.95	24	2.1
DOE 20	0.50	0.95	24	2.1
DOE 21	0.47	0.92	20	1.7
DOE 22	0.47	0.98	20	1.7
DOE 23	0.47	0.92	20	2.5
DOE 24	0.47	0.98	20	2.5
DOE 25	0.47	0.95	20	2.1
DOE 26	0.47	0.95	20	2.1
DOE 27	0.47	0.95	20	2.1

Source: Yan, B. et al., *Phytochemical Analysis*, 25, 59–65, 2014.

purchased from the National Institute for the Control of Pharmaceutical and
Biological Products (Beijing, China).

Design of experiments was conducted to evaluate the effects of input material attributes and process parameters on the CQAs as shown in Figure 14.2.
A four-factor Box-Behnken design with three central points (Table 14.2) was
conducted. As the water content in the concentrate was considered as an
important material attribute (Gong et al. 2010), it was taken as a factor in the
DOE. Three batches of concentrate were adjusted to different water content
(respectively 0.44, 0.47, and 0.50 g/g) by mixing them with certain amounts
of deionized water, and then taken as different input materials in the DOE.

Case Studies

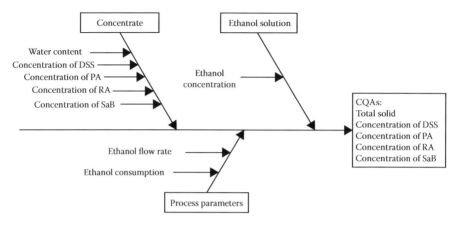

FIGURE 14.2
Ishikawa diagram showing the input material attributes, process parameters and the output CQA of the ethanol precipitation process. DSS, danshensu; PA, protocatechuic aldehyde; RA, rosmarinic acid; SaB, salvianolic acid B.

Ethanol concentration is another important material attribute that fluctuates in industrial production; therefore, it was taken as another factor in the DOE. The ranges of the four DOE factors were set based on historical production experience. Ethanol precipitation experiments were conducted following Table 14.2 in random order. During the process, the ethanol solution of designed concentration was pumped into 150 g of concentrate at a designed flow rate under continuous stirring. The ethanol addition was stopped when the ethanol consumption reached the designed amount. Then the mixture was refrigerated at 5°C for 15 h. Finally, the supernatant was collected. The three batches of concentrates and 27 batches of supernatants were analyzed for determining the concentrations of the phenolic acids and the total solid. The four phenolic acids were determined by high performance liquid chromatography (HPLC) analysis according to the method in the state drug standards (SFDA 2012) with the HPLC system HP1100 series. The concentration of total solid was determined by hot air drying at 105°C for 3 h.

The optimization model for calculating the best process parameters according to the input material attributes was established. The desired values of the CQAs were set as the averages of the CQAs of the three central points in DOE (i.e., DOE 25–27) and the control ranges of the CQAs were set as 90 to 110 percent of the desired values of the CQAs (Table 14.3). The control ranges could be better defined based on the input material requirements of the process following the ethanol precipitation process, or based on the CQAs of historical good batches. However, for the explanatory purpose of this case study, the setting of control ranges was not considered as an important issue. Therefore, the control ranges were set simply as described above. All the w_i in Equation 14.1 were set to 1 because the CQAs were considered as equally

336 Quantitative Methods for Traditional Chinese Medicine Development

TABLE 14.3

Desired Values and Control Limits of the Critical Quality Attributes for Ethanol Precipitation

	y_{TS} (%)	y_{DSS} (mg/g)	y_{PA} (mg/g)	y_{RA} (mg/g)	y_{SaB} (mg/g)
y_{des}	6.360	2.950	0.755	0.646	4.640
Hi_{des}	6.996	3.245	0.831	0.711	5.104
Lo_{des}	5.724	2.655	0.680	0.581	4.760

Source: Yan, B. et al., *Phytochemical Analysis*, 25, 59–65, 2014.

important. $Lo_{z,j}$ and $H_{iz,j}$ in Equation 14.3 were set as the minimum and the maximum of the process parameters used in the DOE.

14.3 Successful TCM Clinical Cases

As indicated earlier, one of major criticisms during TCM development is that relevant clinical data are not scientifically evaluated and documented, especially for those negative outcomes or failures. Thus, the reported relevant clinical data may be biased and hence misleading. In addition, the observed positive results may not reach statistical significance in the sense that they may occur purely by chance alone and hence may not reproducible. In this section, for illustrative purposes, several clinical cases, which indicate that TCM work, as described in the website of http://www.chinese-medicine-work.com/herbal-formula, are briefly discussed below.

14.3.1 Case 1: Power of Chinese Herbal Medicine

This case is a story regarding an infant who experiences seizures treated with Chinese herbal medicine. A baby boy was born at 42 weeks. The baby boy experienced a seizure within his first 24 hours of birth. On his second day of life, he had another seizure. The baby boy was hospitalized for two weeks following his birth. During his hospital stay, an EEG showed edema of the brain, and an MRI revealed moderate damage to the cortex and brain stem. Upon returning home with his parents, The baby boy was unable to nurse after discharge from the hospital. He has become accustomed to a plastic feeding tube. His mother was advised to use a nipple shield, and after one week, the baby was breastfeeding. At the stage of his development, the baby boy was unable to hold up his head longer than a few minutes while resting on his belly, and, if tired, he could not hold his head up for more than a minute. After a few months he gained some strength and was able to lift his head for up to three or four minutes at a time, but his seizures continued to occur at the rate of 6 to 12 a day.

Case Studies 337

After having consulted a Chinese doctor, the baby's parent decided to adopt Chinese herbal medicine in conjunction with weekly acupuncture treatments. The Chinese herbal medicine consists of herbs that themselves are nutritive and also nourish digestive capacity. They stimulate the appetite, enhance nutrient absorption, and may be a helpful adjunct to some nursing babies, giving them greater strength and stamina. Within one week after beginning treatment of Chinese herbal medicine, the infant's seizures completely ceased. He continued taking the Chinese herbal medicine (formula) and ingested a total of 28 ounces of the formula over the course of one month as the baby seems to tolerate the dose (almost an ounce, or 30 ml per day) well. Over the next three months, the baby boy appeared fine, with good reflexes, muscle tone, and a bright spirit. But he began to have petit mal seizures, with 10 recorded during a 24-hour EEG. The results, however, were deemed inconclusive because there was no clearly defined locus of abnormal brain activity to account for the seizures. However, at the end of the second month, he stopped taking the herbs and has not had a single episode of seizure since then. According to the Chinese doctor, the nutritive value of formula is provided by tonic herbs for the Kidney, Spleen and Stomach, *Qi* and Blood (see medical theory of TCM as described in Chapter 1). The herbs in the formula are themselves nutritive and also nourish digestive capacity. They stimulate the appetite, enhance nutrient absorption, and may be a helpful adjunct to some nursing babies, giving them greater strength and stamina. The formula also regulates fluids and strengthens the *Wei* or defensive *Qi*. For children who are vulnerable to frequent colds, flus, allergies, or asthma, prescribing Grow and Thrive when they are well will bolster their resistance to invasions of Wind, Damp, and Cold.

The story of the baby boy born with seizures is a nearly miraculous anecdote that dramatically attests to the power of TCM. That is, the power of an infant to adapt to a severe trauma and developmental challenge; the power of the Chinese medicine mind to recognize the root of a problem and identify a coherent solution; the power of a simple remedy that enables a very small person to overcome a serious and complex malady. Unfortunately, this power is not confirmed by scientific and rigorous clinical evaluation based on conducting an adequate and well-controlled clinical trial.

14.3.2 Case 2: Chinese Herbal Medicine Alleviates Eczema, Allergies, and Stress

This case involves a 36-year-old man with chronic eczema who complained of a red, peeling rash on his neck, forehead, and scalp that had been recurring for many years. His childhood health history revealed many rashes as an infant, asthma treated with bronchodilators and inhaled steroids, and frequent infections treated with antibiotics. In the preceding year, he had received a course of antibiotics for skin infection. However, the stress from work has exacerbated his skin problems, which have a negative impact on his daily life.

The diagnosis from a Chinese doctor indicated that his tongue appeared pale and flabby with thin, yellow fur, which suggests insufficiency of Blood and *Qi* and Heat in the Stomach. Moreover, his pulse did not appear to faithfully reflect Heat signs other than a quality of Blood Heat at the Liver position and a slight pounding quality of the dramatic quality of his symptoms and physical appearance. The Heart position along with frequent changes in intensity (force) indicates possible underlying nervousness and anxiety. The Chinese doctor suspected that this man's early health problems might be due to his chronic dermatitis. His recurrent rash is a signal of an accumulation of Heat and Toxins seeking an exit through the skin. However, his repeated use of antibiotics and inhaled steroids for asthma inhibited his body's efforts to release Heat and Toxins, engendering recurring outbreaks of rashes. Although the course of antibiotics treatment could clear the acute infection, it perpetuated the same pattern of accumulation and unsuccessful elimination of the underlying pathogenic factors.

As indicated by the Chinese doctor, the systemic deficiencies of *Qi* and Blood, the presence of Heat, Blood Heat and Toxins, the notable pounding and changing intensity of the Heart pulse, and the exacerbation of his rash under stress all represented a pattern not only of accumulation of pathogenic factors, but of *Yang* uprising due to deficiency as well as an instability of the Heart and Mind. Thus, the Chinese doctor prescribed herbal remedies (the reader may want to consult with http://www.chinese-medicine-work.com/herbal-formula for more details) for achieving dynamic balances among the affected organs.

Because eczema can be expressed by the Blood-Heat-Toxin, the above herbs were chosen as the primary formula. That is, Tonify Blood will replenish the Blood and *Yin* as the Heat and Toxins are dispelled. In addition, since the man's nervous and excitable nature predisposes him to generate excess Heat, Comfort *Shen* will help to soothe his hyperactive nerves, relax his mind and repress the flaring of Fire. After several weeks of treatment, the man's condition greatly improved and he was experiencing only rare episodes of overheating, sweating, or over excitement. At this point his prescription was modified by deleting Comfort *Shen* and equalizing the proportions of Fire Fighter and Tonify Blood.

In conclusion, not only did the herbal remedies remarkably improve the man's skin, but he also seemed more able to modulate his energy, activity, and excitability. This clinical case indicates the importance of global dynamic balance among organs (the fundamental medical theory of TCM). The signs and symptoms observed are the indications that there are off-balance in certain organs. The use of TCM can help to return to and hopefully maintain global dynamic balance (i.e., health status) of the man.

14.3.3 Case 3: Chinese Herbal Medicine Helps Upper Respiratory Infection with Vertigo

This case is related to a 45-year-old woman who sought treatment for a lingering cough, dyspepsia with gas and bloating, fatigue, and vertigo. The

Case Studies 339

lady complained that these symptoms had persisted for two months. In addition, she indicated that she had been rather stressful in the past few months owing to her recent career move. During clinical evaluation, the Chinese doctor noted that there was a slightly pale tongue with some red papillae at the front quarter, and a thickened, somewhat damp, yellowish-white coating that is an indication that the pathogenic factors were still present in the Lung, Stomach and Intestines. Her pulse had slightly pounding and inflated qualities at the Lung position along with tense, pounding, and slippery qualities at the Stomach position. Thus, the Chinese doctor concluded that her condition was a manifestation of a Wind invasion that had penetrated into the Lung and Stomach because of an insufficiency of *Qi* and *Wei*, resulting in the accumulation of Dampness and Phlegm.

Note that in Chinese medical theory, Wind is an adverse climate that will definitely affect the body like a sudden gust of wind affects the trees, shaking the leaves and branches, wreaking temporary havoc. When a Wind invasion occurs, symptoms of the common cold or flu will present including dizziness and migratory pains in the joints, muscles, and head. Vertigo or respiratory congestion can happen when Wind obstructs circulation.

In order to evict the pathogenic factors, it would be necessary to strengthen the Stomach so that she could generate more *Qi*, which in turn would augment the *Wei* and strengthen the Lung. Thus, the Chinese doctor gave her initial prescription (the reader may want to consult with http://www.chinese-medicine -work.com/herbal-formula for more details) in order to fix the problem.

After returning for a follow-up appointment the next week, the lady reported complete recovery from her symptoms within four days with no recurrence. The Chinese doctor indicated that this was because Grow and Thrive rectifies *Qi* deficiency, harmonizes the Stomach and Spleen, and augments the Defensive *Wei Qi*. Windbreaker clears Wind, Heat, and Phlegm, relieving sniffles, sore throat, earache, fever, and the signs of cold, flu, ear inflammation, or allergic congestion. Along with subduing cough, Chest relief soothes the throat and chest, gently dispels Phlegm, aids expectoration, replenishes moisture, rectifies the *Qi* of the Lung, purges Wind and Heat, and bolsters the Nutritive *Ying* and Defensive *Wei Qi*.

This clinical case indicates that the understanding of medical theory and/ or mechanism behind TCM is extremely important in order to ensure the success of TCM. In practice, rater-to-rater or Chinese doctor-to-Chinese doctor variability is anticipated owing to differences in experience and knowledge of medical theory and mechanism of TCM.

14.3.4 Case 4: Chinese Herbal Medicine Cures Acute Constipation

This case involves a 63-year-old woman who was seeking help with a left-sided abdominal ache and constipation that occurred after eating at a restaurant the day before. This woman previously suffered bouts of intestinal complaints, including diarrhea, following the surgical removal of her thyroid gland due to Graves' Disease. As a result, it is prudent to select a remedy that would be effective without aggravating her gastrointestinal (GI) tract. During the clinical evaluation, the Chinese doctor found that her tongue had a slightly thickened, yellow-white coating consistent with many forms of indigestion. It was also reddened at the lateral edges. The redness of the edges of the tongue was a diagnostically consistent feature that, along with characteristics of her personality and history, distinguished her as a Wood Type with a constitutional pattern of Liver-Spleen and Liver-Lung dishar-mony. In view of these factors and her acute symptoms, the following for-mula was given to harmonize Liver and Stomach (Wood and Earth), regulate the *Qi* of the Stomach, and gently activate the bowel.

On the basis of the above observations and diagnosis, the Chinese doctor prescribed herbal remedies (the reader may want to consult with http://www .chinese-medicine-work.com/herbal-formula for more details) in order to fix the problem. After receiving the Chinese herbal medicine, the patient's indi-cated that she had recovered within 48 hours without any signs, symptoms, and adverse reactions. At that point, the patient was instructed to stop tak-ing the herbal medicine. Under the medical theory/mechanism, harmonize Liver-Spleen disperses *Qi*, Moisture, and Blood, Tonifies Blood, dispels Wind and Heat, activates digestion, and relieves tension. Tummy Tamer relieves indigestion, gas, and bloating due to food accumulation and stagnation of *Qi* and Moisture. Easy going activates the bowels, overcoming constipation due to food stagnation and accumulation.

14.3.5 Remarks

The above isolated successful clinical cases indeed provide evidence that TCM works in certain disease areas. In practice, however, it is not clear how many cases failed in treating similar diseases. Thus, the effects of the pre-scriptions (doses) need to be scientifically evaluated through conducting adequate and well-controlled clinical trials with target patient population (patient population with the diseases under study) for achieving the ultimate goal of modernization and/or Westernization of TCMs. In other words, the development of TCM should switch from experience-based (subjective) clini-cal evaluation to evidence-based (objective) clinical evaluation for scientific validity of the TCM under investigation.

14.4 Case Studies of Chinese Herbal Medicines

As cancers (solid tumors), cardiovascular diseases, and diabetes are consid-ered the top three life-threatening diseases in China, the search for alterna-tive treatments such as Chinese herbal medicines has become the center of

Case Studies 341

attention in public health in China. In this section, we will focus on case studies for these disease areas.

14.4.1 TCM in Cancer Care

TCM has been widely applied for cancer care in China. TCM plays an important role in minimizing disability, protecting cancer patients against suffering from complications, and helping patients to live well (see, e.g., Yoder 2005). Ernst (2009) indicated that TCM may also assist in supportive and palliative care by reducing side effects of conventional treatment or improving quality of life. In the West, there is an increasing trend towards complementary/alternative medicine (TCM) use by breast cancer survivors (Boon et al. 2007).

In their review of controlled clinical studies published in Chinese, Li et al. (2013) revealed that the earliest clinical trial in China started at the end of the 1970s, and the first clinical trial in the TCM area was a study of Chinese herbal injection for angina published in 1983 (see also, Wu et al. 2004). In the past few years, several researchers have conducted systematic reviews on case reports (Liu et al. 2011) and case series (Yang et al. 2012). Although there have been a large number of controlled clinical studies published in Chinese literature since 1984, no systematic searching and analysis has been done until the comprehensive review on controlled clinical studies published in Chinese conducted by Li et al. (2013). Their review is briefly summarized below.

14.4.1.1 Study Selection and Data Extraction

Randomized controlled trials (RCTs) or nonrandomized (clinical) clinical studies (CCSs) with at least one group involving TCM treatment for all types of cancer-related patients including malignant tumor, malignant hematologic disease, and patients with precancerous condition were included. A structured data extraction form was designed to capture bibliometric information, including citation information, publication types, and funding information if available. All the extraction was verified by an independent PI, and any discrepancies were discussed with the other PIs for consensus. As a result, about 2964 controlled clinical studies of TCM for cancer from 1984 to 2011 were systematically identified and analyzed for current evidence of clinical benefits of controlled clinical studies of TCM for cancer care.

14.4.1.2 TCM Intervention

As indicated in the work of Li et al. (2013), TCM interventions reported in the total 2964 studies were classified into herbal medicine, acupoint stimulation, dietary therapy, massage, TCM psychological intervention, TCM five element music therapy and qigong. Herbal medicine, including oral decoction, injection, external usage, perfusion, aerosol inhalation, mouth rinsing, and

342   *Quantitative Methods for Traditional Chinese Medicine Development*

nasal feeding, were the most frequently applied interventions in both treatment group (2667 studies, 89.98 percent) and control group (327 studies, 11.03 percent). Among all the types of herbal medicine, more than half (1145 out of 1720, 66.57 percent) of decoctions were individualized in most of the studies. On the other hand, conventional treatment reported, in the 2964 studies included chemotherapy, Western medicine as routine treatment, radiotherapy, interventional therapy, and surgery. Chemotherapy was the dominating conventional treatment in both treatment group (1170 studies, 54.98 percent in the 2128 studies reporting TCM plus conventional medicine) and control group (1328 studies, 47.87 percent in the 2774 studies reporting TCM plus conventional medicine or conventional medicine only), followed by Western medicine or other routine treatments.

14.4.1.3 Randomization

Li et al. (2013) pointed out that among the 2385 RCTs, about 16.5 percent (394 out of 2385) employed randomization methods, such as random table, computer software randomization, drawing lots, and tossing a coin. There were 33 studies used traditional envelope method (or random envelop) as the randomization method. These methods may not be rigorous; however, Li et al. (2013) considered them adequate randomization methods. In this case study, an interesting finding is that conference proceedings and dissertations had a higher rate of reporting randomization methods among those studies mentioning randomization.

14.4.1.4 Blinding

Blinding seems to be an issue in clinical trials for TCM. In this case study, only a small portion of studies (63 studies) reported the use of blinding with the participants. Among these 63 studies, only 40 studies (63.5 percent) indicated that participants who were blinded including patients, physicians, raters (outcome measurers) and biostatisticians. The other 23 studies just mentioned blinding, single blinding, or double blinding without providing any detailed information regarding how the blinding were done. Similar to randomization, conference proceedings and dissertations reported participants who were blinded more frequently when blinding was mentioned.

14.4.1.5 Outcome Measurement

The most frequently reported outcome measurement in this case study was clinical symptom (1667 studies, 56.2 percent), followed by laboratory indices or test results (1270 studies, 42.9 percent), quality of life (1129 studies, 38.1 percent), chemo/radiotherapy induced side effects (1094, 36.9 percent), tumor size (869 studies, 29.3 percent), and safety (547 studies, 18.5 percent). These outcome measures, however, are different from Western well-established

Case Studies 343

endpoints such as response rate, time to disease progression, and overall survival. In this case study, survival was reported in 433 (14.6 percent) studies while metastasis and relapse were reported in 109 (3.9 percent) studies and 101 (3.4 percent) studies, respectively. Among the total 1129 studies reporting quality of life as the outcome measurement, Karnofsky score was applied in most of the studies (942 studies, 83.4 percent). There were 41 studies reported quality of life measured by QOL score without providing detailed information regarding what instruments for QOL assessment were used and their validation. In addition, about 17.4 percent (a total of 516 studies) reported clinical effectiveness levels graded by combined several outcomes without giving adequate information for each of the original outcome.

14.4.1.6 Significant Evidence

As far as Li et al. (2013) are concerned, in this case study, there were only five well-designed randomized clinical trials with positive survival findings using Chinese herbal medicine. One study used herbal extract granules, another used a herbal capsule, and three used conventional Chinese herbal decoctions. Two of the studies reported TCM alone as the treatment intervention and the other three involved integrative TCM and conventional medicine.

14.4.1.7 Overall Conclusion/Recommendation

Among the 2964 studies, Li et al. (2013) summarized the conclusions/recommendations as described in the individual studies. They found that 756 (25.5 percent) studies recommended the test treatment under study to a broader community based on the observed treatment effectiveness. The most commonly seen conclusion and/or recommendation is that the test treatment is very effective with good safety and is very suitable for generalization to clinical applications.

14.4.1.8 Remarks

This case study reveals the following issues for TCM in cancer care. First, clinical studies still focused on experience based rather than evidence based. Second, the outcome measurements are not objective and not validated. Third, most clinical studies are not considered adequate and well-controlled clinical studies. For example, randomization and blinding were not employed to minimize possible bias. As indicated earlier, substantial evidence regarding effectiveness and safety can only be provided through conducting adequate and well-controlled clinical studies. However, there is an indication that TCM in cancer care is moving toward the right direction such as from experience-based clinical investigation to evidence-based clinical investigation. Most clinicians begin to receive good clinical practice (GCP) training for conducting

344   *Quantitative Methods for Traditional Chinese Medicine Development*

randomized clinical trials for assessment of effectiveness and safety of Chinese herbal medicines. For example, Peking University Clinical Research Institute (PUCRI) offers clinical trial training to clinicians at least twice a year in the area of the City of Beijing.

14.4.2 Case Study: Modeling of Hypertension Prescriptions

Like TCM in cancer care discussed in the previous section, similar issues, drawbacks, and problems are seen in most clinical studies conducted for assessment of effectiveness and safety of Chinese herbal medicines for treating cardiovascular diseases such as hypertension. Hypertension is a complex chronic disorder in which the patient's blood pressure is elevated abnormally. Although many Western medicines are available for treating hypertension, the results are not satisfactory with some undesirable effects due to the limitations caused by their complex pathogeneses. As a result, many patients seek alternative treatments such as TCM. As indicated by Shi et al. (2004) and Wang (2008), various TCM treatments for treating hypertension have been developed and proved to be effective. Thus, in this section, we will focus on a case study conducted by Xu et al. (2011) regarding the development, validation, and demonstration of the usefulness of some formula descriptors for hypertension prescriptions through so-called quantitative formula–activity relationship (QFAR) model. To introduce the QFAR model for hypertension prescriptions, we need to have a good understanding of herb properties in terms of their natures and actions for achieving global dynamic balance among the organs in the body.

14.4.2.1 Herb Properties and Medical Practice

As indicated earlier, in TCM theory and practice, the basic properties of an herb include four natures and five flavors, the lifting, lowering, floating, and sinking (LLFS), meridian affinity, and toxicity (see also, Xu et al. 2011). The four natures refer to Cold, Hot, Warm, and Cool, which are derived from the effects of herbal actions on the organic body. For example, an herb that acts to eliminate or reduce Heat nature is Cold or Cool nature, where the cool nature is weaker than the Cold nature. The five flavors in TCM are acrid, sweet, sour, bitter, and salty. Herbs with similar flavors tend to have similar actions. Xu et al. (2011) indicated that many illnesses have a tendency for movement upward (e.g., vomiting and cough), downward (e.g., diarrhea and rectal prolapse), outward (e.g., spontaneous sweating), or inward (e.g., unresolved exterior symptoms extending to the interior). LLFS properties reflect an herb's ability to reverse or eliminate such tendencies. For example, lifting is opposite to lowing, while floating is opposite to sinking. Meridian affinity refers to which meridian is associated with each visceral organ and its branches. For example, for all herbs of Cold nature that can eliminate or reduce Heat, herbs that are more effective at reducing Heat from the lung/

Case Studies 345

liver are said to have a lung/live affinity. Toxicity of an herb, on the other hand, is referred to as its undesirable effects on the human body. Table 14.4 provides 24 features concerning the properties of single herbs.

In practice, prescribing an herbal formula is the most commonly used method in TCM for treating patients with various diseases. A formula usually consists of various selected herbs with suitable doses based on syndrome diagnosis for etiology and the composition of therapies according to the principles of herb combination. In recent years, herb formulas for treating various diseases have been designed, reported, and validated. These herb formulas are then improved or adjusted by subsequent Chinese doctors based on their own clinical judgment/experience. As a result, there exist tens of thousands of effective herbal formulas for treating various diseases proposed in Chinese literatures, which are considered validated by both TCM theory and successful clinical cases.

TABLE 14.4

Basic Herbal Properties by Features

Properties	No.	Features	Extents
Natures	1	Cold	Strongly/moderately/mildly/not
	2	Hot	Strongly/moderately/mildly/not
	3	Warm	Moderately/mildly/not
	4	Cool	Moderately/mildly/not
	5	Neutral	Moderately/not
Flavors	6	Sour	Moderately/mildly/not
	7	Bitter	Moderately/mildly/not
	8	Sweet	Moderately/mildly/not
	9	Acrid	Moderately/mildly/not
	10	Salty	Moderately/mildly/not
Meridian affinity	11	Spleen affinity	Yes/no
	12	Stomach affinity	Yes/no
	13	Lung affinity	Yes/no
	14	Kidney affinity	Yes/no
	15	Heart affinity	Yes/no
	16	Pericardium affinity	Yes/no
	17	Large intestine affinity	Yes/no
	18	Small intestine affinity	Yes/no
	19	Bladder affinity	Yes/no
	20	Gallbladder affinity	
	21	Sanjian affinity	Yes/no
	22	Liver affinity	Yes/no
Toxicity	23	Toxicity	Strongly/moderately/mildly/not
LLFS	24	LLFS	Sinking and lowering/lifting and floating/not obvious

Source: Reproduced from Xu, L. et al., *Chemometrics and Intelligent Laboratory Systems*, 109, 186–191, 2011.

346   *Quantitative Methods for Traditional Chinese Medicine Development*

14.4.2.2 Least Squares Support Vector Machine

Xu et al. (2011) proposed to study these formulas by examining the relationships between the formulas and their corresponding activities. For the purpose of illustration, Table 14.5 lists possible principal actions or effects of single herbs. As a result, Xu et al. (2011) proposed the concept of quantitative formula–activity relationship (QFAR) to model formula activities by considering different information at various levels contained in a formula. Under the QFAR model, a least squares support vector machine (LS-SVM) proposed by Suykens and Vandewalle (1999) is employed to not only to classify effective/negative formulas (based on some pre-specified criteria on herbal properties and principal actions or effects of herbs) but also to minimize risk. The LS-SVM is briefly summarized below.

Xu et al. (2011) considered the following the simplest method to generate formula descriptors:

$$X = CS^T,$$

where C and S are dose matrix and feature matrix of single herbs, whose columns contain the doses of an herb in different formulas and the features (e.g., properties and principal actions) of the herb, respectively. Suppose that we are interested in discriminating the effective formulas from the negative ones. Under the equality type of constraints in the formulas, we denote one class (effective formulas) as +1 and the other class (negative formulas) as −1, then the support vector machine (SVM) classifier can be constructed as follows

$$w^T \phi(x_k) + b \geq 1 \quad \text{if} \quad y_k = +1, \quad k = 1,\ldots,n$$

$$w^T \phi(x_k) + b \leq 1 \quad \text{if} \quad y_k = -1, \quad k = 1,\ldots,n$$

where x_k and y_k are the kth input vector and the kth output value, respectively, w and b are the model parameters to be estimated and n is the number of objects, ϕ is a function that maps the input space into another high-dimensional space. Thus, LS-SVM can be formulated as follows:

$$\min_{w,b,e} f(w,b,e) = \frac{1}{2} w^T w + \gamma \frac{1}{2} \sum_{k=1}^{n} e_k^2$$

subject to the following equality constraints:

$$y_k [w^T \phi(x_k) + b] = 1 - e_k, \quad k = 1,\ldots,n.$$

Case Studies

TABLE 14.5

List of Possible Principal Actions of Single Herbs

No.	Features	Action Values (Yes = 1/No = 0)
1	Warm-acrid herbs, release exterior	1/0
2	Cool-acrid herbs, release exterior	1/0
3	Cool heat and purge fire	1/0
4	Cool heat and dry dampness	1/0
5	Cool heat and detoxify position	1/0
6	Cool heat and cool blood	1/0
7	Cool endogenous heat	1/0
8	Offensive purgative effect	1/0
9	Lubricant laxation	1/0
10	Drastic water-expelling	1/0
11	Dispel wind-dampness and cold	1/0
12	Dispel wind-dampness and clear heat	1/0
13	Dispel wind-dampness, strength sinew-bone	1/0
14	Aromatic herbs, dissipate dampness	1/0
15	Drain water and disperse swelling	1/0
16	Diuretics, dredge stranguria	1/0
17	Dispel dampness, retire icterus	1/0
18	Warm interior	1/0
19	Regulate *Qi*	1/0
20	Relieve food retention	1/0
21	Expel parasites	1/0
22	Cool blood, stop bleeding	1/0
23	Stop bleeding, resolve stasis	1/0
24	Astringing hemostasis	1/0
25	Warm meridian, stop bleeding	1/0
26	Stimulate blood circulation, analgesic herbs	1/0
27	Stimulate blood circulation, regulate menstruation	1/0
28	Stimulate blood circulation, cure wound	1/0
29	Remove blood stasis, eliminate masses	1/0
30	Warm herbs, dissolve phlegm	1/0
31	Clear and resolve heat-phlegm	1/0
32	Stop cough, relieve asthma	1/0
33	Tranquilizer mind	1/0
34	Nourish heart, calm mind	1/0
35	Calm liver, repress Yang	1/0
36	Anticonvulsants, extinguish wind	1/0
37	Aromatic herbs, open orifices	1/0
38	Reinforce *Qi*	1/0
39	Tonify Yang	1/0
40	Enrich the blood	1/0

(*Continued*)

TABLE 14.5 (CONTINUED)

List of Possible Principal Actions of Single Herbs

No.	Features	Action Values (Yes = 1/No = 0)
41	Tonify Yin	1/0
42	Secure exterior, stop sweating	1/0
43	Astringe the lung and the intestine	1/0
44	Control nocturnal emission, polyuria and leukorrhagia	1/0
45	Induce vomiting	1/0
46	Detoxify, expel parasite, relieve itching	1/0
47	Draw out toxin and suppuration, promote granulation	1/0

Source: Reproduced from Xu, L. et al., *Chemometrics and Intelligent Laboratory Systems*, 109, 186–191, 2011.

Thus, the Lagrangian cane be defined as

$$L(w,b,e;\alpha) = f(w,b,e) - \sum_{k=1}^{n} \alpha_k \left\{ y_k \left[w^T \phi(x_k) + b \right] - 1 + e_k \right\}$$

where α_k are Lagrangian multipliers. The optimal conditions can be deduced by taking derivatives with respect to w, b, e_k, and α_k and set them be equal to 0, which result in the following equations:

$$w = \sum_{k=1}^{n} \alpha_k y_k \phi(x_k),$$

$$\sum_{k=1}^{n} \alpha_k y_k = 0,$$

$$\alpha_k = \gamma e_k, \quad k = 1,2,\ldots,n,$$

$$y_k \left[w^T \phi(x_k) + b \right] - 1 + e_k = 0, \quad k = 1,2,\ldots,n.$$

As a result, the solution of LS-SVM can be obtained by solving the following equations:

$$\begin{bmatrix} 0 & -y^T \\ y & ZZ^T + \dfrac{1}{\gamma} I \end{bmatrix} \begin{bmatrix} b \\ \alpha \end{bmatrix} = \begin{bmatrix} 0 \\ 1 \end{bmatrix},$$

Case Studies 349

where $= [\phi(x_1)y_1; \phi(x_2)y_2; \ldots; \phi(x_n)y_n]$, $I = [1;1;\ldots;1]$, $e = [e_1; e_2; \ldots; e_n]$, and $\alpha = [\alpha_1; \alpha_2; \ldots; \alpha_n]$. Now, consider Gaussian nonlinear transformation (i.e., radical basis function). The input matrix X is then replaced by an $n \times n$ kernel matrix K given below

$$K = \begin{bmatrix} k_{11} & \cdots & k_{1n} \\ \vdots & \ddots & \vdots \\ k_{n1} & \cdots & k_{nn} \end{bmatrix},$$

where k_{ij} $(k = 1, \ldots, n)$ is defined by the radical basis function as

$$k_{ij} = \exp\left(\frac{-\left\|x_i - x_j\right\|^2}{\sigma^2}\right).$$

Note that when training the LS-SVM classification model based on the radical basis function transformation, only two parameters (i.e., γ and σ) need to be optimized. The kernel width parameter (i.e., σ) is related to the confidence in the data as the magnitude of σ also influences the nonlinear nature of the regression. In other words, as σ decreases, the kernel becomes narrower, which forces the model toward a more complex solution. The regularization parameter γ, on the other hand, controls the trade-off between maximizing the margin and minimizing the training error. Too small a value of γ will result in an underfitted model, while too large a value of γ will lead to an overfit of the training data and the model will have poor prediction performance. Therefore, it is suggested that γ should be optimized together with the kernel width parameter σ at the same time.

14.4.2.3 An Example

Xu et al. (2011) conducted a case study by collecting 235 TCM formulas for treating hypertension. These 235 formulas composed of 1 to 18 individual herbs have been collected from official databases and literature, see, e.g., http://www.tcm120.com/1w2k or http://www.cintcm/opencms/index.html. As indicated by Xu et al. (2011), these formulas have been shown to be effective in treating hypertension and the data sources are reliable. On the basis of properties of single herbs (Table 14.4) and principal actions or effects of single herbs (Table 14.5), the data were analyzed using the LS-SVM model. The purpose is not only to discriminate the effective formulas from the negative ones but also to optimize the two parameters in LS-SVM and avoid overfitting. To build a robust and reliable classification model, detection of outliers in the effective formulas was performed using robust principal component analysis (Hubert et al. 2009). After removal of outliers, the remaining 229 effective formulas split

350   *Quantitative Methods for Traditional Chinese Medicine Development*

to form a test set (containing 200 formulas) and a validation set (containing 29 most active formulas). For a robust and reliable model, the optimal parameters are determined to be $\sigma^2 = 0.55$ and $\gamma = 10$. With the optimized parameters, LS-SVM model is built to predict the classes of test samples. The results indicate that samples 1 through 29 are effective formulas while 30 through 229 are negative formulas. The analysis results also indicate that 2 out of 29 (6.9 percent) effective formulas are misclassified and 7 out of 200 (3.5 percent) negative formulas are wrongly predicted. The prediction accuracy for positive and negative formulas are 93.1 percent (27/29) and 96.5 percent (193/2000), respectively.

14.4.2.4 Remarks

In the case study by Xu et al. (2011), it was shown that QFAR model for hypertension formulas through the application of LS-SVM model with the new formula descriptors can discriminate effective formulas from negative formulas with a high accuracy. However, not much detail regarding the interpretation of the model is provided.

14.4.3 Case Study: Acupuncture for Treating Diabetes

14.4.3.1 TCM Classification of Diabetes

In Chinese, diabetes is known as Xiao-ke (wasting and thirsting) or Tang-niao-bing (sugar urine illness). According to TCM theory and practices, diabetes is classically divided into three types: upper, middle, and lower Xiao-ke. Each has characteristic symptoms. The upper type is characterized by excessive thirst, the middle by excessive hunger, and the lower by excessive urination. These types are closely associated with the lungs, stomach, and kidneys, respectively (see also, Covington 2001).

14.4.3.2 Diagnosis and Treatment

For evaluation of patients with a chronic illness of diabetes, Chinese doctors often take a detailed, multisystem case history with observations by the Chinese four diagnostic techniques that give information about the state of the patient's health. These observations include the shape, color, and coating of the tongue, the color and expression of the face, the odor of the breath and body, and the strength, rhythm, and quality of the pulse. One of the most common ways of differentiating symptoms and syndromes in TCM is according to the eight principles: Yin and Yang, Interior and Exterior, Cold and Heat, and Deficiency and Excess. These characteristics are summarized in Table 14.6 (Heat/Cold, Excess/Deficiency) and Table 14.7 (Yin and Yang), respectively.

Unlike Western medicine, TCM is not concerned with measuring and monitoring blood glucose levels in diabetic patients. TCM focuses on treatment of individual patient's deficiency and disharmony (among related

Case Studies

TABLE 14.6

Summary of Heat/Cold and Excess/Deficiency Signs

General Signs	Description	Tongue	Pulse
Heat patterns	Red face High fever Dislike of heat Cold reduces discomfort Rapid movement Outgoing manner Thirst or desire for cold drinks Dark urine Constipation	Red material Yellow moss	Rapid
Cold patterns	Pale White face Limbs cold Fear of cold Heat reduces discomfort Slow movement Withdrawn manner No thirst or a desire for hot drinks Clear urine Watery stool	Pale material White moss	Slow
Excess patterns	Ponderous Heavy movement Heavy, coarse respiration Pressure and touch increase 　discomfort	Thick moss	Strong
Deficiency patterns	Frail, weak movement Tiredness Shortness of breath Pressure relieves discomfort Inactive Passive appearance Low voice Dizziness Little appetite	Pale material Thin moss	Weak

Source: Reproduced from Covington, M.B., *Diabetes Spectrum*, 14, 154–159, 2001.

organs). Acupuncture and moxibustion have been used in treating diabetic patients to reduce blood glucose levels and normalize endocrine function. In practice, many clinical studies have demonstrated that acupuncture has a beneficial effect on lowering serum glucose levels (see, e.g., Mao 1984; Chen et al. 1994).

14.4.3.3 Successful Examples

Covington (2001) presented two successful examples concerning using acupuncture in the treatment of diabetes. As indicated in the work of

352 *Quantitative Methods for Traditional Chinese Medicine Development*

TABLE 14.7

Signs of Yin and Yang Patterns

Examination	Signs of Yin	Signs of Yang
Looking	Quiet	Agitated, restless, active manner
	Withdrawn	Rapid, forceful movement
	Slow, frail manner	Red face
	Patient is tired and weak, like to lie down curled up	Patient likes to stretch when lying down
	No spirit	Tongue material is red or scarlet, and dry
	Excretions and secretions are watery and thin	Tongue moss is yellow and thick
	Tongue materials is pale, puffy and moist	
	Tongue moss is think and white	
Listening and smelling	Voice is low and without strength	Voice is coarse, rough, and strong
	Few words	Patient is talkative
	Respiration is shallow and weak	Respiration is full and deep
	Shortness of breath	Putrid odor
	Acrid odor	
Asking	Feels cold	Patient feels hot
	Reduced appetite	Dislike heat or touch
	No taste in mouth	Constipation
	Desires warmth and touch	Scanty, dark urine
	Copious and clear urine	Dry mouth
	Pressure relieves discomfort	Thirst
	Scanty pale menses	
Touching	Frail, minute, thin, empty, or otherwise week pulse	Full, rapid, slippery, wiry, floating, or otherwise strong pulse

Source: Reproduced from Covington, M.B., *Diabetes Spectrum*, 14, 154–159, 2001.

Covington (2001), the first successful example concerning a study of 46 patients with painful peripheral neuropathy evaluated acupuncture analgesia to determine its short- and long-term efficacy (Abuaisha et al. 1998). For the short-term efficacy, the results indicated that about 77 percent (34 out of 46) patients experienced significant improvement in their symptoms. For the long-term efficacy, after a follow-up period of up to 52 weeks, 67 percent were able to stop or significantly reduce their pain medication. About 21 percent (7 out of 46 subjects) indicated that their symptoms had disappeared completely. The second successful example is related to a randomized, sham-controlled, crossover study of 50 subjects with type 2 diabetes for evaluation of the effectiveness of percutaneous nerve stimulation (PENS) therapy for treating neuropathic pain (Hamza et al. 2000). The results showed that active PENS treatment improved neuropathic pain symptoms in all patients. In addition to reducing pain, the treatment helps in improving physical activity levels, sense of well-being, and quality of life.

Case Studies 353

14.4.4 Case Study: Treatment for Multiple Sclerosis

14.4.4.1 Diseases

As described in Wikipedia (http://www.en.wikipedia.org), multiple sclerosis (MS) is an inflammatory disease in which the insulating covers of nerve cells in the brain and spinal cord are damaged. This damage disrupts the ability of parts of the nervous system to communicate, resulting in a wide range of signs and symptoms including physical, mental, and sometimes psychiatric problems. Thus, MS, sometimes, is also known as disseminated sclerosis or encephalomyelitis disseminate. MS takes several forms, with new symptoms either occurring in isolated attacks (relapsing forms) or building up over time (progressive forms). Between attacks, symptoms may disappear completely; however, permanent neurological problems often occur, especially as the disease advances.

Multiple sclerosis is the most common autoimmune disorder affecting the central nervous system. While the cause is not clear, a number of new treatments and diagnostic methods are under development (e.g., Venditti et al. 1956; Vickers and Dharmananda 1996). The underlying mechanism is thought to be either destruction by the immune system or failure of the myelin-producing cells. Proposed causes for this include genetics and environmental factors such as infections. MS is usually diagnosed based on the presenting signs and symptoms and the results of supporting medical tests. There is no known cure for multiple sclerosis. Treatments attempt to improve function after an attack and prevent new attacks. Medications used to treat MS while modestly effective can have adverse effects and be poorly tolerated. Many people pursue alternative treatments, despite a lack of evidence. The long-term outcome is difficult to predict, with good outcomes more often seen in women, those who develop the disease early in life, those with a relapsing course, and those who initially experienced few attacks. Life expectancy is on average 5 to 10 years lower than that of an unaffected population.

14.4.4.2 Chinese Herbal Therapy

The recommended traditional herb formula for treatment of the liver/kidney deficiency type *Wei* syndrome is *Hu Qian Wan* (Huang and Wang 1993). The Chinese name may be roughly translated as Pill of Tiger's Walk; it refers to the well-controlled movements a tiger makes from a place of hiding while stalking a prey. The tiger also represents the yin: a tiger in hiding has great potential for expressing its power, and that hidden potential is yin. The herb formula has the therapeutic action of nourishing yin. As with other traditional treatments, the formula may be modified somewhat according to clinical presentation, especially at the initiation of therapy. For long-term applications, it is considered a well-balanced prescription.

Hu Qian Wan is a formula devised by Zhu Danxi (1280–1358 A.D.) that was recorded in his book *Dan Xi Xin Fa* (Dan Xi's Theories). Zhu Danxi was originally known as Zhu Zhenheng, and he lived in Danxi (Zhejiang Province). He became known as the renowned physician of Danxi and was thus given the name Zhu Danxi thereafter. Zhu is known as leader of one of the four schools of Chinese medical disease etiology and treatment that evolved during the period of 1150–1350 A.D.; Zhu's was the last of these schools and one of the most influential in subsequent centuries (see, e.g., Yakazu 1985a,b). The four schools of thought were labeled according to the type of therapy that was predominantly advocated: cooling, purgation, spleen/stomach tonification, and yin nourishing. In modern practice, the latter two tonification-based schools remain dominant forces, joined by the late 19th century "school" of vitalizing blood circulation.

14.4.4.3 Multiple Sclerosis Clinical Trial

The largest study of Chinese medical treatment for multiple sclerosis was carried out by Lu and Wang (1990) at the Departments of Neurology and Traditional Chinese Medicine in Fujian. Patients were first divided into four groups for differential treatment, two groups with deficiency-type syndrome and two groups with excess-type syndrome. The categories and treatments were:

1. Liver/kidney yin deficiency: raw and cooked rehmannia, lycium fruit, anemarrhena, salvia, peony, cornus, ligustrum, deer horn glue, tortoise plastron glue, achyranthes (*chuanniuxi*), tang-kuei, and licorice. This is a modification of the traditional Left Restoring Pill (*Zuo Gui Wan*) with the addition of anemarrhena, ligustrum, salvia, tang-kuei, and peony; it is somewhat similar to *Hu Qian Wan*. Each herb is used in a dosage of 10–12 grams per day, except licorice (5 grams).

2. Spleen-stomach weakness: astragalus, salvia, codonopsis, atractylodes, hoelen, pinellia, citrus, jujube, and licorice. This is a modification of the traditional Major Six Herbs Combination (*Liu Junzi Tang*) with astragalus and salvia added. Each herb is used in a dosage of 8–15 grams per day, except jujube (12 pieces) and licorice (4 grams).

3. *Qi* and blood stasis syndrome: astragalus, codonopsis, salvia, rehmannia (raw), peony (red and white), bupleurum, tang-kuei, scute, cnidium, pinellia, and licorice. This formula combines Minor Bupleurum Combination (*Xiao Chaihu Tang*) with three herbs for promoting blood circulation—salvia, peony (red and white), and cnidium—plus astragalus. Each herb is present in the amount of 9–15 grams per day, except licorice (4 grams).

4. Damp-heat syndrome: ching-hao, talc, peony, scute, bupleurum, bamboo, akebia, hoelen, chih-shih, pinellia, rhubarb, jujube. This formula

Case Studies 355

is similar to treatments for febrile diseases described in previous centuries, such as the Ching-hao and Scute Combination (*Hao Jin Qingtan Tang*). Each herb is present in the amount of 8–12 grams, except jujube (12 pieces).

The formulas would be modified for certain presenting symptoms. For example, for urinary incontinence, add cuscuta, alpinia, and rose fruit; for constipation, add ho-shou-wu, persica, cistanche, and rhubarb; for mental fogginess, add schizandra; for abdominal distention, add magnolia bark and chih-shih; for muscular atrophy, add tang-kuei, gelatin, and dipsacus.

The decoctions were consumed as a cooling drink (rather than hot; because many MS patients have an aversion to heat), once per day. Anti-inflammatory Western drugs (dexamethasone or prednisone) were given during acute active periods. Thirty-five patients were treated and except for three that discontinued treatment within the first ten days, some improvement was found. Two cases were deemed basically cured after taking 45 and 68 doses; 15 were markedly improved and another 15 somewhat improved, most of them taking 20 to 40 doses. Eleven of the patients had tried corticosteroids unsuccessfully before switching to the traditional herb combinations; of these, seven were markedly improved, three improved, and only one failed to respond.

These researchers followed up their work with an attempt to prevent exacerbations (Lu et al. 1995). They prescribed *Ping Fu Tang* (Pacify Relapse Decoction) to 30 patients over a period of 3 to 13 years (average of 6 years). The formula contained astragalus, codonopsis, hoelen, atractylodes, pinellia, licorice, jujube, bupleurum, scute, tortoise shell, ligustrum, tang-kuei, peony, ophiopogon, rehmannia, lycium, and anemarrhena. The prescription basically has the effect of tonifying qi, yin, and blood, and clearing deficiency heat. It can be seen that this prescription is derived from the first two formulas listed in the previous article for treatment of multiple sclerosis, based on deficiencies of liver, kidney, and spleen (it also has some herbs of Minor Bupleurum Combination, as mentioned below). The preventive therapy was basically a tonic formula. It was prescribed in the form of a decoction, taken in 2 to 3 daily doses, using 8 to 15 grams of each herb (except smaller amounts of licorice and jujube). According to the researchers, relapses were prevented except for two patients who each experienced only one minor exacerbation, each event following a viral infection (common cold). A control group of MS patients not treated by this remedy was monitored for three years: they suffered from exacerbations at the rate of 1 to 4 times per year.

Ping Fu Tang included rehmannia, tortoise shell, peony, and anemarrhena, ingredients of *Hu Qian Wan*, which have the functions of nourishing yin and blood and cleansing deficiency fire. In addition, they added ligustrum, lycium fruit, and ophiopogon to nourish yin. A strategy for nourishing blood and essence is to tonify the qi so that more nutrients are obtained from the food. The formula included astragalus, codonopsis, hoelen, atractylodes, licorice, and jujube toward this end (these herbs also enhance immune

356 *Quantitative Methods for Traditional Chinese Medicine Development*

functions to aid resistance to infections that induce exacerbations). Because the point of the treatment was not to rectify flaccidity but rather to prevent flaccidity by preventing exacerbations, the herbs for treating flaccidity in the legs, such as tiger bone and cynomorium found in *Hu Qian Wan* were not included. Also, as the patients are being treated continuously with the yin-nourishing tonics, it is not necessary to strongly inhibit deficiency fire, so phellodendron is not essential to the prescription (anemarrhena, unlike phellodendron, has the secondary property of being a yin tonic). Thus, the treatment largely reflects the principles of *Zhu Danxi* in relation to understanding the cause of a flaccidity syndrome. The doctors explained that part of their thinking in developing the formula was based on the current understanding of autoimmunity, which explains the presence of so many qi tonics and the herbs of Minor Bupleurum Combination (*Xiao Chaihu Tang*), such as pinellia, bupleurum, and scute, which is believed to be helpful in chronic inflammatory diseases.

If a T-cell attack against myelin sheaths is initiated by influenza, common cold, sinusitis, or other infections, ability to prevent such infections or halt their progress would be one obvious key step in preventing damage due to the usual sequence of events in an exacerbation. Protection from transmissible viral infections, such as staying away from those who are currently suffering from the infection, is one method of prevention. Enhancing the immune system functions with tonic herbs is another method. Many Westerners are led to believe, by poorly written articles on immune disorders, that enhancing immune system vigilance would worsen any autoimmune disease; however, this would only be a potential problem during an exacerbation; even then, other components of the immune system that help to shut down the autoimmune attack may be coaxed into activity with proper immune-regulating herbal treatment strategies.

14.4.4.4 Amyotrophic Lateral Sclerosis and Progressive Spinal Muscular Atrophy Studies

Case studies of ALS were reported by Lin (1983). In one case, the primary formula combined tonic herbs: astragalus, tang-kuei, peony, rehmannia, aconite, cinnamon bark, and lycium fruit, with several herbs used to promote circulation of blood and relieve spasms (the spasms being a significant problem in many cases of ALS): centipede, scorpion, persica, carthamus, morus twig, and clematis. These herbs were made as a decoction taken in divided doses 3 times daily for several days. In addition, a small amount of powder made from strychnos and musk (0.25 grams of each, 3 times daily) was given. As follow-up, the decoction formula was modified (cnidium, platycodon, chih-ko, tiger bone, deer antler, and zaocys were added; morus twig and clematis were deleted) and made into pills instead of decoction, to be taken 18 grams per day—the musk and strychnos powders were included in the pills. The pills were taken for two years until the disease was resolved. A

Case Studies 357

follow-up after three years with no further medication showed that the disease had remitted. A similar approach was used with a second patient who consumed a decoction made with astragalus, atractylodes, cinnamon twig, tang-kuei, persica, carthamus, centipede, eupolyphaga, fenugreek, aconite (*chuanwu*), licorice, and zaocys. After using this decoction for several days, the pill described above was used for long-term medication and a clinical cure was obtained, with a follow-up after five years confirming the satisfactory result.

The third case emphasized treatment of yin deficiency fire, using a decoction with phellodendron, raw rehmannia, moutan, alisma, anemarrhena, hoelen, stephania, coix, chin-chiu, dipsacus, achyranthes, centipede, and scorpion. This decoction was given for more than two months and then modified, taking out stephania, coix, and chin-chiu, and adding dipsacus, deer antler, epimedium, tang-kuei, cnidium, and carthamus. This formula was then used for more than three months. Finally, the above mentioned pill was again used for long-term therapy, and a cure was obtained, with no relapse by the end of two years without the medication.

Kang (1985) reported two cases of progressive spinal myoatrophy where the main prescriptions given were variations of *Shengji Yisui Tang* (Decoction for Generating Muscles and Benefiting Marrow). One such prescription contained tang-kuei, lycium fruit, atractylodes, ophiopogon, tortoise shell, achyranthes, phellodendron, alisma, chaenomeles, and licorice for a yin deficiency case and deer antler, eucommia, atractylodes, astragalus, psoralea, malt, crataegus, pinellia, codonopsis, sinapis, hoelen, alisma, chaenomeles, achyranthes, and cinnamon twig for a yang deficiency case with weak digestion and phlegm accumulation. Treatment time was six months and included acupuncture and massage therapy. Long-term follow-up showed persisting benefits of the treatment, with normal nerve conduction and physical activities.

In a study of 15 patients with progressive ALS, a significantly expanded version of *Hu Qian Wan* was employed (Xie 1985). This contained astragalus, epimedium, deer antler, syngnathus, sea horse, ginseng, tortoise shell glue, tang-kuei, peony, rehmannia, lycium fruit, eucommia, dipsacus, cuscuta, cynamorium, atractylodes, coix, citrus, achyranthes, chaenomeles, chin-chiu, agkistrodon, tiger bone, psoralea, anemarrhena, phellodendron, cinnamon twig, chiang-huo, tu-huo, and siler. The formula was based on the traditional prescription *Jian Bu Hu Qian Wan* (Step Reinforcing Tiger's Walk Pill). The pills were taken in a dosage of 3 to 9 grams at a time, 2 to 3 times per day depending on the person's constitution and severity of the disease, but were not to be used by patients showing yin deficiency fire syndrome. Two of the patients were said to be cured and five improved. The pills were to be used on a regular basis over a period of several years.

Strychnos is sometimes mentioned as part of ALS treatments. A muscle-invigorating combination known as Mobilizing Powder may produce temporary alleviation of flaccidity. The combination includes strychnos, musk, and centipede. Strychnos in small doses tones the muscles and in large doses paralyzes them. It is used in the treatment of other autoimmune disorders, including MG and rheumatoid arthritis. Unfortunately, this herb cannot enter into Western treatments for autoimmune diseases because of concerns over the toxicity of strychnine, one of the main active components.

A large-scale study of progressive spinal muscular atrophy (80 cases) and ALS (30 cases) was described by Huo (1985). The primary formula used for treatment was *Yisui Tang*, made with codonopsis, atractylodes, astragalus, rehmannia, psoralea, dipsacus, cuscuta, achyranthes, cibotium, tang-kuei, peony, millettia, tortoise shell, deer antler gelatin (each herb 9 to 15 grams in decoction), with 5 grams each phellodendron and anemarrhena. This formula is a substantial modification of *Hu Qian Wan*, utilizing several yang tonic herbs to replace the tiger's bone of the ancient prescription. According to the report, 59 cases were considered cured (symptoms alleviated, muscles regenerated, and muscular function restored), 18 markedly improved, 25 improved, and 8 showed no improvement.

14.4.4.5 Case Study for Myasthenia Gravis

Yakazu (1985a,b) reported that formulas containing ma-huang, such as Pueraria Combination (*Gegen Tang*) and Minor Blue Dragon Combination (*Xiao Qinglong Tang*), were repeatedly found to improve symptoms, at least for short-term treatment, in patients with MG. He attributes this effect to the active component ephedrine, which was previously reported to be effective for myasthenia by Dr. Nabi Ryoken in his book The Revised Practical Medical Service. Ma-huang is traditionally used in the treatment of muscular aching and ephedrine is known to promote circulation through the striated muscles. Yakazu also recommended the use of peony and licorice, stating that this combination "adjusts the tenseness" of the muscles. Licorice also has cortisone-like action. These two herbs are frequently used to relieve muscle spasms, perhaps with better effect in patients suffering from deficiency syndromes. In like manner, he thought that pueraria, traditionally used to relax tense muscles in the neck and shoulders, might help to treat flaccidity of these same muscles when given to patients with MG. In the case study of early MG presented by Shao Nianfang, pueraria was included.

In a study of treatments for MG, Qiu (1986) reported that eight patients received capsules containing strychnos (0.2 grams per capsule), gradually increasing the daily dosage to reach seven capsules each time, three times daily. In addition, the patients were treated with decoctions according to the classification of underlying syndrome. For those with spleen deficiency, Ginseng and Astragalus Combination (*Buzhong Yiqi Tang*) plus epimedium were given. For spleen and kidney deficiency, a decoction of astragalus, epimedium, tang-kuei, atractylodes, codonopsis, rehmannia, dioscorea, curculigo, anemarrhena, and morinda was given; in cases of more severe yang deficiency and cold, cinnamon twig, aconite, and deer antler glue were

Case Studies 359

added. As a result of these therapies, 5 of the 8 patients noted significant improvements.

Li (1986) reported on the cumulative results of treating 250 patients over a period of five years. He claimed that long-term ingestion of herbs that tonify the spleen and kidney could lead to a clinical cure in nearly half the patients. The duration of therapy necessary was 3 to 5 months for the eye-muscle type (which was easier to cure) and 6 to 8 months for the general type. Domei Yakazu believed that those not cured by tonification therapies might benefit from the ma-huang formulas.

14.4.4.6 Remarks

Formal clinical trials involving several patients rather than individual case studies began in 1975 and have included only few hundred patients. Because the Western medical knowledge of the diseases was limited and advanced equipment often not available, the early research was based almost entirely on traditional analysis of treating flaccidity syndrome and guesses as to the treatment of autoimmunity. The claimed positive results, ranging from a high proportion of persons with marked improvements to a substantial number of cases declared cured, were often a consequence of treating patients with different formulas according to diagnostic categories and with changes in prescription during the first few weeks or months of therapy. Tonification of spleen, kidney, and liver are the prominent methods of therapy. It was common to combine decoctions and pills and to use pills as long-term therapy, which sometimes lasted for two years. In some cases, acupuncture, Western medicine, and other therapies were said to be used: undoubtedly, in most trials the patients received the therapeutic interventions that the physicians felt were necessary within the limitations of what could be offered.

14.5 Concluding Remarks

In this chapter, several individual successful cases and case studies for cancer care, hypertension prescriptions, acupuncture treatment for diabetes, and TCM treatment for multiple sclerosis are presented. These case studies do provide evidence that TCM is effective for treating various critical diseases. However, it is a concern whether the observed cases are isolated cases that may have selection bias (i.e., only successful cases are reported) and/or may not have any statistical meaning (i.e., the observed treatment effects may be due to chance and hence may not be reproducible). In other words, the successful cases may not constitute so-called substantial evidence for efficacy and safety of TCM under investigation, especially when majority of clinical studies were not randomized clinical trials and did not employ randomization and/or blinding for preventing bias. Most importantly, the majority of clinical studies are not in compliance with good clinical practices for clinical investigation.

In recent years, however, the majority of clinical studies for clinical investigation of TCM in treating various diseases conducted in China have begun to adopt the concept of randomized clinical trials including valid study design, power analysis for sample size calculation, randomization/blinding, appropriate statistical methods for data analysis, and valid statistical/clinical interpretation of clinical results in order to provide substantial evidence of effectiveness and safety of the TCM under investigation.

15

Current Issues and Recent Developments

15.1 Introduction

In recent years, as more and more innovative drug products have gone off patents, the search for new or alternative medicines such as botanical drug products that can treat critical and/or life-threatening diseases has become the center of attention of many pharmaceutical companies and research organizations such as the US NIH. Botanical drug products are often referred to as TCM. This leads to the development of TCM, especially for those intended for treating critical and/or life-threatening diseases such as cancer. The use of TCM in humans for treating various diseases has a history of a few thousand years, although not much convincing scientific evidence (documentation) regarding clinical safety and efficacy is available. Thus, how to effectively and scientifically develop a promising TCM the Western way has become an important issue in public health.

A Western medicine (WM) (e.g., a small molecular chemical drug product) often contains a single active ingredient, while a TCM (e.g., a botanical drug product) usually consists of multiple active and inactive components. These multiple active and inactive components may not be characterized, and their relationships are usually unknown. Thus, in practice, it is of great concern whether a TCM can be scientifically evaluated the Western way owing to some fundamental differences between a WM and a TCM. These fundamental differences include differences in medical theory, mechanism and practice, techniques of diagnostic procedure (i.e., inspection, auscultation and olfaction, interrogation, and pulse taking and palpation), criteria for evaluation of safety and efficacy in clinical trials, and treatment (i.e., fixed dose for a Western medicine versus a flexible dose for a TCM).

The purpose of this chapter is multifold. First, it is to provide a comparison between a WM (e.g., chemical drug product) and a traditional TCM (e.g., botanical drug product) in terms of the fundamental differences. Second, it is to provide an overview of regulatory requirements for botanical drug product development based on a guidance published in 2004 (FDA 2004). Finally, it is to discuss critical scientific and/or regulatory issues that are

361

362   *Quantitative Methods for Traditional Chinese Medicine Development*

commonly encountered during the development of a botanical drug product or TCM. These issues include, but are not limited to, intellectual property (IP), variation (or consistency) in raw materials, component-to-component interactions, animal studies, matching placebo and calibration of study endpoints in clinical trials, packaging insert, and transition from experience-based to evidence-based clinical practice.

The remainder of this chapter is organized as follows. In Section 15.2, critical issues that are commonly encountered during the development of a TCM will be briefly described. Section 15.3 provides frequently asked questions (from regulatory perspectives) for development of a TCM in the United States. Recent development of TCMs is discussed in Section 15.4. Concluding remarks are provided in Section 15.5.

15.2 Critical Issues in TCM Development

In this section, a number of critical issues that are often encountered during the development of a TCM are briefly discussed.

15.2.1 Intellectual Property

Song (2011) indicated that innovation of TCM can be divided into two categories: one is the self-innovation of TCM and the other is innovation based on knowledge and techniques of TCM. Both innovations have been presented with different questions of intellectual property (IP) derived from past events. As Song (2011) pointed out, under market economy conditions where private rights are legitimate and interests must be maximized, a proper intellectual property legal system should be established for the protection of the innovation of TCM. Hence, not only rules of market economy but also intellectual property law must be complied with. However, the majority of people involved in self-innovation of TCM generally do not seek the protection of IP due to the nature of conservativeness of Chinese people and most importantly lack of confidence in the current patent system for IP protection.

15.2.1.1 Patentability Requirements

Hsiao (2007) pointed out that in the current patent system, an invention has to satisfy the examiner in many aspects including its novelty, inventive steps, industrial applicability, and enablement. An invention has to pass the novelty test before proceeding to other steps. Failure to satisfy the novelty requirement will render the invention nonpatentable. In the past several decades, novelty has barred many Chinese herbal medicines (products) from patentability because they are either based on traditional formulas or have the same

Current Issues and Recent Developments   363

medicinal use and are already available to the public. In practice, some interventions are considered non-novel and hence not patentable. These situations include (1) when the claimed medical uses can be deduced from prior work based on a common mode of action, and (2) when the claimed medical uses can be ascribed to pharmacological effects closely related to those in prior work.

As indicated by the Taiwan Intellectual Property Office (TIPO) Guidelines for Patent Examination, an invention is referred to as any creation of technical concepts by utilizing the rules of nature. Thus, inventions that are mere discovery, against the rule of nature, not using the rule of nature, or nontechnical in character are not considered as inventions. TIPO adopts the standard of absolute novelty in the sense that an invention has to be new and nothing similar to those that have appeared before the date of filing, for those are available to the public are considered as prior work. Note that in patent law, novelty reflects the basic principle in property law that ownership of an intervention is acquired by being the first in time to possess it. In order to transform something belonging to nature or the public domain, the discoverer has to transform the discovery into an invention to demonstrate possession. To assist examiners to search for prior work in relation to Chinese herbal medicines, TIPO has established a database of classics and traditional formulas that are in the public domain. Along this line, there are several possible types of end products of traditional Chinese medicine deriving from traditional knowledge, methods of treatments, products, and processes are patentable (Koon et al. 1999). The first two, however, are not considered inventions under the current Taiwan Patent Law. In Taiwan, invention refers to the creation of technical concepts by utilizing the rule of nature; therefore, it needs to have some degree of technical characteristic. Despite the controversies of patenting traditional medicines, the patenting of products and processes of Chinese herbal inventions is not a novel idea.

15.2.1.2 Complexities of Patent Application

In current practice, the dominant Western drug discovery process from natural products has the following goals that (1) it is to isolate bioactive compounds for direct use as drugs, (2) it is to produce bioactive compounds of novel or known structures as lead compounds for semi-synthesis to produce patentable entities of higher activity and/or lower toxicity, (3) it is to use agents as pharmacologic tools, and (4) it is to use the whole plant or part of the plant as a herbal remedy (Fabricant and Farnsworth 2001). In practice, if the Chinese herbal invention is not a pure compound, then there are some complexities in filing a patent application. The first complexity is the difference in the names used in the classics. Many plants have different names especially they are from different sources. The lack of uniformity has not only create confusion but also result in inconsistency for the development of TCM. For example, *Smallanthus Sonchifloius* in the folk medicine and *Saussyrea Lanicep Hand-Mazz* in the classics are two different types of plants

364 Quantitative Methods for Traditional Chinese Medicine Development

with very different pharmacological uses, but their names are similar in terms of Chinese language. The second complexity relates to the crude materials and the difficulties in allocating the effective active ingredients. The third complexity is that unlike chemical compounds (which could be identically reproduced), plants are living organisms that vary in characteristics even within the same variety of plants. Another complexity is that impure substances are abundant in plants. Last, it is difficult to prove the pharmacological efficacy of Chinese herbal medicine.

15.2.2 Variation in Raw Materials

One of the critical issues in TCM manufacturing is variation in raw materials. The variation in raw materials, which may be due to the fact that they come from different regions, climates, and time of harvest, could have a negative impact on the quality of the TCM and consequently the safety and efficacy of the TCM. Yan and Qu (2013) indicated that the efficacy of a TCM depends on the combined effects of its components. Variation in chemical composition between batches of TCM has been always the deterring factor of achieving consistency in efficacy. These components, however, may or may not be correlated and may have component-to-component interaction that will have an impact on achieving the optimal therapeutic effect of the TCM. In practice, unfortunately, the correlations among the components and their relative ratios for achieving the optimal therapeutic effect are often unknown.

15.2.2.1 Utilization Ratio of Extracts

Yan and Qu (2013) indicated that batch mixing process can significantly reduce the batch-to-batch variation in TCM extracts by mixing them in a well-designed proportion, which is referred to as utilization ratio of the extracts (URE). Yan and Qu (2013) suggested an innovative and practical batch mixing method for achieving an acceptable efficiency for manufacturing of TCM products by using a minimum number of batches of extracts to meet the content limits under an acceptable URE. Yan and Qu (2013) indicated that URE is affected by the correlation between the contents of components. In practice, URE decreases with the increase in the number of targets and the relative standard deviations of the contents. URE could be increased by increasing the number of storage tanks. Thus, to achieve an acceptable URE, it is desirable to use up some batches of extracts in one mixing to reduce the number of residual batches. These findings provide reference standards for designing the batch mixing process.

15.2.2.2 Batch Mixing Optimization Model

Yan and Qu (2013) proposed a batch mixing optimization model to reduce variation in raw materials and improve the quality of the TCM under development. Their method is briefly described below. Suppose that there are t (target) components with controlled contents in the mixture. Let s be the number of storage tanks, i.e., the maximum number of batches of extracts that can be stored. Also let $x = (x_1, x_2, ..., x_s)$ be the amounts of each stored batch of extract used for mixing and $u = (u_1, u_2, ..., u_s)$, the amounts of each batch of extract stored. Define $a_k = (a_{1k}, a_{2k}, ..., a_{tk})'$, the contents of the constituents in the kth batch of extract stored. For unidentified constituents, test values such as peak areas on the chromatographic fingerprint obtained by certain analytical methods can be used. Thus, we have $A = (a_1, a_2, ..., a_s)$, a $t \times s$ matrix that consists of the contents of the components in the batches of extracts stored. Now, let b be the amount of mixture needed in each batch and (L_i, U_i) be the minimum and maximum content limits of the ith component. Yan and Qu (2013) proposed to maximize

$$\max \sum_{i=1}^{s} x_i^2, \tag{15.1}$$

which maximizes the sum of squares of the used amounts of each batch. Therefore, the optimization model in this study is to maximize the value of Equation 15.1 under the following constraints:

$$\sum_{i=1}^{s} x_i = b, \tag{15.2}$$

where Equation 15.2 determines the amount of mixture needed for the follow-up process. The contents of the constituents in the mixture are assumed to be the weighted average of the contents in the extracts, where the weights are the amounts of each batch used for mixing;

$$\min L' \le \frac{A \cdot x'}{b} \le \max U', \tag{15.3}$$

where $\max U = (\max U_1, \max U_2, ..., \max U_t)$, the maximum content limits for the components in the mixtures and $\min L = (\min L_1, \min L_2, ..., \min L_t)$, the minimum content limits for the constituents in the mixtures. Equation 15.3 ensures that the contents are in the range of their limits, and,

$$0 \le x' \le u', \tag{15.4}$$

where Equation 15.4 is the maximum amount of each batch that can be used for mixing. Note that the above optimization model can be solved by quadratic programming algorithm. In TCM manufacturing, batch mixing can

366 *Quantitative Methods for Traditional Chinese Medicine Development*

be conducted with the extracts obtained from previous processes like decoction, concentration, and purification. The extracts created are first stored in the storage tanks. Batch mixing ratios are calculated according to the optimization model and mixtures are created for the follow-up process.

15.2.2.3 Remarks

The batch mixing process can significantly reduce the variation in the quality of TCM extracts among different batches by mixing them in a well-designed URE. The batch mixing method proposed in this work uses a minimum number of batches of extracts to meet the content limits, which is more practical in industrial production. The impacts of the important factors on URE were studied by simulations, which provide a reference for designing the batch mixing process. The results of the study have demonstrated that batch mixing is a valuable method to improve the batch-to-batch quality consistency of TCM and may contribute to the increase in consistency of the efficacy of TCM.

15.2.3 Component-to-Component Interactions

Unlike most Western medicines, TCM often consists of a number of components whose pharmacological activities may or may not be quantitatively characterized. Besides, the relative proportions (ratios) of the components for achieving optimal therapeutic effect are also unknown in addition to possible component-to-component (drug-to-drug) interaction among these components. Thus, the study to determine the relative ratios of components for achieving the optimal therapeutic effect has become the key to the success of TCM development. To study the main effects and interactions of these components, some commonly employed designs are briefly described below.

15.2.3.1 Factorial Design

A full factorial design is a design that consists of all possible different combinations of one level from each factor. If there are l_k levels for the kth factor X_k, the corresponding full factorial design is called a general $l_1 l_2, \ldots, l_k$ factorial design. For example, when $l_i = 2$ (or 3) for all i, the general factorial design is called a 2^K (or 3^K) factorial design. A 2^K (or 3^K) factorial design denotes a full factorial design at two levels (or at three levels). In practice, a factorial design is expressed in terms of a number of arrays (or runs) that indicate the levels of each factor. For example, for a typical 2^4 factorial design, the arrangement of the arrays is given in the following standard order (see Table 15.1). The first column of the design matrix consists of successive minus (−) and plus (+) signs, the second column of successive pairs of (−) and (+) signs, the third column of four (−) signs followed by four (+) signs, and so on. In general, the Kth column consists of 2^{K-1} (−) signs followed by 2^{K-1} (+) signs. In this 2^4 factorial

Current Issues and Recent Developments

TABLE 15.1

A Full 2^4 Factorial Design

	Design Matrix				
Run	X_1	X_2	X_3	X_4	Y
1	−	−	−	−	Y_1
2	+	−	−	−	Y_2
3	−	+	−	−	Y_3
4	+	+	−	−	Y_4
5	−	−	+	−	Y_5
6	+	−	+	−	Y_6
7	−	+	+	−	Y_7
8	+	+	+	−	Y_8
9	−	−	−	+	Y_9
10	+	−	−	+	Y_{10}
11	−	+	−	+	Y_{11}
12	+	+	−	+	Y_{12}
13	−	−	+	+	Y_{13}
14	+	−	+	+	Y_{14}
15	−	+	+	+	Y_{15}
16	+	+	+	+	Y_{16}

design, there are four factors at two levels, with a total of $N = 2^4 = 16$ runs. The two levels of each factor are conventionally denoted by (+) and (−) (they are sometimes denoted by 1 and −1). If a variable is continuous, the two levels, (+) and (−), denoted the high and low levels. If a variable is qualitative, the two levels may denote two different types or the presence and absence of the variable. Each row represents a different combination of one level from each factor. A full factorial design provides estimates not only for main effects but also for interactions with maximum precision. The main effects and interaction effects can easily be obtained using a table of contrast coefficients and/ or Yate's algorithm (see, e.g., Myers 1976; Hicks 1982).

15.2.3.2 Fractional Factorial Design

A fractional factorial design is a design that consists of s fraction of a full factorial experiment. For example, a $(1/2)^P$ fraction of a 2^K factorial design is called a 2^{K-P} fractional factorial design. When $P = 1$, a full factorial design reduces to a one-half factorial design. For a full 2^4 factorial design, there are 16 effects, including grand average, four main effects, six two-factor interactions, four three-factor interactions, and a single four-factor interaction. The full 2^4 factorial design contains 16 observations, which provide independent estimates for each of these 16 effects. However, if we consider only a one-half fraction (i.e., only eight observations available), due to limited

TABLE 15.2

A 2^{4-1} Fractional Factorial Design

	Design Matrix				
Run	X_1	X_2	X_3	$X_4 = X_1X_2X_3$	Y
1	$-$	$-$	$-$	$-$	Y_1
2	$+$	$-$	$-$	$+$	Y_2
3	$-$	$+$	$-$	$+$	Y_3
4	$+$	$+$	$-$	$-$	Y_4
5	$-$	$-$	$+$	$+$	Y_5
6	$+$	$-$	$+$	$-$	Y_6
7	$-$	$+$	$+$	$-$	Y_7
8	$+$	$+$	$+$	$+$	Y_8

resources available, it is impossible to obtain 16 independent estimates. For a 2^{4-1} fractional factorial design, the eight observations cannot provide independent estimates for the 16 effects alone but for some confounding effects, such as the sum of a main effect and a three-factor interaction that are confounded with each other. In practice, however, the three-factor or higher-factor interactions are usually negligible (see Table 15.2). In this case, a fractional factorial design is useful in estimating the main effects. In practice, a fractional factorial design is useful when there are many factors to be studied because it is almost impossible to perform a full factorial design even at two levels.

15.2.3.3 Central Composite Design

A central composite design is a full factorial design or a fractional factorial design augmented by a $\pm \alpha$ level at each of the K factors and n central points. The central composite design consists of one center point, eight points on the cube (a 2^3 factorial arrangement), and six star points. It should be noted that a central composite design with $K = 2$, $\alpha = 1$, and $n = 1$ reduces to a 3^2 factorial design (see Table 15.3). For a full 2^K factorial design, although the design provides independent estimates for the $2^K - 1$ effects, it does not give an estimate of the experimental error unless some runs are repeated. Unlike the full 2^K factorial design, the central composite design provides an estimate of the experimental error. The experimental error is usually estimated based on n observations at the central point.

15.2.3.4 Remarks

In addition to the factorial design, the fractional factorial design, and the central composite design, other designs such as the classical Plackett and Burman design (Plackett and Burman 1946) and the factorial or fractional factorial in randomized block design are also useful.

TABLE 15.3

Central Composite Design for $K = 3$ and $n = 1$

Run	X_1	X_2	X_3
1	−1	−1	−1
2	1	−1	−1
3	−1	1	−1
4	1	1	−1
5	−1	−1	1
6	1	−1	1
7	−1	1	1
8	1	1	1
9	0	0	0
10	α	0	0
11	$-\alpha$	0	0
12	0	α	0
13	0	$-\alpha$	0
14	0	0	α
15	0	0	$-\alpha$

15.2.4 Animal Studies

As indicated earlier, the use of TCM in treating critical and life-threatening diseases has had a long and noble history. It has been actively practiced nowadays in many parts of the world. Because TCM often consists of multiple components, it is unquestionable that many components are successful in suppressing different types of diseases in humans. However, there does not appear to be any evidence (e.g., scientific documentation) that meets stringent Western criteria for safely and efficacy to support their use in humans. Thus, in pharmaceutical development, animal studies such as mice, rats, rabbits, dogs, or monkeys for testing toxicity and evaluation of efficacy are required for regulatory review and approval before they can be used in humans.

However, there are tremendous debates regarding whether animal studies are necessary for the development of TCM, especially for those that have been used for thousands of years. Most Chinese doctors suggest that it would be better to focus on clinical development, instead of going back to animal studies to obtain evidence for a precise pharmacological profile. It would be better to focus on safety and efficacy by starting with clinical trials. It is also suggested that studies on mechanisms and active ingredients should be conducted after safety and efficacy have been confirmed.

For development of Western medicines, animal studies (models) are often used to screen experimental drugs before they enter human trials. Animal models can provide pharmaceutical scientists insight into how the drugs work in the living system and evaluate the toxicity at various doses assuming

370 Quantitative Methods for Traditional Chinese Medicine Development

that the animal model is predictive of the human model. Although there have been controversial debates over which diseased animal models should be used to screen new drugs before they can proceed to the clinical trials, certain animal models in different therapeutic areas maintain good standards for drug screening used in the pharmaceutical industry, for example, the subcutaneous, xenografts in cancer drug screening. Although animal models used in the preclinical test do provide valuable information (if they are predictive of human models), one of the concerns is apparent physiological and genetic differences between human and animals, which clearly indicate that the diseased models are different from the human equivalent.

15.2.5 Matching Placebo in Clinical Trials

In recent years, randomized controlled trials (RCTs) have been recognized as the gold standard in clinical trials for evaluation of safety and efficacy of a test compound under investigation. One of the important components in RCTs is blinding. The ultimate goal of clinical trials is to achieve a double-blind design to avoid any possible operational bias due to the knowledge of the treatment assignment. Qi et al. (2008) conducted a comprehensive review on the validity of matching placebo used in blind clinical trials for Chinese herbal medicine in recent years and related patents. The review was conducted based on a database called the *Wanfang Database*, which contains a total of 827 Chinese journals of medicine and/or pharmacy, from 1999 to 2005 and 598 full-length articles related to clinical trials utilizing matching placebo. A total of 77 blind clinical trials utilizing matching placebo for Chinese medicine were extracted manually from the 598 articles. After reviewing the 77 full-length articles, it was found that nearly half of the clinical trials did not pay attention to the physical quality of the testing drug and matching placebo and whether they were comparable in terms of physical quality. The rest provided very limited information regarding the preparation of matching placebo. Thus, the integrity of blinding is questionable. Among the 598 articles, unfortunately, only two articles specifically validated the comparability between the test drug and the matching placebo. On the basis of this review, Qi et al. (2008) concluded that researchers in Chinese medicine commonly ignored the quality of the matching placebo in comparison to the test drug. This may have led to substantial bias in clinical trials. As a result, Qi et al. (2008) urged that quality specifications and evaluation of the matching placebo must be developed and carefully evaluated in order to reduce possible bias in randomized controlled TCM trials.

As indicated by Qi et al. (2008), only a small number of randomized controlled trials in traditional Chinese medicine have been reported, most of them are of poor quality in methodology including placebo preparation and verification. Fai et al. (2011) also pointed out that in many clinical trials of Chinese herbal medicines, it is very difficult to make a quality matching placebo to achieve the purpose of blinding. Ideally, the characteristics of the test

Current Issues and Recent Developments

drug and matching placebo should be identical in color, appearance, smell and taste. The quality matching placebo should be identical to the test drug in physical form, sensory perception, packaging, and labeling, and it should have no pharmaceutical activity. For this purpose, Fai et al. (2011) developed a placebo capsule to match a herbal medicine in terms of its physical form, chemical nature, appearance, packaging, and labeling. On the basis of the assessment results, the developed placebo capsule assessment results suggested that the placebo was found satisfactory in these aspects. Thus, Fai et al. (2011) concluded that a matching placebo could be created for a RCT involving herbal medicine. In addition, Fai et al. (2011) also discussed the means to acquire a patent for a developed matching placebo.

It should be noted that the preparation of matching placebo is extremely important to maintain the integrity of blinding to avoid any possible operational bias that may be introduced owing to the knowledge of the treatment assignment. The oral dosage form of capsule is often considered for preparation of matching placebo for clinical trials involving Chinese herbal medicines as it may remove the strong smell and taste of the herbal medicines. However, one of the major challenges is that patients or clinicians will reveal the treatment assignments if they break the capsules. Thus, standard operating procedures for preventing patients and clinicians from breaking the capsules are necessary developed.

15.2.6 Calibration of Study Endpoints

Unlike WMs, the primary study endpoints for assessment of safety and effectiveness of a TCM are usually assessed by a quantitative instrument or the four diagnostic procedures (as discussed in Chapter 1) by experienced Chinese doctors. The assessment by a quantitative instrument has been criticized in many ways. First, it may not capture the true health of status of the patients with diseases under study (e.g., by asking wrong questions). Second, it may not detect the effect of the test treatment under investigation. As an example, consider a quantitative instrument with possible scores from 0 (perfect health) to 100 (worst possible disease status). Suppose the scores can be classified into the following categories of health status: Health (0–25), Mild (26–50), Moderate (51–75), and Severe (76–100). In this case, there is significant difference between a patient with a score of 25 (Health) and a patient with a score of 26 (Mild) despite they only differ by one point. On the other hand, a patient with a score of 26 and a patient with a score of 50 are both considered having Mild disease status although they differ by 24 points. Thus, the assessment based on a quantitative instrument by experienced Chinese doctors is not only subjective but also lack of validity. Consequently, the reliability of the assessment is a concern, especially when there is evidence of large rater-to-rater variability.

Thus, although the quantitative instrument is developed by the community of Chinese doctors and is considered a gold standard for assessment of safety and effectiveness of the TCM under investigation, it may not be accepted by

372   *Quantitative Methods for Traditional Chinese Medicine Development*

the Western clinicians not only due to the lack of validity and reliability, but also the interpretation of the assessment (or translation of assessment to well-established and widely accepted clinical endpoints). In practice, it is very difficult for a Western clinician to conceptually understand the clinical meaning of the difference detected by the subjective Chinese quantitative instrument due to fundamental differences in medical theory, perception and practice.

Thus, for modernization or Westernization of TCMs, whether the subjective quantitative instrument can accurately and reliably assess the safety and effectiveness of the TCM is a concern for development of TCM. In practice, it is then suggested that a clinical trial be conducted to calibrate the subjective quantitative assessment against either life events or well-established clinical endpoints that are commonly used in assessment of Western medicines. The clinical trials should consist of two arms: one arm will include subjects with diseases under study diagnosed by the subjective quantitative instrument and the other arm will include subjects diagnosed by Western diagnostic or testing procedures. Each subject post-treatment will be assessed by both Chinese doctors using the quantitative instrument and Western clinicians based on the well-established and widely accepted study endpoints (Hsiao et al. 2009).

15.2.7 Package Insert

One of questions that are commonly asked in the development of a TCM is that the developed TCM is intended for use by Chinese doctors only, Western doctors only, or both. The answer to this question has an impact on the preparation of package insert. As discussed in the previous section, the translation between Chinese study endpoints and Western study endpoints is not clear. As a result, it is difficult to conceptually determine the observed treatment effect (based on Chinese study endpoints) is of clinically relevance or importance.

If the TCM is intended for use by Western doctors, it must be developed under the review and approval pathway of Western medicines such as the pathway of IND/NDA of US FDA. On the other hand, if the TCM is intended for use by Chinese doctors, it will be developed under the review and approval pathway of TCMs such as regulatory requirements set forth by Taiwan Food and Drug Administration (TFDA) or China Food and Drug Administration (CFDA). In this case, the preparation of package insert is very different from that of Western medicines. If the TCM is intended for use by both Chinese doctors and Western doctors, then the calibration between Chinese study endpoints and Western study endpoints discussed in the previous section is essential.

15.2.8 Transition from Experience-Based
to Evidence-Based Clinical Practice

As indicated earlier, TCMs have been in practice for thousands of years. Many of the commonly used TCMs were found safe and efficacious. However, evidence of safety and efficacy of these TCM were not documented for scientific

Current Issues and Recent Developments 373

evaluation. Unlike evidence-based clinical data, the experience-based clinical information has been criticized for lacking of scientific validity and reliability for assessment of safety and efficacy of the TCMs (currently being used or under development). As an example, Chinese patients are likely to report only successful cases, while those patients who fail (which may be due to severe adverse events or lack of efficacy) are likely seeking for alternatives and then lost to follow-up. As a result, experience-based clinical information is considered not only subjective but also biased (due to selection bias) and misleading.

In practice, how to collect relevant and important clinical data from experience-based clinical practice is then of particular interest to clinical scientists for development of TCMs. Most Chinese doctors resist to (1) collect clinical data that they are not familiar with and (2) cooperate with Western doctors to collect further information from their patients owing to fundamental differences in culture and clinical theory, perception, and practice. Thus, the transition from experience-based clinical practice to evidence-based clinical practice requires careful communication and planning. This transition is essential for achieving the ultimate goal of modernization and/or Westernization of TCMs.

15.2.9 Prescription versus Dietary Supplement

One of the most controversial issues in the development of TCMs is that the pharmaceutical development of a TCM which has been available in the market place as a lawful dietary supplement. As is well recognized, the TCM will become a prescription drug once it is approved by the regulatory agency. In other words, the TCM (in the form of dietary supplement) needs to be withdrawn from the market place. This may have created problems for those subjects who have used the TCM as a dietary supplement for years.

15.3 Frequently Asked Questions from a Regulatory Perspective

The following is a list of some selected questions and answers from the FDA guidance on botanical drug products (FDA 2014). Some comments from the author are included whenever appropriate.

15.3.1 Are INDs Required for Clinical Studies of Botanical Products That Are Lawfully Marketed as Dietary Supplements in the United States?

FDA's Response: It depends on what the botanical product is being studied. If a lawfully marketed botanical dietary supplement is studied for dietary supplement use, i.e., effect on the structure and/or a function of the body, an IND is not required (see final rule on "Structure and Function Claims

374 *Quantitative Methods for Traditional Chinese Medicine Development*

for Dietary Supplements," 65 FR 1000, January 6, 2000). Although an IND is not legally required for such a study, CDER encourages sponsors to submit one. If you have questions on how to design such a study, FDA would be willing to review and provide advice on protocols. You may contact CDER's Botanical Review Team at 301-827-2250 or botanicalteam@cder.fda.gov. If a botanical preparation is being studied for its effects on a disease in the proposed investigation (i.e., to cure, treat, mitigate, prevent, or diagnose disease, including its associated symptoms), it is considered a new drug and will need to be studied under an IND (see section 312.2).

Author's Comments: A controversial issue is encountered. Suppose that an IND of a TCM (botanical product) is also a lawfully marketed product as a dietary supplement in the United States. In this case, it is very controversial that a drug product under investigation be available to the general public. Moreover, it will become unavailable to the general public after it is approved (i.e., it becomes a prescription drug product) by the regulatory agency.

15.3.2 Are INDs Required for Clinical Studies on Marketed Dietary Supplements for Research Purposes Only?

FDA's Response: It depends on the use. If the intent is to study the effect of the product on the structure and/or a function of the body, no IND is needed. If the study is to assess the effects on disease, an IND is needed.

15.3.3 Is There Any Other Setting in Which an IND Is Not Required for the Botanical Study?

FDA's Response: When a nonmarketed botanical preparation is studied in the United States for a dietary supplement use, an IND is not required. In addition, clinical studies conducted in foreign countries require no IND. However, FDA will accept an IND for either kind of study. In the absence of an IND, an investigational new drug intended for export for the purpose of clinical investigation must comply with the requirements set forth in section 312.110(b)(2) unless the new drug has been approved or authorized for export under section 802 of the Act (21 U.S.C. 382).

15.3.4 May a Sponsor Submit an IND for a Phase 3 Study of a Botanical Product Not Previously Studied under an IND?

FDA's Response: Yes. Clinical data collected from phase 1 and phase 2 studies conducted without an IND can be used to support a phase 3 study involving the same drug substance if they are adequately designed and conducted. The formulation/dosage form of the botanical product used in the proposed phase 3 study ideally would be the same as that of the product used in phase 1 and 2 studies as well as in the preclinical (nonclinical) studies. If the product is different, additional studies may be appropriate.

Current Issues and Recent Developments 375

Author's Comments: FDA seems to accept clinical data collected from previous studies not under an IND provided that they are adequately designed and conducted. Although it is always a good idea to collect more relevant clinical data to support a phase 3 study, there are potential risks of (1) selection bias, (2) study-by-study variability, and (3) possible treatment-by-study interaction. Thus, it is suggested that a meta-analysis of clinical data collected from previous studies not under an IND be conducted to summarize similarities and dissimilarities of these studies for a systematic review of these relevant data to determine whether these clinical data are relevant and can be used to support the proposed phase 3 study.

15.3.5 For NDA Approvals of Botanical Drug Products, Must All Studies Be Carried Out under INDs?

FDA's Response: No. FDA does not require that all studies submitted in an NDA be conducted under an IND. Clinical studies need not necessarily be conducted under an IND (i.e., if they are carried out abroad). The clinical data generated from these studies conducted without an IND can be used to support an NDA if the studies were adequately designed and conducted under good clinical practices. Although an IND is not required by law in all cases, the sponsor is encouraged to go through the IND process. Compliance with the IND requirements will help to ensure that an adequate pharmaceutical product development program is in place so that the material will meet the quality standards not only for various phases of clinical trials but also for eventual marketing. It will also help to ensure that the clinical trials will be well designed so that data generated can be persuasive.

Author's Comments: FDA will only accept clinical data generated from these studies conducted abroad without an IND to support an NDA if the studies were adequately designed and conducted under good clinical practices. Most clinical data collected abroad (especially China) were not adequately designed and in compliance with good clinical practices according to FDA standards. Some of these data may be accepted and some not if data quality and integrity of the studies are in serious doubt. It will be very helpful if a set of acceptance criteria for clinical data generated abroad can be developed to avoid subjective judgment and unnecessary argument regarding the acceptance of these relevant clinical data.

15.3.6 It Appears That the Changes in Regulatory Approaches Described in the Guidance on Botanical Drug Products Concern Only IND Applications. How Will These Changes Be Applied to the NDA Requirements for Botanical Drugs?

FDA's Response: To facilitate the clinical development of botanical drugs, FDA decided to focus initially on guidance for INDs, especially the early

376 *Quantitative Methods for Traditional Chinese Medicine Development*

phases of clinical study. The standards for the safety and efficacy required for marketing approval of a botanical drug are the same as those required for a conventional chemical drug for the same indication. However, the product quality standards for a botanical drug can be different from those for a purified chemical drug. The Botanical Drug Products guidance contains recommendations for establishing appropriate quality standards for botanical drugs.

15.3.7 Some Botanical Preparations Are Not Administered Orally, e.g., Intravenous, Topical, and Inhalation Products. How Are These Non-Oral Formulations Considered in the Guidance?

FDA's Response: The guidance applies to all dosage forms of botanical products. All parenteral, topical, inhalation, or other non-orally administered botanical products are considered to be drugs, not dietary supplements, and must be studied under an IND for any use (see section 201(ff) of the Act). Just as for purified chemical drugs, the type of quality testing varies from dosage form to dosage form. For example, all injectables are required to be sterile and pyrogen-free (211.165(b) and 211.167 and 314.50(d) (1)(ii)(b)); oral tablets are not. In addition, dietary supplements are orally ingested and the human experience of an orally administered botanical dietary supplement may not be applicable to the same botanical product given through other routes.

15.3.8 In Terms of IND Requirements and Regulatory Review by the Agency, Is There Any Difference between a Commercial Development Program and an Academic Research Project?

FDA's Response: No. The Agency applies the same standards to both commercial and academic sponsors when evaluating the safety and quality of human studies proposed in INDs.

15.3.9 Intellectual Property Rights Are a Difficult Issue for Developing New Drugs from Well Known Botanical Preparations. How Does FDA Protect the Confidentiality of a Sponsor's Submission? What Kind of IND/NDA Data May FDA Release without Prior Permission from the Sponsor?

FDA's Response: IND information generally is not publicly available (see sections 312.130 and 314.430). Once an NDA is approved, FDA may release certain safety and efficacy information (section 314.430(e)). Manufacturing information (including information related to growers and suppliers) provided in an NDA or a Drug Master File (DMF) is considered proprietary and may not be released (21 U.S.C. 331(j); 21 CFR 20.61).

Current Issues and Recent Developments 377

15.3.10 How Does FDA Ensure That the New Botanical Drug Products Guidance Will Be Implemented Consistently across the Different New Drug Review Divisions?

FDA's Response: FDA will provide reviewers in all divisions with training on how to implement the guidance.

15.3.11 One of the Major Premises of the New Guidance Is That Because Many Botanical Products Have Been Used by a Large Population for a Long Period of Time, They Are Presumed to Be Safe Enough to Be Studied in Clinical Trials without First Undergoing Conventional Nonclinical Studies. What Kind of Documentation Should a Sponsor Submit to Demonstrate Prior Human Experience with the Sponsor's Product?

FDA's Response: The Agency recognizes that prior human experience with a botanical product can be documented in many different forms and sources, some of which may not meet the quality standards of modern scientific testing. The sponsor is encouraged to provide as much data as possible, and the review team for the botanical drug IND generally will accept all available information for regulatory consideration. FDA will assess the quality of the submitted data on a case-by-case basis. It should be emphasized that, in reviewing botanical drugs, the Agency does not lower or raise the safety and efficacy standards for marketing approval that apply to purified chemical drugs. The guidance simply recommends the use of different types of data for preliminary safety consideration of human trials (e.g., large quantities of mostly anecdotal human data instead of animal studies).

15.3.12 In Many Cases, Botanical Therapies Are Highly Individualized with Variations in Relative Contents of Multiple Plant Ingredients Tailored for Each Patient. Must a Sponsor Submit a Separate IND for Every Change in Composition, If Similar Patients Are Being Treated for the Same Indication?

FDA's Response: Studies can be designed to take into account individualized treatments. Multiple formulations can be included in one IND if they are being studied under a single clinical trial. It is important that the IND provide the rationale for using multiple formulations and the criteria used to assign patients to different treatment regimens.

15.3.13 Many Medicinal Plants with Therapeutical Potential Are Quite Toxic. Does the New Guidance Address the Study of Such Botanicals?

FDA's Response: The guidance discusses this issue in the sections addressing botanical drug products with known safety issues (e.g., section VI.A).

378 *Quantitative Methods for Traditional Chinese Medicine Development*

Well-known examples of safety issues concerning botanicals include the nephrotoxicity associated with herbal preparations containing aristolochic acid and the hepatotoxicity associated with comfrey products containing pyrrolizidine alkaloid. Other examples include the cardiovascular and central nervous system effects associated with yohimbe and the hepatotoxicity associated with germander and chaparral. In such cases, FDA will evaluate the known risk and the potential benefit of an investigational drug for its intended use. When the potential benefit of an investigational drug outweighs its risk in the intended patient population, clinical trials may be allowed to proceed under an IND (see section 312.42). For example, FDA will accept a relatively higher level of toxicity of an investigational drug when studied to treat terminally ill cancer patients. However, additional nonclinical studies may be appropriate to adequately characterize the toxicity (e.g., can a dose be identified that would not be expected to produce toxicity?) and/or additional monitoring may be appropriate during the clinical trial. Also, FDA may recommend against human studies (e.g., bioavailability, clinical pharmacology) in healthy volunteers.

15.3.14 There Is a Concern That If a Botanical Is Being Studied under an IND or Is Approved as a New Drug in an NDA, Its Subsequent Status as a Dietary Supplement May Be Jeopardized. Is This True?

FDA's Response: No, it is generally not true for products already on the market before approval of an NDA. It is also generally not true for products marketed before authorization of an IND for which substantial clinical investigations have been instituted and the existence of such investigations has been made public (see section 201(ff)(3) of the Act).

Author's Comments: FDA's response on this question is somewhat confusing if the botanical being studied under an NDA is identical to the dietary supplement in the marketplace. There must be a distinction between an approved botanical drug product and a dietary supplement with identical components (ingredients). See also author's comments on question described in the first question in this FAQ.

15.3.15 What Is FDA's Advice on the Initial Approach for Sponsors Not Familiar with New Drug Development and Regulatory Processes?

FDA's Response: A sponsor should first consult the guidance. If there are questions concerning the guidance document or other questions about the submission of INDs for botanical drugs, consult the appropriate CDER review division for the therapeutic class of the sponsor's product. CDER also grants pre-IND meetings with sponsors.

Author's Comments: The current guidance is similar to the guidances for chemical drug products with single active ingredient. It should be noted that most botanical drug products consist of multiple components. Thus, some of

Current Issues and Recent Developments 379

the guidances for chemical drug products with single active ingredients cannot be applied directly. For example, for stability testing for establishment of drug expiration dating period (or shelf life), it is not clear how to determine the shelf life of botanical drug products with multiple components.

15.3.16 The Guidance States That the Submission of an NDA for a Drug Derived From Plants Taken from the Wild Is an Extraordinary Circumstance Requiring the Submission of an Environmental Assessment (EA) under Section 25.21. Are Plants Maintained in Their Native Setting on Private Land Considered Wild?

FDA's Response: Yes. Plants that are obtained from their native setting on either public or private land are considered to be taken from the wild. Cultivated plants are considered those that are grown collectively in controlled settings such as plantations, farms, or greenhouses, i.e., purposely segregated from wildlife to the extent practicable.

Author's Comments: Should the wildness be judged based on their variability associated with the measurement? Variation in raw (source) materials has a great impact on the development of botanical products.

15.3.17 Is a Drug Made with a Commercially Available Crude Extract Viewed the Same as a Drug Derived from Plants Taken from the Wild for Purposes of Determining the Need for an EA?

FDA's Response: Yes. If an NDA is submitted for a drug made from a crude extract or intermediate from a plant taken from the wild, an EA is required under section 25.21. This is true whether or not the extract or intermediate is commercially available. As for an IND for a drug made from a crude extract or intermediate from a plant taken from the wild, the FDA will decide on a case-by-case whether an EA is required.

Author's Comments: Case-by-case often indicates that there are no standards but based on reviewers' preferences. Thus, it is suggested an objective guideline or guidance be developed so that the sponsors can follow without any arguments.

15.3.18 What Is the GMP Status of Botanical Raw Materials (Starting Materials) in Terms of Compliance and Inspection?

FDA's Response: Starting materials of botanical origin that are used to produce a botanical drug substance should be evaluated for quality. The use of appropriate starting materials and the drug substance manufacturer's ability to control the source depend on appropriate specifications (tests, analytical procedures, and acceptance criteria). In addition to establishing specifications, manufacturers can achieve adequate quality control of starting materials by applying the principles outlined in FDA's botanical guidance and by following good agricultural and good collection practice for starting

380 *Quantitative Methods for Traditional Chinese Medicine Development*

materials of herbal origin (e.g., European Medicines Evaluation Agency *HMPWP/31/99*). Upon receipt of the starting materials at a processing facility, it is the responsibility of the drug substance manufacturer to determine the suitability of these raw materials before use. This can be accomplished by examining and/or testing to ensure that the acceptance criteria are met and by documenting the quality control for the processing of the starting materials. FDA will review the inspection and examination of starting materials upon receipt when conducting a current good manufacturing practice (CGMP) inspection of a drug substance manufacturer.

Author's Comments: In addition the quality and consistency of starting (raw) materials, the quality and consistency of in-process materials and end-products should also be considered. Because botanical drug products often consist of multiple components. The pharmacological activities of some of these components are usually unknown and their relative relationships (proportions) are not clear. In other words, appropriate (acceptable) specifications for quality assurance and control may not be available. Thus, studies for establishment of reference standards (specifications) for each components are recommended. Without well-established specifications, content uniformity testing, disintegration testing, dissolution testing, and stability testing as described in the U.S. Pharmacopeia (USP) cannot be performed.

15.3.19 Will FDA Assign the Same Level of Priority to Botanical Drug Products as to Other Drug with Respect to Meeting with IND Sponsors and NDA Applicants?

FDA's Response: Yes, FDA treats botanical and purified chemical drugs the same.

Author's Comments: Because there are not too many regulatory submissions for botanical drug products at this time, one of the major concerns is that whether FDA has sufficient man power (e.g., medical and statistical reviewers) who are familiar with botanical drug products to meet the need if the volume of submissions grows substantially in the near future. More data need to be collected in order to confirm FDA's response.

15.4 Recent Developments

15.4.1 Development of Diagnostic Checklist

15.4.1.1 Criticisms of Chinese Diagnostic Procedures

As indicated in Chapter 1, the Chinese diagnostic procedure for patients with certain diseases consists of four major techniques, namely, inspection, auscultation and olfaction, interrogation, and pulse taking and palpation.

Current Issues and Recent Developments 381

One of the major criticisms of Chinese diagnostic procedures is subjectivity. The accuracy and reliability of the diagnosis rely on the experience of the Chinese doctor who conducts the diagnosis. These experience-based diagnostic procedures are considered subjective and not scientifically valid in rigorous clinical research. In addition, we may expect a relatively high doctor-to-doctor variability, which definitely will have a negative impact on the evaluation of the safety and efficacy of TCM under investigation. These are obstacles for the modernization of TCM. Thus, there is need for a search for objective diagnostic procedures in TCM clinical research.

15.4.1.2 Objective Diagnostic Checklist

Without loss of generality, consider the disease of psoriasis. Psoriasis is a chronic inflammatory skin disease with a genetic basis. Its ill-defined causes make it difficult to diagnose. According to modern TCM diagnosis, it is recognized that psoriasis is due to (1) the invasion of pathogenic wind that incubates in the *yin* and blood, or (2) the accumulation and stagnation of *qi* (vital energy) and blood caused by emotional upset. It may also be caused by impairment or disharmony in the functioning or other organs and energy pathway channel (see, e.g., Jiang et al. 2012). Yang et al. (2013) indicated that generally topical treatment, oral medication, and advice on lifestyle and environment are prescribed to relieve the lesions and the impairment or disharmony of the body. TCM treatment is based on *Zheng* composition rather than disease definition (Lu et al. 2004; Xu and Jiao 2005). Thus, for the same disease, there are varieties of syndromes related to different climates and geographical locations. As a result, developing a consensual checklist of TCM symptoms and signs to assist identifying and classifying psoriasis would be useful for TCM clinical practice and scientific research.

For illustrative purposes, consider the example given by Yang et al. (2013) for development of a diagnostic checklist of traditional Chinese medicine signs and symptoms for psoriasis. As indicated by Yang et al. (2013), a Delphi study was conducted with three rounds to develop a checklist from a consensus of well-recognized experts in psoriasis in China. The Delphi method attempts to assess the extent of agreement (consensus development) and to resolve disagreement (consensus development) in medical and health-related research. The Delphi technique can be performed in three steps. First, the opinions of a group of experts are sought based on an anonymous self-administered questionnaire to eliminate the influence of peer pressure. Second, a feedback system is used to allow the respondents to compare their opinion against a statistical summary of the whole group. Finally, this process is repeated until the opinions are stable. Thus, using the Delphi method, experts can participate without geographic limitations, offer their opinions independently and confidentially without face-to-face meetings and change their assessment based on the systematic feedback from the results of the previous rounds in consecutive stages of the process.

382 *Quantitative Methods for Traditional Chinese Medicine Development*

The Delphi study started with the formation of a selection committee, which consisted of four key opinion leaders of the TCM Dermatology Association in psoriasis research: two from Beijing area (representing northern China) and two from Yunnan province (representing southern China). The selection committee is responsible for formulating the panel and item selection criteria. The initial checklist was derived from the literature review. Each item in the checklist has one of the following scores: (1) strongly agree, (2) disagree, (3) neutral, (4) agree, and (5) strongly disagree. The items covered eight domains including color, characteristic, and shape of the skin lesions, associated factors, physical expression, tongue and its coating, pulse, and living environment.

A survey was then conducted in three rounds to obtain consensus from an expert panel which consisted of 16 experts on psoriasis who were selected from the Beijing area and Yunnan province. Experts were asked to rate each item. Additional items may be added if deemed appropriate by the experts. At each round, mean and standard deviation of each item were calculated. Items with a mean score below three were removed from the checklist. These removed items and the newly added items were then sent to the experts for reevaluation at the next round. The process was repeated until the final round. At the final run, a checklist containing 96 items of eight domains was developed for classifying psoriasis with TCM signs and symptoms (see Table 15.4). The developed checklist was validated using intraclass correlation coefficient (ICC) to test its agreement and consistency among the experts across rounds.

15.4.1.3 Remarks

The development of a checklist from a consensus of experts has significant impact on TCM research and modernization. First, it allows further research studies and clinical practice to be standardized. On the basis of a standard list of signs and symptoms, diagnosis, and treatment of patients with certain diseases (such as psoriatic patients) may be unified. In addition, variations in clinical practice among Chinese doctors can be minimized. Most importantly, the development of a diagnostic checklist helps move experience-based (subjective) research toward evidence-based (objective) research to achieve the ultimate goal of the modernization of TCM.

15.4.2 Unified Approach for Assessing Health Profile

As pointed out in the preface of this book, in recent years, as more and more innovative drug products have gone off patent, the search for new medicines that treat critical and/or life-threatening diseases such as cardiovascular diseases and cancer has become the center of attention of many pharmaceutical companies and governmental research organizations such as US NIH. This leads to the study of promising TCM. Chinese doctors believe that all of the

Current Issues and Recent Developments

TABLE 15.4

Checklist of Signs and Symptoms for Psoriasis

Domain	Signs and Symptoms
Skin lesion color	Full red, red, garnet, pink, darker skinned
Type of skin lesion	Papule, scaling, crust, pustule, cracking, erythema
Shape of skin lesion	Scattered, guttate, ostaceous, plaque, map, shape, generalized lesion, annular, thickness, hyperpigmentation, depigmentation, rough surface, infiltration, thin scale, thick scale, easy scaly exfoliation, dry scale
Associate factors	*Trigger factors*: overexertion, depression, stirring *Aggravating factors*: smoking, drinking alcohol, hot water, stimulating medicine, infection, during menstruation, postpartum *Predilection diet*: heavy and greasy, pungent, cold and raw *Stool*: less stool, constipation *Mental irritation*: sense of distress in the chest, anxiety and irritability *Itching degree*: severe, mild, slight, absent *Itching frequency*: continuous, intermittent *Fever*: fever, hot palms, soles and heart *Urine*: scanty dark urine *Muscle and joint*: muscles and joint pain, stiffness with bending limitation *Mouth*: dry mouth and thirsty, dry mouth and not thirsty, bitter taste, fetid breath, sticky taste *Sleep*: insomnia, frequent dreams *Complexion*: flushed *Nail manifestation*: nails not lustrous *Menstruation*: scanty menstruation, crimson color, blood clot *Throat*: sore throat, redness of pharyngeal portion, tonsil suppuration
Tongue and its coating	*Substance*: pale, red, maroon, dark purple tongue or tongue with petechiae, thin delicate, enlarged tongue fissured *Coating*: white, yellow, greasy, glossy, rough, less, peeling, sublingual varicose veins and bluish purple
Pulse	Moderate, slippery, rapid, string, deep, thread, hesitant
Living environment	Humid, dry, hot, cold

Source: Modified from Yang, X. et al., *Chinese Medicine*, 8, 10. Table 2, 2013.

organs within a healthy subject should reach the so-called global dynamic balance or harmony among organs to maintain health. Once the global balance is broken at certain sites such as heart, liver, or kidney, some signs and symptoms will then appear to reflect the imbalance at these sites. An experienced Chinese doctor usually assess the causes of global imbalance before a TCM with flexible doses is prescribed to fix the problem. This approach is sometimes referred to as a personalized (or individualized) medicine approach. In practice, TCM consider inspection, auscultation and olfaction, interrogation, and pulse taking and palpation as the primary diagnostic procedure. The scientific validity of these subjective and experience-based diagnostic procedures has been criticized due to (1) lack of reference standards and (2) anticipated large doctor-to-doctor variability

384   *Quantitative Methods for Traditional Chinese Medicine Development*

Cheng and Chow (2015) proposed a unified approach for developing a composite health index for diagnosis of illness based on a number of indices collected from a given subject under the concept of global dynamic balance among organs. Dynamic balance among organs can be defined as follows. Following the concept of testing bioequivalence or biosimilarity, if the 95 percent confidence of a given index is totally within some balance limits, e.g., (δ_L, δ_U), we conclude that there is dynamic balance among organs of the subject. If we fail to reject the null hypothesis, we conclude that there is a signal of illness. In practice, these signals of illness can be grouped to diagnose specific diseases based on some pre-specified reference standards for diseases status of specific diseases which are developed based on indices related to specific organs (or diseases). Statistical validity of Cheng and Chow's (2015) unified approach, however, requires further research.

15.4.3 Bridging Traditional Chinese Medicine

As indicated by Wang et al. (2005), the introduction of the concept of systems biology, enables the study of living systems from a holistic perspective based on the profiling of a multitude of biochemical components. It opens up a unique and novel opportunity to reinvestigate natural products. In the study of their bioactivity, the necessary reductionistic approach on single active components has been successful in the discovery of new medicines, but at the same time the synergetic effects of components were lost.

Systems biology, and especially metabolomics, is the ultimate phenol-typing. It opens up the possibility of studying the effect of complex mixtures, such as those used in TCM, in complex biological systems; abridging it with molecular pharmacology. This approach is considered to have the potential to revolutionize natural product research and to advance the development of scientific based herbal medicine.

15.5 Concluding Remarks

As indicated in the preface of this book, as more and more innovative drug products are going off patent, the search for new medicines that treat critical and/or life-threatening diseases has become the center of attention of many pharmaceutical companies and research organizations such as the NIH. This leads to the study of promising traditional Chinese (herbal) medicines (TCM), especially for those intended for treating critical and/or life-threatening diseases such as cardiovascular, diabetes, and cancer. The development of promising TCMs will benefit patients with critical or life-threatening diseases by providing an alternative for treatment and hopefully for cure. The development of promising TCMs will also enhance the search

Current Issues and Recent Developments 385

for personalized medicine since it focuses the minimization of intrasubject variability for achieving the optimal therapeutic effect. The development of new treatments (focusing on efficacy) in conjunction with TCMs (focusing on the reduction of toxicity) will be the direction of future clinical research for treating critical or life-threatening diseases of many pharmaceutical companies and clinical research organizations.

The process for pharmaceutical/clinical research and development of Western medicines (WM) is well established, and yet it is a lengthy and costly process. This lengthy and costly process is necessary to ensure the efficacy, safety, quality, stability and reproducibility of the drug product under investigation. For pharmaceutical/clinical research and development of a TCM the Western way, one may consider directly applying this well-established process to the TCM under investigation. However, this process may not be feasible due to some fundamental differences between a TCM and a WM. These fundamental differences include (1) medical theory/mechanism, and practice, (2) techniques of diagnosis, and (3) treatments are briefly described in the subsequent subsections (see also Table 1.2).

As a result, FDA has similar but different review and approval processes for regulatory submission of TCM. The FDA draft guidance on botanical drug products is a milestone for modernization (Westernization) of TCM development. Owing to fundamental differences between Western medicines and TCMs, practical (controversial) issues in the process of evaluation, review, and approval inevitably arise. Some of these issues are related to statistical methods for assessment of (1) quality and consistency of raw, in-process, and end-product, (2) analytical method development and validation for quantitative assessment of individual components, (3) the establishment of reference standards or specifications for individual components, (4) validation and QA/QC of a manufacturing process for TCM, (5) stability testing for determination of drug shelf-life, and (6) issues (e.g., preparation of matching placebo, calibration of study endpoint, and interpretation of results) in conducting randomized controlled clinical trials. Many of these issues remain unsolved. More methodology research is needed in order to address these issues.

One of the key issues in botanical drug product or TCM development is to clarify the difference between Westernization of TCM and modernization of TCM. For Westernization of TCM, we follow regulatory requirements at critical stages of the process for pharmaceutical development including drug discovery, formulation, laboratory development, animal studies, clinical development, manufacturing process validation and quality control, regulatory submission, review, and process despite the fundamental differences between WM and TCM. For modernization of TCM, it is suggested that regulatory requirements should be modified in order to account for the fundamental differences between WM and TCM. In other words, we still ought to be able to see if TCM is really working with modified regulatory requirements using Western clinical trials as a standard for comparison.

In practice, it is recognized that WMs tend to achieve the therapeutic effect sooner than that of TCMs for critical and/or life-threatening diseases. TCMs are found to be useful for patients with chronic diseases or non-life-threatening diseases. In many cases, TCMs have been shown to be effective in reducing toxicities or improving safety profile for patients with critical and/or life-threatening diseases. As a strategy for TCM research and development, it is suggested that (1) TCM be used in conjunction with a well-established WM as a supplement to improve its safety profile and/or enhance therapeutic effect whenever possible, and (2) TCM should be considered as the second line or third line treatment for patients who fail to respond to the available treatments. However, some sponsors are interested in focusing on the development of TCM as a dietary supplement due to (1) the lack or ambiguity of regulatory requirements, (2) the lack of understanding of the medical theory/mechanism of TCM, (3) the confidentiality of nondisclosure of the multiple components, and (4) the lack of understanding of pharmacological activities of the multiple components of TCM.

Because TCM consists of multiple components which may be manufactured from different sites or locations, the post-approval consistency in quality of the final product is both a challenge to the sponsor and a concern to the regulatory authority. As a result, some post-approval tests, such as tests for content uniformity, weight variation, and/or dissolution and (manufacturing) process validation, must be performed for quality assurance before the approved TCM can be released for use.

References

Aarons, L. (1991). Population pharmacokinetics: Theory and practice. *British Journal of Clinical Pharmacology*, 32, 669–670.

Abdel-Rahman, A., Anyangwe, N., Carlacci, L. et al. (2011). The safety and regulation of natural products used as foods and food ingredients. *Toxicological Sciences*, 123, 333–348.

Abdi, H. (2007a). Singular Value Decomposition (SVD) and Generalized Singular Value Decomposition (GSVD). In: *Encyclopedia of Measurement and Statistics*, Ed. Salkind, N.J. Sage Publications, Thousand Oaks, CA, 907–912.

Abdi, H. (2007b). Eigen-decomposition: Eigenvalues and eigenvectors. In: *Encyclopedia of Measurement and Statistics*, Ed. Salkind, N.J. Sage Publications, Thousand Oaks, CA, 304–308.

Abdi, H. and Williams, L. (2010). Principal component analysis. *WILEs Computational Statistics*, 2, 433–459.

Abeni, D., Picardi, A., Pasquini, P., Melchi, C.F. and Chren, M.M. (2002). Further evidence of the validity and reliability of the Skindex-29. *Dermatology*, 204, 43–49.

Abuaisha, B.B., Boulton, A.J. and Costanzi, J.B. (1998). Acupuncture for the treatment of chronic painful peripheral diabetic neuropathy: A long-term study. *Diabetes Research and Clinical Practice*, 39, 115–121.

AI (1989). Die junge Generation wendet sich den Naturheilmitteln zu. *Allensbacher Berichte*, Nr. 17.

Al-Banna, M.K., Kelman, A.W. and Whiting, B. (1990). Experimental design and efficient parameter estimation in population pharmacokinetics. *Journal of Pharmacokinetics and Biopharmaceutics*, 18, 347–360.

Balant, L.P. (1991). Is there a need for more precise definitions of bioavailability? *European Journal of Clinical Pharmacology*, 40, 123–126.

Bartholomew, D.J. (1981). Posterior analysis of the factor model. *British Journal of Mathematical and Statistical Psychology*, 34, 93–99.

Bartlett, M.S. (1954). A note on the multiplying factors for various χ^2 approximations. *Journal of Royal Statistical Society, Serious. B*, 16, 296–298.

Beal, S.L. and Sheiner, L.B. (1980). The NONMEM system. *American Statistician*, 34, 118–119.

Beal, S.L. and Sheiner, L.B. (1982). Estimating population pharmacokinetics. *Critical Reviews in Biomedical Engineering*, 8, 195–222.

Beal, S.L. and Sheiner, L.B. (1989). *NONMEM, User's Guide, NONMEM Project Group*. University of California San Francisco, San Francisco.

Berger, R.L. (1982). Multiparameter hypothesis testing and acceptance sampling. *Technometrics*, 24, 295–300.

Bergner, M., Bobbitt, R.A., Carter, W.B. and Gilson, B.S. (1981). The sickness impact profile: Development and final revision of a health status measure. *Medical Care*, 19, 787–805.

Bergum, J.S. (1990). Constructing acceptance limits for multiple stage tests. *Drug Development and Industrial Pharmacy*, 16, 2153–2166.

388   *References*

Boon, H.S., Olatunde, F. and Zick, S.M. (2007). Trends in complementary/alternative medicine use by breast cancer survivors: Comparing survey data from 1998 and 2005. *BMC Womens Health*, 30, 4.

Box, G.E.P. and Draper, N.R. (1987). *Empirical Model-Building and Response Surface*. Wiley, Hoboken, NJ.

Burt, T. (2011). Microdosing and phase 0. Presented at Duke Clinical Research Unit, Duke University Medical Center, Durham, NC, September 15.

Carter, W.H. and Wampler, G.L. (1986). Review of the application of response surface methodology in the combination therapy of cancer. *Cancer Treatment Reports*, 70, 133–140.

Carter, W.H., Wampler, G.L., Stablein, D.M. and Campbell, E.D. (1982). Drug activity and therapeutic synergism in cancer treatment. *Cancer Research*, 42, 2963–2971.

Chen, M.L. (1995). Individual bioequivalence. Invited presentation at International Workshop: Statistical and Regulatory Issues on the Assessment of Bioequivalence, Dusseldorf, Germany, October 19–20.

Chen, M.L. (1997). Individual bioequivalence—A regulatory update. *Journal Biopharmaceutical Statistics*, 7, 5–11.

Chen, D.C., Gong, D.Q. and Zhai, Y. (1994). Diabetes acupuncture research. *Journal of Traditional Chinese Medicine*, 14, 163–166.

Chen, K. (2002). Personal communication. Victoria, B.C., September, 2002.

Chen, K.W., Li, G. and Chow, S.C. (1997). A note on sample size determination for bioequivalence studies with higher-order crossover designs. *Journal of Pharmacokinetics and Biopharmaceutics*, 25, 753–765.

Chen, M.L., Lesko, L. and Williams, R.L. (2001). Measures of exposure versus measures of rate and extent of absorption. *Clinical Pharmacokinetics*, 40, 565–572.

Cheng, B. and Chow, S.C. (2015). A unified approach for assessment of traditional Chinese medicine clinical trials. Unpublished manuscript.

Chew, V. (1966). Confidence, prediction, and tolerance regions for the multivariate normal distribution. *Journal of American Statistics Association*, 61, 605–617.

Chow, S.C. (1992). Statistical Design and Analysis of Stability Studies. Presented at the 48th Conference on Applied Statistics, Atlantic City, NJ.

Chow, S.C. (1997a). Good statistics practice in drug development and regulatory approval process. *Drug Information Journal*, 31, 1157–1166.

Chow, S.C. (1997b). Pharmaceutical validation and process controls in drug development. *Drug Information Journal*, 31, 1195–1201.

Chow, S.C. (1999). Individual bioequivalence—A review of the FDA draft guidance. *Drug Informational Journal*, 33, 435–444.

Chow, S.C. (2007). Statistical Design and Analysis of Stability Studies. Chapman and Hall/CRC Press, Taylor & Francis, New York, New York.

Chow, S.C. and Chang, M. (2006). *Adaptive Design Methods in Clinical Trials*. Chapman and Hall/CRC Press, Taylor & Francis, New York.

Chow, S.C. and Ki, F. (1994). On statistical characteristics of quality of life assessment. *Journal of Biopharmaceutical Statistics*, 4, 1–17.

Chow, S.C. and Ki, F. (1996). Statistical issues in quality of life assessment. *Journal of Biopharmaceutical Statistics*, 6, 37–48.

Chow, S.C. and Ki, F. (1997). Statistical comparison between dissolution profiles of drug products. *Journal of Biopharmaceutical Statistics*, 7, 241–258.

Chow, S.C. and Liu, J.P. (1994). Recent statistical development in bioequivalence trials—A review of FDA guidance. *Drug Information Journal*, 28, 851–864.

References

Chow, S.C. and Liu, J.P. (1995). *Statistical Design and Analysis in Pharmaceutical Science: Validation, Process Control, and Stability.* Marcel Dekker, Inc., New York.

Chow, S.C. and Liu, J.P. (1997). Meta analysis for bioequivalence review. *Journal of Biopharmaceutical Statistics,* 7, 97–111.

Chow, S.C. and Liu, J.P. (1998). *Design and Analysis of Animal Studies in Pharmaceutical Development.* Marcel Dekker, Inc., New York.

Chow, S.C. and Liu, J.P. (2000). *Design and Analysis of Clinical Trials.* John Wiley & Sons, New York.

Chow, S.C. and Liu, J.P. (2004). *Design and Analysis of Clinical Trials,* 2nd Edition. John Wiley & Sons, New York.

Chow, S.C. and Liu, J.P. (2008). *Design and Analysis of Bioavailability and Bioequivalence Studies,* 3rd Edition. Chapman and Hall/CRC Press, Taylor & Francis, New York.

Chow, S.C. and Liu, J.P. (2013). *Design and Analysis of Clinical Trials,* 3rd Edition. John Wiley & Sons, New York.

Chow, S.C. and Shao, J. (1989). Test for batch-to-batch variation in stability analysis. *Statistics in Medicine,* 8, 883–890.

Chow, S.C. and Shao, J. (1990). An alternative approach for the assessment of bioequivalence between two formulations of a drug. *Biometrical Journal,* 32, 969–976.

Chow, S.C. and Shao, J. (1991). Estimating drug shelf-life with random batches. *Biometrics,* 47, 1071–1079.

Chow, S.C. and Shao, J. (2002). *Statistics in Drug Research—Methodologies and Recent Development.* Marcel Dekker, Inc., New York.

Chow, S.C. and Shao, J. (2003). Stability analysis with discrete responses. *Journal of Biopharmaceutical Statistics,* 13, 451–462.

Chow, S.C. and Shao, J. (2007). Stability analysis for drugs with multiple ingredients. *Statistics in Medicine,* 26, 1512–1517.

Chow, S.C. and Tse, S.K. (1990). Outlier detection in bioavailability/bioequivalence studies. *Statistics in Medicine,* 9, 549–558.

Chow, S.C. and Tse, S.K. (1991). On the estimation of total variability in assay validation. *Statistics in Medicine,* 10, 1543–1553.

Chow, S.C., Shao, J. and Wang, H. (2002a). Probability lower bounds for USP/NF tests. *Journal of Biopharmaceutical Statistics,* 12, 79–92.

Chow, S.C., Shao, J. and Wang, H. (2002b). *Sample Size Calculation in Clinical Research.* Marcel Dekker, Inc., New York.

Chow, S.C., Shao, J. and Wang, H. (2002c). Individual bioequivalence testing under 2x3 designs. *Statistics in Medicine,* 21, 629–648.

Chow, S.C., Shao, J. and Wang, H. (2003). Statistical tests for population bioequivalence. *Statistica Sinica,* 13, 539–554.

Chow, S.C., Chang, M. and Pong, A. (2005). Statistical consideration of adaptive methods in clinical development. *Journal of Biopharmaceutical Statistics,* 15, 575–591.

Chow, S.C., Pong, A. and Chang, Y.W. (2006). On traditional Chinese medicine clinical trials. *Drug Information Journal,* 40, 395–406.

Chow, S.C., Endrenyi, L., Lachenbruch, P.A., Yang, L.Y. and Chi, E. (2011). Scientific factors for assessing biosimilarly and drug interchangeability of follow-on biologics. *Biosimilars,* 1, 13–26.

Church, J.D. and Harris, B. (1970). The estimation of reliability from stress-strength relationships. *Technometrics,* 12, 49–54.

Coste, J., Fermanian, J. and Venot, A. (1995). Methodological and statistical problems in the construction of composite measurement scales: A survey of six medical and epidemiological journals. *Statistics in Medicine*, 14, 331–345.

Covington, M.B. (2001). Traditional Chinese medicine in the treatment of diabetes. *Diabetes Spectrum*, 14, 154–159.

Cui, Y., Song, X.L., Reynolds, M., Chuang, K. and Xie, M.L. (2012). Interdependence of drug substance physical properties and corresponding quality control strategy. *Journal of Pharmaceutical Sciences*, 101, 312–321.

Davidian, M. and Gallant, A.R. (1993). The nonlinear mixed effects model with a smooth random effects density. *Biometika*, 80, 475–488.

Davidian, M. (2003). What's in between dose and response? Lecture notes. Myrto Lefkopoulou Lecture.

Davidian, M. and Giltinan, D.M. (1995). *Nonlinear Models for Repeated Measurement Data*. Chapman and Hall, London.

Davit, B.M., Conner, D.P., Fabian-Fritsch, B. et al. (2008). Highly variable drugs: Observations from bioequivalence data submitted to the FDA for new generic drug applications. *The AAPS Journal*, 10, 148–156.

Dempster, A.P., Laird, N.M. and Rubin, D.B. (1977). Maximum likelihood from incomplete data via EM algorithm. *Journal of the Royal Statistical Society, Series B*, 39, 1–38.

de lemos, M. (2002). Herbal supplement PC-Spes for prostate cancer. *Ann. Pharmacother.*, 36, 921–926.

DOH (2004a). *Draft Guidance for IND of Traditional Chinese Medicine*. Department of Health, Taipei, Taiwan.

DOH (2004b). *Draft Guidance for NDA of Traditional Chinese Medicine*. Department of Health, Taipei, Taiwan.

Draper, N.R. and Smith, H. (1980). *Applied Regression Analysis*. Wiley, New York.

Duchesne, C. and Macgregor, J.F. (2004). Establishing multivariate specification regions for incoming materials. *Journal of Quality Technology*, 36, 78–94.

Dziuban, C.D. and Harris, C.W. (1973). On the extraction of components and the applicability of factor analytic techniques. *American Educational Research Journal*, 10, 93–99.

EC (1975a). Council Directive 75/318/EEC of 20 May 1975 on the approximation of the laws of Member States relating to analytical, pharmacotoxicological and clinical standards and protocols in respect of the testing of proprietary medicinal products. *Official Journal of the European Communities*, June 1975.

EC (1975b). Council Directive 75/319/EEC of 20 May 1975 on the approximation of provisions laid down by law, regulation or administrative action relating to proprietary medicinal products. *Official Journal of the European Communities*, June 1975.

EC (1989). Quality of herbal remedies. In: *The Rules governing Medicinal Products in the European Community, Vol. III. Guidelines on the Quality, Safety and Efficacy of Medicinal Products for Human Use*. Office for Official Publications of the European Communities, Luxembourg.

EC (1991). Commission Directive 91/507/EEC of 19 July 1991 modifying the Annex to Council Directive 75/318/EEC on the approximation of the laws of Member States relating to analytical, pharmacotoxicological and clinical standards and protocols in respect of the testing of medicinal products. *Official Journal of the European Communities*, 270/32 of 26 September 1991.

References 391

EC (1993). Council Directive 93/39/EEC of 14 June 1993 amending Directives 65/65/EEC, 75/318/EEC and 75/319/EEC in respect of medicinal products. *Official Journal of the European Communities*, 214 of 24 August 1993.

Edler, L. (1998). List of PK-PD software packages. http://dkfz-heidelberg.de/biostatistics/pkpd/pkcompl/html, Heidelberg, Germany.

EMA (2010). Concept paper on similar biological medicinal products containing recombinant follicle stimulation hormone. A/CHMP/BMWP/94899/2010. London.

Endrenyi, L., Fritsch, S. and Yan, W. (1991). (Cmax)/AIIC is a clearer measure than (Cmax) for adsorption rates in investigations of bioequivalence. *International Journal of Clinical Pharmacology, Theraphy and Toxicology*, 29, 394–399.

Enis, P. and Geisser, S. (1971). Estimation of the Probability that Y<X. *Journal of American Statistical Association*, 66, 162–168.

Eriksson, L., Johansson, E., Kettaneh-Wold, N. and Wold, S. (2001). *Multi- and Megavariate Data Analysis: Principles and Applications*. Umetrics, Umea, Sweden.

Ernst, E. (2009). Complementary and alternative medicine (CAM) and cancer: The kind face of complementary medicine. *International Journal of Surgery*, 7, 499–500.

ESCOP (1990). Bieldermann, BJ. Phytopharmaceuticals—The growing European market? Presentation at the ESCOP Symposium "European Harmony in Phytotherapy," Institut für Medizinische Statistik, October 20.

Ette, E.L., Sun, H. and Ludden, T.M. (1994). Design of population pharmacokinetic studies. *Proceedings of the Biopharmaceutical Section of the American Statistical Association*, Alexandria, VA, pp. 487–492.

Everitt, B.S. (1984). *An Introduction to Latent Variable Models*. Chapman and Hall, New York.

Fabricant, D.S. and Farnsworth, N.R. (2001). The value of plants used in traditional medicine for drug discovery. *Environmental Health Perspectives*, 109, 69–75.

Fai, C.K., Qi, G.D., Wei, D.A. and Chung, L.P. (2011). Placebo preparation for the proper clinical trial of herbal medicine—Requirements, verification and quality control. *Recent Pat Inflamm Allergy Drug Discov*, 5, 169–174.

FDA (1987). *Guideline for Submitting Documentation for the Stability of Human Drugs and Biologics*. Center for Drugs and Biologics, Office of Drug Research and Review, Food and Drug Administration, Rockville, MD.

FDA (1988). *Guideline for the Format and Content of the Clinical and Statistical Sections of New Drug Applications*. The United States Food and Drug Administration, Rockville, MD.

FDA (1991). *Guidance for Conjugated Estrogen Tablets—In Vivo Bioequivalence and In Vitro Drug Release*. Center for Drug Evaluation and Research, Food and Drug Administration, Rockville, MD.

FDA (1992). *Guidance on Statistical Procedures for Bioequivalence Using a Standard Two-treatment Crossover Design*. Division of Bioequivalence, Office of Generic Drugs, Centre for Drug Evaluation and Research, U.S. Food and Drug Administration, Rockville, MD.

FDA (1995). *Guidance for Industry—Immediate Release Solid Oral Dosage Forms Scale-up and Postapproval Changes* (SUPAC): *Chemistry, Manufacturing, and Controls, In Vitro Dissolution Testing and In Vivo Bioequivalence Documentation*. Division of Bioequivalence, Office of Generic Drugs, Food and Drug Administration, Rockville, MD.

FDA (1998). *Guidance for Industry: Stability Testing of Drug Substances and Drug Products (draft guidance)*. The United States Food and Drug Administration, Rockville, MD.

FDA (2000). *Guidance for Industry: Analytical Procedures and Methods Validation (draft guidance)*. The United States Food and Drug Administration, Rockville, MD.

FDA (1999). *Guidance for Industry—Population Pharmacokinetics*. Center for Drug Research and Evaluation, the United States Food and Drug Administration, Rockville, MD.

FDA (2001a). *Guidance for Industry on Statistical Approaches to Establishing Bioequivalence*. Center for Drug Evaluation and Research, Food and Drug Administration, Rockville, MD.

FDA (2001b). *Guidance for Industry—Bioanalytical Method Validation*. The United States Food and Drug Administration, Rockville, MD.

FDA (2003a). *Guidance on Bioavailability and Bioequivalence Studies for Orally Administrated Drug Products—General Considerations*. Center for Drug Evaluation and Research, the US Food and Drug Administration, Rockville, MD.

FDA (2003b). *Guidance on Bioavailability and Bioequivalence Studies for Nasal Aerosols and Nasal Sprays for Local Action*. Center for Drug Evaluation and Research, Food and Drug Administration, Rockville, MD.

FDA (2003c). *Guidance for Industry—INDs for Phase 2 and Phase 3 Studies, Chemistry, Manufacturing, and Controls Information*. Center for Drug Evaluation and Research, Food and Drug Administration, Rockville, MD.

FDA (2004). *Guidance for Industry—Botanical Drug Products*. The United States Food and Drug Administration, Rockville, MD.

FDA (2010). *Draft Guidance for Industry—Adaptive Design Clinical Trials for Drugs and Biologics*. The United State Food and Drug Administration, Rockville, MD.

Feeny, D.H. and Torrance, G.W. (1989). Incorporating utility-based quality-of-life assessment measures in clinical trials. *Medical Care*, 27, S198–S204.

Feller, W. (1968). *An Introduction to Probability and Its Applications*, Vol. I, 3rd Edition. John Wiley & Sons, New York.

Finlay, A.Y. and Khan, G.K. (1994). Dermatology Life Quality Index (DLQI): A simple practical measure for routine clinical use. *Clinical and Experimental Dermatology*, 19, 210–216.

Fuchs, C. and Kenett, R.S. (1987). Multivariate tolerance regions and F-tests. *Journal of Quality Technology*, 19, 122–131.

Garcia-Munoz, S. (2009). Establishing multivariate specifications for incoming materials using data from multiple scales. *Chemometrics and Intelligent Laboratory Systems*, 98, 51–57.

Gibson, J.M. and Overall, J.E. (1989). The superiority of a drug combination over each of its components. *Statistics in Medicine*, 8, 1479–1484.

Gill, J.L. (1988). Repeated measurements, split-plot trend analysis versus of first differences. *Biometrics*, 44, 289–297.

Gong, X.C., Yan, B.J. and Qu, H.B. (2010). Correlations of three important technological parameters in first ethanol precipitation of Danshen. *China Journal of Chinese Materia Medica*, 35, 3274–3277.

Gong, X.C., Wang, S.S. and Qu, H.B. (2011). Comparison of two separation technologies applied in the manufacture of botanical injections: Second ethanol precipitation and solvent extraction. *Industrial & Engineering Chemistry Research*, 50, 7542–7548.

References

Gould, S.J. (1981). The real error of Cybil Burt: Factor analysis and the reification of intelligence. In: *The Mismeasure of Man*. Ed. Gould S.J. W.W. Norton and Company Inc., New York, 234–320.

Guilford, J.P. (1954). *Psychometric Methods*, 2nd Edition. McGraw-Hill, New York.

Guttman, I. (1970). Construction of β-content tolerance regions at confidence level γ for large samples from the k-variate normal distribution. *Annals of Mathematical Statistics*, 41, 376–400.

Guyatt, G.H., Veldhuyen Van Zanten, S.J.O., Feeny, D.H. and Patric, D.L. (1989). Measuring quality of life in clinical trials: A taxonomy and review. *Canadian Medical Association Journal*, 140, 1441–1448.

Haidar, S.H., Davit, B.M., Chen, M.L. et al. (2008a). Bioequivalence approaches for highly variable drugs and drug products. *Pharmaceutical Research*, 25, 237–241.

Haidar, S.H., Makhlouf, F., Schuirmann, D.J., Hyslop, T., Davit, B., Conner, D. and Yu, L.X. (2008b). Evaluation of a scaling approach for the bioequivalence of highly variable drugs. *The AAPS Journal*, 10, 450–454.

Hall, I.J. and Sheldon, D.D. (1979). Improved bivariate normal tolerance regions with some applications. *Journal of Quality Technology*, 11, 13–19.

Hamza, M.A., White, P.F., Craig, W.F. et al. (2000). Percutaneous electrical nerve stimulation: A novel analgesic therapy for diabetic neuropathic pain. *Diabetes Care*, 23, 365–370.

Hashimoto, Y. and Sheiner, L.B. (1991). Designs for population pharmacodynamics: Value of pharmacokinetic data and population analysis. *Journal of Pharmacokinetics and Biopharmaceutics*, 19, 333–353.

Hauschke, D., Steinijans, V.W., Diletti, E. and Durke, M. (1992). Sample size determination for bioequivalence assessment using a multiplicative model. *Journal of Pharmacokinetics and Biopharmaceutics*, 20, 557–561.

He, P., Deng, K., Liu, Z., Liu, D., Liu, J.S. and Geng, Z. (2012). Discovering herbal functional groups of traditional Chinese medicine. *Statistics in Medicine*, 31, 636–642.

Hendrickson, A.E. and White, P.O. (1964). Promax: A quick method for rotation to orthogonal oblique structure. *British Journal of Statistical Psychology*, 17, 65–70.

Henley, A.J., Festa, A., D'Agostino, R.B. et al. (2004). Metabolic and inflammation variable clusters and prediction of type 2 diabetes: Factor analysis using directly measured insulin sensitivity. *Diabetes*, 53, 1773–1781.

Hicks, C. (1982). *Fundamental Concepts in the Design of Experiments*, 3rd Edition. CBS College Publishing, New York.

Hollenberg, N.K., Testa, M. and Williams, G.H. (1991). Quality of life as a therapeutic endpoint—An analysis of therapeutic trials in hypertension. *Drug Safety*, 6, 83–93.

Hsiao, J.I.H. (2007). Patent protection for Chinese herbal medicine product invention in Taiwan. *The Journal of World Intellectual Property*, 10, 1–21.

Hsiao, C.F., Tsou, H.H., Pong, A., Liu, J.P., Lin, C.H., Chang, Y.J. and Chow, S.C. (2009). Statistical validation of traditional Chinese diagnostic procedure. *Drug Information Journal*, 43, 83–95.

Hu, J. and Liu, B. (2012). The basic theory, diagnostic, and therapeutic system of traditional Chinese medicine and the challenges they bring to statistics. *Statistics in Medicine*, 31, 602–605.

Huang, B. and Wang, Y. (1993). *Thousand Formulas and Thousand Herbs of Traditional Chinese Medicine*, Vol. 2. Heilongjiang Education Press, Harbin, China.

Huang, H.X. and Qu, H.B. (2011). In-line monitoring of alcohol precipitation by near-infrared spectroscopy in conjunction with multivariate batch modeling. *Analytica Chimica Acta*, 707, 47–56.

Hubert, M., Rousseeuw, P.J. and Verdonck, T. (2009). Robust PCA for skewed data and its outlier map. *Computational Statistics & Data Analysis*, 53, 2264–2274.

Hung, H.M.J. (1992). On identifying a positive dose-response surface for combination agents. *Statistics in Medicine*, 11, 703–711.

Hung, H.M.J. (1993). Two-stage tests for studying monotherapy and combination therapy in two-by-two factorial trials. *Statistics in Medicine*, 12, 645–660.

Hung, H.M.J. (1996). Global tests for combination drug studies in factorial trials. *Statistics in Medicine*, 15, 233–247.

Hung, H.M.J. (2000). Evaluation of a combination drug with multiple doses in unbalanced factorial design clinical trials. *Statistics in Medicine*, 19, 2079–2087.

Hung, H.M.J. (2010). Combination drug clinical trial. In: *Encyclopedia of Biopharmaceutical Statistics*, Ed. Chow, S.C. Informa Healthcare, Taylor & Francis, London, 324–326.

Hung, H.M.J., Ng, T.H., Chi, G.Y.H. and Lipicky, R.J. (1989). Testing for the existence of a dose combination beating its components. In *Proceedings of Biopharmaceutical Section of the American Statistical Association*, Alexandria, VA, pp. 53–59.

Hung, H.M.J., Ng, T.H., Chi, G.Y.H. and Lipicky, R.J. (1990). Response surface and factorial designs for combination antihypertensive drugs. *Drug Information Journal*, 24, 371–378.

Hung, H.M.J., Chi, G.Y.H. and Lipicky, R.J. (1993). Testing for the existence of a desirable dose combination. *Biometrics*, 49, 85–94.

Hung, H.M.J., Chi, G.Y.H. and Lipicky, R.J. (1994). On some statistical methods for analysis of combination drug studies. *Communications in Statistics—Theory and Methods, A*, 23, 361–376.

Huo, Y. (1985). Treatment of myodystrophy with Chinese herbs. *Tianjin Journal of Traditional Chinese Medicine*, 6.

Hyslop, T., Hsuan, F. and Holder, K.J. (2000). A small-sample confidence interval approach to assess individual bioequivalence. *Statistics in Medicine*, 19, 2885–2897.

ICH (1993). Stability testing of new drug substances and products. *Tripartite International Conference on Harmonization Guideline Q1A*, Geneva, Switzerland.

ICH (1996). Validation of analytical procedures: Methodology. *Tripartite International Conference on Harmonization Guideline*, Geneva, Switzerland.

ICH (1997). E5 Guideline on ethnic factors in the acceptability of foreign data. *The U.S. Federal Register*, 83, 31790–31796.

ICH (1998). E9 Guideline for statistical principles for clinical trials. *Tripartite International Conference on Harmonization Guideline*, Geneva, Switzerland. Available at http://www/ich.org/LOB/media/MEDIA485.pdf.

ICH Q1A (1993). *Stability Testing of New Drug Substances and Products*. Tripartite International Conference on Harmonization Guideline Q1A, Geneva.

ICH Q1D (2003). *Guidance for Industry: Q1D Bracketing and Matrixing Designs for Stability Testing of New Drug Substances and Products*. Center for Drug Evaluation and Research and Center for Biologics Evaluation and Research, Food and Drug Administration, Rockville, MD.

ICH Q1E (2004). *Evaluation of Stability Data*. Tripartite International Conference on Harmonization Guideline Q1E, Geneva.

References

395

ICH (2009). Tripartite International Conference on Harmonization Guideline Guidance on nonclinical safety studies for the conduct of human clinical trials and marketing authorization for pharmaceuticals, Geneva, Switzerland.

Ikawa, T. and Imayama, S. (1983). The effect of Toukiinnshi (Tsumura) for pruritis. *Journal of Pharmaceutical Sciences*, 9, 653–657.

Inagi, I. (2003). Jumihaidokutou. *Kanpo-Igaku*, 27, 180–183.

Jelliffe, R.W., Gomis, P. and Schumitzky, A. (1990). A population model of gentamicin made with a new nonparametric EM algorithm. Technical Report 90–94, University of Southern California, Los Angeles.

Jiang, M., Zhang, C., Zheng, G. et al. (2012). Traditional Chinese medicine Zheng in the era of evidence-based medicine: A literature analysis. *Evidence-Based Complementary and Alternative Medicine*, 2012, 409568. doi:10.1155/2012/409568.

John, S. (1963). A tolerance region for multivariate normal distributions. *Sankhya, Series A*, 25, 363–368.

Johnson, N.L. and Kotz, S. (1970). *Continuous Univariate Distributions—1*. John Wiley & Sons, New York.

Johnson, R.A. and Wichern, D.W. (1992). *Applied Multivariate Statistical Analysis*, 5th Edition. Prentice Hall, Englewood Cliffs, NJ.

Johnson, N.E., Wade, J.R. and Karlson, M.O. (1996). Comparison of some practical sampling strategies for population pharmacokinetic studies. *Journal of Pharmacokinetics and Biopharmaceutics*, 24, 245–272.

Jones, B. and Kenward, M.G. (1989). *Design and Analysis of Cross-over Trials*. Chapman and Hall, London, 140–188.

Johnson, R.A. and Wichern, D.W. (1998). *Applied Multivariate Statistical Analysis*, 3rd ed. Prentice Hall, Upper Saddle River, NJ.

Ju, H.L. and Chow, S.C. (1995). On stability designs in drug shelf-life estimation. *Journal of Biopharmaceutical Statistics*, 5, 201–214.

Kaiser, H.F. (1958). The varimax criterion for analytic rotation in factor analysis. *Psychometrika*, 23, 187–200.

Kaiser, H.F. (1959). Computer program for varimax rotation in factor analysis. *Educational and Psychological Measurement*, 27, 155–162.

Kaiser, H.F. (1960). The application of electronic computers to factor analysis. *Educational and Psychological Measurement*, 20, 141–151.

Kang, Y. (1985). Case reports of flaccid complexes: Successful treatment of two cases of progressive spinal myoatrophy. *American College of Traditional Chinese Medicine*, 4, 59–63.

Kaplan, R.M., Bush, J.W. and Berry, C.C. (1976). Health status: Types of validity and index of well-being. *Health Services Research*, 4, 478–507.

Karlsson, M.O. and Sheiner, L.B. (1993). The importance of modeling interoccasion cariability in population pharmacokinetic analyses. *Journal of Pharmacokinetics and Biopharmaceutical*, 21, 735–750.

Ki, F.Y.C. and Chow, S.C. (1994). Analysis of quality of life with parallel questionnaires. *Drug Information Journal*, 28, 69–80.

Ki, F.Y.C. and Chow, S.C. (1995). Statistical justification for the use of composite scores in quality of life assessment. *Drug Information Journal*, 29, 715–727.

Kimura, T., Yoshiike, T., Tsuboi, R. et al. (1985). Clinical effect of Jumihaidokuto (Tsumura) on eczema. *Juntendo Medical Journal*, 31, 584–587.

Ko, F.S., Tsou, H.H., Liu, J.P. and Hsiao, C.F. (2010). Sample size determination for a specific region in a multi-regional trial. *Journal of Biopharmaceutical Statistics*, 20, 870–875.

Kondoh, A., Ohta, Y., Yamamoto, K., Iwashita, K., Umezawa, Y., Matsuyama, T., Ozawa, A. and Shinohara, Y. (2005). Feasibility of modified DLQI-based questionnaires for evaluation of clinical efficacy of herbal medicine in chronic skin disease. *Tokai Journal of Experimental and Clinical Medicine*, 30 (2), 97–102.

Koon, W.S., Lo, M.W., Marsden, J.E. and Ross, S.D. (1999). The genesis trajectory and heteroclinic connections. *AAS/AIAA Astrodynamics Specialist Conference, Girdwood, Alaska, 1999*, AAS99-451.

Krishnamoorthy, K. and Mathew, T. (1999). Comparison of approximation methods for computing tolerance factors for a multivariate normal population. *Technometrics*, 41, 234–249.

Krishnamoorthy, K. and Yu, J. (2004). Modified Nel and van der Merwe test for the multivariate Behrens-Fisher problem. *Statistics and Probability Letters*, 66, 161–169.

Krishnamoorthy, K. and Mondal, S. (2006). Improved tolerance factors for multivariate normal distributions. *Communications in Statistics-Simulation and Computation*, 35, 461–478.

Laden, F., Neas, L.M., Dockery, D.W. and Schwartz, J. (2000). Association of fine particulate matter from different sources with daily mortality in six US cities. *Environmental Health Perspectives*, 108, 941–947.

Lai, Y.H. and Hsiao, C.F. (2013). Using a tolerance region approach as a statistical quality control process for traditional Chinese medicine. *The 3rd International Conference on Applied Mathematics and Pharmaceutical Sciences*, Singapore, April 29–30, 346–349.

Lao, L., Huang, Y., Feng, C., Berman, B.M. and Tan, M.T. (2012). Evaluating traditional Chinese medicine using modern clinical trial design and statistical methodology: Application to a randomized controlled acupuncture trial. *Statistics in Medicine*, 31, 619–627.

Laska, E.M. and Meisner, M.J. (1989). Testing whether an identified treatment is best. *Biometrics*, 45, 1139–1151.

Laska, E.M. and Meisner, M.J.C. (1990). Hypothesis testing for combination treatment. In Statistical Issue in Drug Research and Development, edited by Peace, K.L. Dekker, New York, pp. 276–284.

Laska, E.M., Tang, D.I. and Meisner, M.J. (1992). Testing hypotheses about an identified treatment when there are multiple endpoints. *Journal of American Statistical Association*, 87, 825–831.

Laska, E.M., Meisner, M.J. and Tang, D.I. (1997). Classification of the effectiveness of combination treatments. *Statistics in Medicine*, 16, 2211–2288.

Lehmann, E.L. (1952). Testing multiparameter hypotheses. *Annals of Mathematical Statistics*, 23, 541–552.

Lehmann, E.L. (1986). *Testing Statistical Hypotheses*, 2nd Edition. Wiley, New York.

Li, G. (1986). Discussion about myasthenia gravis and the spleen-kidney theory, *Journal of Traditional Chinese Medicine*, 6 (1), 48–51.

Li, Y., Yi, D., Zhang, H. and Qin, Y. (2012). Syndrome evaluation in traditional Chinese medicine using second-order latent variable model. *Statistics in Medicine*, 31, 672–680.

Li, X., Yang, G., Li, X. et al. (2013). Traditional Chinese medicine in cancer care: A review of controlled clinical studies published in Chinese. *PLoS One*, 8 (4), e60338. doi:10.1371/journal.pone.0060338.

Lin, T. (1983). Treatment of amyotrophic lateral sclerosis with a series of proved formulas, *Guangxi Journal of Traditional Chinese Medicine*, 6 (2), 22–23.

References

397

Lin, M., Chu, C.C., Chang, S.L. et al. (2001). The origin of Minnan and Hakka, the so-called "Taiwanese," inferred by HLA study. *Tissue Antigen*, 57, 192–199.

Lindsey, J.K. (1993). *Models for Repeated Measurements*. Oxford Science Publications, Oxford, UK.

Lindstrom, M.J. and Bates, D.M. (1990). Nonlinear mixed effects models for repeated measures data. *Biometrics*, 46, 673–687.

Liu, J.P. (1995). Use of repeated crossover designs in assessing bioequivalence. *Statistics in Medicine*, 14, 1067–1078.

Liu, J.P. and Weng, C.S. (1991). Detection of outlying data in bioavailability/bioequivalence studies. *Statistics in Medicine*, 10, 1375–1389.

Liu, J.P. and Chow, S.C. (1992). On power calculation of Schuirmann's two one-sided tests procedure in bioequivalence. *Journal of Pharmacokinetics and Biopharmaceutics*, 20, 101–104.

Liu, J.P. and Weng, C.S. (1994). Estimation of log-transformation in assessing bioequivalence. *Communication is Statistics–Theory and Methods*, 23, 421–434.

Liu, J.P. and Weng, C.S. (1995). Bias of two one-sided tests procedures in assessment of bioequivalence. *Statistics in Medicine*, 14, 853–861.

Liu, J.P. and Chow, S.C. (1996). Statistical issues on FDA conjugated estrogen tablets guideline. *Drug Information Journal*, 30 (4), 881–889.

Liu, J.P. and Chow, S.C. (1997). Some thoughts on individual bioequivalence. *Journal of Biopharmaceutical Statistics*, 7, 41–48.

Liu, W. and Gong, C. (2015). Acupuncture: Ancient therapeutics for stroke. http://www/acufinder.com/Acupuncture+Information/Detail/Acupuncture+Ancient+Therapeutics+for+Stroke.

Liu, J., Li, X., Liu, J., Ma, L., Li, X. and Fønnebø, V. (2011). Traditional Chinese medicine in cancer care: A review of case reports published in Chinese literature. *Forsch Komplementmed*, 18, 257–263.

Liu, B., Zhou, X., Wang, Y. et al. (2012). Data processing and analysis in real-world traditional Chinese medicine clinical data: Challenges and approaches. *Statistics in Medicine*, 31, 653–660.

Lu, X. and Wang, Y. (1990). Thirty-five cases of multiple sclerosis treated by traditional Chinese medical principles using differential diagnosis. *Chinese Journal of Integrated Traditional and Western Medicine*, 10 (3), 174–175.

Lu, X., Li, Z. and Wang, H. (1995). Research on the prevention of multiple sclerosis relapse with traditional Chinese medicine. *Journal of Traditional Chinese Medicine*, 36 (7).

Lu, A.P., Jia, H.W., Xiao, C. and Lu, Q.P. (2004). Theory of traditional Chinese medicine and therapeutic method of diseases [in Chinese]. *World J Gastroenterol*, 10, 1854–1856.

Lu, Q., Chow, S.C. and Tse, S.K. (2007). Statistical quality control process for traditional Chinese medicine with multiple correlative components. *Journal of Biopharmaceutical Statistics*, 17, 791–808.

Lyden, P., Lu, M., Jackson, C., Marler, J., Kothari, R., Brott, T. and Zivin, J. (1999). NINDS tPA Stroke Trial Investigators. Underlying structure of the National Institutes of Health Stroke Scale: Results of a factor analysis. *Stroke*, 30, 2347–2354.

Mahoney, F. and Barthel, D. (1965). Functional evaluation: The Barthel Index. *Maryland State Medical Journal*, 14, 61–65.

Mallet, A. (1986). A maximum likelihood estimation method for random coefficient regression models. *Biometrika*, 73, 645–656.

Mao, L.Q. (1984). The treatment of diabetes by acupuncture. *Journal of Chinese Medicine*, 15, 3–5.

MAPP (2004). *CDER/FDA Manual of Policies and Procedures (MAPP): Review of Botanical Drug Products*. Center for Drug Evaluation and Research, Food and Drug Administration, Rockville, MD, June, 2004.

Mazzo, D.J. (1998). *International Stability Testing*. Interpharm Press, Buffalo Grove, IL.

Mellon, J.I. (1991). Design and Analysis Aspects of Drug Stability Studies When the Product is Stored at Several Temperatures. Presented at the 12th Annual Midwest Statistical Workshop, Muncie, IN.

MOPH (1984). *Drug Administration Law of the People's Republic of China*, Beijing, China, September 20.

MOPH (1992). The approval of new pharmaceuticals (concerning the revision and the additional regulations on the sections on Chinese Traditional Medicine). Implemented on 1 September 1992. Ministry of Health of the People's Republic of China.

MOPH (2002). *Guidance for Drug Registration*. Ministry of Public Health, Beijing, China.

Morrison, D.F. (1976). *Multivariate Statistical Methods*, 2nd Edition. McGraw-Hill Book Company, New York.

Müller, P. and Rosner, G.L. (1997). A Bayesian population model with hierarchical mixture priors applied to blood count data. *Journal of American Statistical Association*, 92, 1279–1292.

Muteki, K. and MacGregor, J.F. (2008). Optimal purchasing of raw materials: A data-driven approach. *AIChE Journal*, 54, 1554–1559.

Murphy, J.R. and Weisman, D. (1990). Using random slopes for estimating shelf-life. *Proceedings of the Biopharmaceutical Section of the American Statistical Association*, Alexandria, VA, pp. 196–203.

Murphy, J.R. (1996). Uniform matrix stability study designs. *Journal of Biopharmaceutical Statistics*, 6, 477–494.

Myers, R.H. (1976). *Response Surface Methodology*. Allyn and Bacon, Boston.

NCCLS (2001). *User Demonstration of Performance for Precision and Accuracy*. Approved Guidance, NCCLS document EP15-A, National Committee for Clinical Laboratory Standards, Wayne, PA.

Nedelman, J.R. (2005). On some disadvantages of the population approach. *The AAPS journal*, 7, E374–E382.

Nel, D.G. and van der Merwe, C.A. (1986). A solution to the multivariate Behrens-Fisher problem. *Communication in Statistics—Theory and Methods*, 15, 3719–3735.

Nordbrock, E. (1992). Statistical comparison of stability designs. *Journal of Biopharmaceutical Statistics*, 2, 91–113.

Nordbrock, E. (1994). Design and analysis of stability studies. *Proceedings of the Biopharmaceutical Section of the American Statistical Association*, Alexandria, VA, pp. 291–294.

Nordbrock, E. (2000). Stability matrix design. In *Encyclopedia of Biopharmaceutical Statistics*, S. Chow, Ed. Marcel Dekker, New York, pp. 487–492.

Olschewski, M. and Schumacher, M. (1990). Statistical analysis of quality of life data in cancer clinical trials. *Statistics in Medicine*, 9, 749–763.

Patel, H.I. (1991). Comparison of treatments in a combination therapy trial. *Journal of Biopharmaceutical Statistics*, 1, 171–183.

Patel, H.I. (1994). Dose-response in pharmacokinetics. *Communications in Statistics, Theory and Methods*, 23, 451–465.

References 399

PDR (1998). *Physicians' Desk Reference for Herbal Medicines*. Medical Economics Company, Montvale, NJ.

Peabody, F. (1927). The care of the patient. *JAMA*, 88, 877.

Peace, K.E. (1990). Response surface methodology in the development of antianginal drugs. In: *Statistical Issues in Drug Research and Development*, Ed. Peace, K. Dekker, New York, 285–301.

Phillips, K.F. (1990). Power of the two one-sided tests procedure in bioequivalence. *Journal of Pharmacokinetics and Biopharmaceutics*, 18, 137–144.

Phillips, J.A., Cairns, V. and Koch, G.G. (1992). The analysis of a multiple-dose, combination-drug clinical trial using response surface methodology. *Journal of Biopharmaceutical Statistics*, 2, 49–67.

Ping, S., Zhou, X.H., Lao, L. and Li, X. (2012). Issues of design and statistical analysis in controlled clinical acupuncture trials: An analysis of English-language reports from Western journals. *Statistics in Medicine*, 31, 606–618.

Pinheiro, J.C. and Bates, D.M. (1995). Approximations to the log likehood function in the nonlinear mixed effects model. *Journal of computational and Graphical Statistics*, 4, 12–35.

Pinheiro, J.C. and Bates, D.M. (2000). *Mixed Effects Models in S and S-Plus*. Springer, New York.

Plackett, R.L. and Burman, J.P. (1946). The design of optimum multifactorial experiments. *Biometrika*, 33, 305–325.

Pong, A. and Raghavarao, D. (2000). Comparison of bracketing and matrixing designs for a two-year stability study. *Journal of Biopharmaceutical Statistics*, 10, 217–228.

Pong, A. and Raghavarao, D. (2001). Shelf-life estimation for drug products with two components. *Proceedings of the Biopharmaceutical Section of the American Statistical Association*, Alexandria, VA.

Pong, A. and Raghavarao, D. (2002). Comparing distributions of drug shelf lives for two components in stability analysis for different designs. *Journal of Biopharmaceutical Statistics*, 12, 277–293.

Pong, A. and Chow, S.C. (2010). *Adaptive Design in Pharmaceutical Research and Development*. Taylor & Francis, New York.

Purich, E. (1980). Bioavailability/bioequivalence regulations: An FDA perspective. In: *Drug Absorption and Disposition: Statistical Considerations*, Ed. Albert, K.S. American Pharmaceutical Association, Academy of Pharmaceutical Sciences, Washington, DC, 115–137.

Qi, G.D., We, D.A., Chung, L.P. and Fai, C.K. (2008). Placebos used in clinical trials for Chinese herbal medicine. *Recent Patents on Inflammation & Allergy Drug Discovery*, 2, 123–127.

Qiu, C. (1986). Strychnos used in treating myasthenia gravis. *Zhejiang Journal of Traditional Chinese Medicine*, 21 (1).

Quan, H., Zhao, P.L., Zhang, J., Roessner, M. and Aizawa, K. (2009). Sample size considerations for Japanese patients based on MHLW guidance. *Pharmaceutical Statistics*, 9, 100–112.

Racine-Poon, A. (1985). A Bayesian approach to nonlinear random effects models. *Biometrics*, 41, 1015–1023.

Racine-Poon, A. and Smith, A.M.F. (1990). Population models, In: *Statistical Methodology in Pharmaceutical Sciences*, Berry, D.A. (Ed.), Dekker, New York, pp. 139–162.

Roy, A. and Ette, E.I. (2005). A pragmatic approach to the design of population pharmacokinetic studies. *The AAPS Journal*, 7, E408–E419.

Ruberg, S.J. and Hsu, J.C. (1992). Multiple comparison procedures for pooling batches in stability studies. *Proceedings of the Biopharmaceutical Section of the American Statistical Association*, Alexandria, VA, pp. 205–209.

Sammel, M.D. and Ryan, L.M. (1996). Latent variable models with fixed effects. *Biometrics*, 52, 650–663.

Sammel, M.D. and Ryan, L.M. (2002). Effects of covariance misspecification in a latent variable model for multiple outcomes. *Statistica Sinica*, 12 (4), 1207–1222.

Sammel, M.D., Ratcliffe, S.J. and Leiby, B.E. (2010). Factor analysis. In *Encyclopedia of Biopharmaceutical Statistics*, 3rd Edition, Ed. Chow, S.C. Taylor and Francis, New York.

Sarkar, S.K., Snapinn, S.M. and Wang, W. (1993). On improving the min test for the analysis of combination drug trials. *Proceedings of the Biopharmaceutical Section of the American Statistical Association*, 212–217.

Satoh, S., Nomura, K., Hashimoto, I. et al. (1995). The effect of Toukiinshi for senile pruritis. *Kanpo-Igaku*, 19, 153–155.

Schuirmann, D.J. (1987). A comparison of the two one-sided tests procedure and the power approach for assessing the equivalence of average bioavailability. *Journal of Pharmacokinetics and Biopharmaceutics*, 15, 657–680.

Schumitzky, A. (1990). Nonparametric EM algorithms for estimating prior distributions. Technical Reports, University of Southern California, Los Angeles, California, 90–92.

Schwabe, U. and Paffrath, D. (1995). Arzneiverordnungs-Report 1995. Gustav Fischer Verlag, Stuttgart.

Searle, S.R., Casella, G. and McCulloch, C.E. (1992). *Variance Components*. Wiley, New York.

Serfling, R. (1980). *Approximation Theorems of mathematical Statistics*. John Wiley & Sons, New York.

SFDA (2012). State drug standards (No. WS3-B-3766-98-2011). State Food and Drug Administration of China, Beijing, China. *Drug Stand China*, 13, 298–300.

Shao, J. and Chow, S.C. (1994). Statistical inference in stability analysis. *Biometrics*, 50, 753–763.

Shao, J. and Chen, L. (1997). Prediction bounds for random shelf-lives. *Statistics in Medicine*, 16, 1167–1173.

Shao, J. and Chow, S.C. (2001a). Two-phase shelf life estimation. *Statistics in Medicine*, 20, 1239–1248.

Shao, J. and Chow, S.C. (2001b). Drug shelf life estimation. *Statistica Sinica*, 11, 737–745.

Sheiner, L.B. (1997). Learning vs confirming in clinical drug development. *Clinical Pharmacology and Therapeutics*, 61, 275–291.

Sheiner, L.B. and Beal, S.L. (1983). Evaluation of methods for estimating population pharmacokinetic parameters, III. Monoexponential model and routine clinical data. *Journal of Pharmacokinetics and Biopharmaceutics*, 11, 303–319.

Sheiner, L.B., Rosenberg, B. and Melmon, K.L. (1972). Modelling of individual pharmacokinetics for computer-aided drug dosage. *Computer and Biomedical Research*, 5, 441–459.

Sheiner, L.B., Rosenberg, B. and Marathe, V.V. (1977). Estimation of population characteristics of pharmacokinetic parameters from routine clinical data. *Journal of Pharmacokinetics and Biopharmaceutics*, 5, 445–479.

References

Shi, Z.X., Lei, Y., Chen, H., Liu, H.X. and Wang, Z.T. (2004). Optimal approach in treating and controlling hypertension. *Chinese Journal of Integrative Medicine*, 10, 2–9.

Simon, L.J., Landis, J.R., Tomaszewski, J.E. and Nyberg, L.M. (1997). *The ICDB Study Group. The Interstitial Cystitis Data Base (ICDB) Study. Interstitial Cystitis.* Lippincott-Raven Press, Philadelphia, PA, 17–24.

Siotani, M. (1964). Tolerance regions for a multivariate normal population. *Annals of the Institute of Statistical Mathematics*, 16, 135–153.

Smith, N. (1992). FDA perspectives on quality of life studies. Presented at DIA Workshop, Hilton Head, SC.

Snapinn, S.M. (1987). Evaluating the efficacy of a combination therapy. *Statistics in Medicine*, 6, 657–665.

Snapinn, S.M. and Sarkar, S.K. (1995). A note on assessing the superiority of a combination drug with a specific alternative. *Proceedings of the Biopharmaceutical Section of the American Statistical Association*, 20–25.

Song, X. (2011). New problems of intellectual property during innovation of traditional Chinese medicine. *World Science and Technology*, 13 (3), 466–469.

Spearman, C. (1904). General intelligence objectively determined and measured. *American Journal of Psychology*, 15, 201–293.

Steimer, J.L., Mallet, A., Golmard, J.F. and Boisvieux, J.F. (1984). Alternative approaches to estimation of population pharmacokinetic parameters; comparison with the nonlinear mixed effect model. *Drug Metabolism Reviews*, 15, 265–292.

Steinhoff, B. (1993). New developments regarding phytomedicines in Germany. *British Journal of Phytotherapy*, 3, 190–193.

Sun, Y., Chow, S.C., Li. G. and Chen, K.W. (1999). Assessing distributions of estimated drug shelf-lives in stability analysis. *Biometrics*, 55, 896–899.

Sun, H., Ette, E.L. and Ludden, T.M. (1996). On the recording of sampling times and parameter estimation from repeated measures of pharmacokinetic data. *Journal of Pharmacokinetics and Biopharmaceutics*, 24, 637–650.

Suykens, J.A.K. and Vandewalle, J. (1999). Least square support vector machine classifiers. *Neural Processing Letters*, 9, 293–300.

Suzugamo, Y., Takahashi, N., Nakamura, M. et al. (2004). A psychometrical appraisal of Japanese DLQI and Skindex-29. *Japanese Journal of Dermatology*, 114, 658.

Takane, Y. (2002). Relationships among various kinds of eigenvalue and singular value decompositions. In: *New Developments in Psychometrics*, Eds. Yanai, H., Okada, A., Shigemasu, K., Kano, Y. and Meulman, J. Springer Verlag, Tokyo, 45–56.

Tandon, P.K. (1990). Applications of global statistics in analyzing quality of life. *Statistics in Medicine*, 9, 819–827.

Testa, M.A. (1987). Interpreting quality of life clinical trial data for use in clinical practices of antihypertensive therapy. *Journal of Hypertension*, 5, S9–S13.

Testa, M.A., Anderson, R.B., Nackley, J.F. and Hollenberg, N.K. (1993). Quality of life and antihypertensive therapy in men: A comparison of Captopril with Enalapril. *New England Journal of Medicine*, 328, 907–913.

Tomaszewski, J.E., Landis, J.R., Russack, V. et al. (2001). The Interstitial Cystitis Database Group. Biopsy features are associated with primary symptoms in interstitial cystitis: Results from the Interstitial Cystitis Database study. *Urology*, 57 (Suppl 6A), 67–81.

Torrance, G.W. (1976). Toward a utility theory foundation for health status index models. *Health Services Research*, 4, 349–369.

Torrance, G.W. (1987). Utility approach to measuring health-related quality of life. *Journal of Chronic Diseases*, 40, 593–600.

Torrance, G.W. and Feeny, D.H. (1989). Utilities and quality-adjusted life years. *International Journal of Technology Assessment in Health Care*, 5, 559–575.

Tothfalusi, L., Endrenyi, L. and Arieta, A.G. (2009). Evaluation of bioequivalence for highly variable drugs with scaled average bioequivalence. *Clinical Pharmacokinetics*, 48, 725–743.

Tse, S.K. and Chow, S.C. (1995). On model selection for standard curve in assay development. *Journal of Biopharmaceutical Statistics*, 5, 285–296.

Tse, S.K., Chang, J.Y., Su, W.L., Chow, S.C., Hsiung, C. and Lu, Q.S. (2006). Statistical quality control process for traditional Chinese medicine. *Journal of Biopharmaceutical Statistics*, 16, 861–874.

Tsong, Y. (1995). Statistical assessment of mean differences between two dissolution data sets. Presented at the 1995 Drug Information Association Dissolution Workshop, Rockville, MD.

Uesaka, H. (2009). Sample size allocation to regions in multiregional trial. *Journal of Biopharmaceutical Statistics*, 19, 580–594.

USP/NF (2000). *The United States Pharmacopeia XXIV and the National Formulary XIX*. The United States Pharmacopeial Convention, Inc., Rockville, MD.

USP/NF (2012). *United States Pharmacopeia 35—National Formulary 30*. United States Pharmacopeia Convention, Rockville, MD.

Velicer, W.F. and Jackson, D.N. (1990). Component analysis versus common factor analysis: Some issues in selecting an appropriate procedure. *Multivariate Behavioral Research*, 25, 1–28.

Venditti, J.M., Humphreys, S.R., Mantel, N. and Goldin, A. (1956). Combined treatment of advanced leukemia (L1210) in mice with amethopterin and 6-mercaptopurine. *Journal of the National Cancer Institute*, 17, 631–658.

Vickers, N.D. and Dharmanonda, S. (1996). Traditional Chinese medicine and multiple sclerosis: A patient guide. ITM, Portland, Oregon, 1996.

Vonesh, E.F. (1996). A note on the use of Laplace's approximation for nonlinear mixed-effects models. *Biometrika*, 83, 447–452.

Vonesh, E.F. and Chinchilli, V.M. (1997). *Linear and Nonlinear Models for the Analysis of Repeated Measurements*. Marcel Dekker, New York.

Wagner, J.G. (1975). *Fundamentals of Clinical Pharmacokinetics*. Drug Intelligence Publications, Hamilton, IL.

Wakefield, J. (1996). The Bayesian analysis of population pharmacokinetic models. *Journal of American Statistical Association*, 91, 62–75.

Wald, A. (1942). Setting of Tolerance Limits when the sample is large. *Annals of Mathematical Statistics*, 13, 389–399.

Wang, X. (1991). Traditional herbal medicines around the globe: Modern perspectives. China: Philosophical basis and combining old and new. *Proceedings of the 10th General Assembly of WFPMM*, Seoul, Korea, October 16–18. Swiss Pharma 1991; 13 (11a):68–72.

Wang, L.Y. (2008). Clinical research of different syndromes of hypertension treated by acupuncture. *Journal of Acupuncture and Tuina Science*, 6, 230–231.

Wang, J. and Endrenyi, L. (1992). A computationally efficient approach for the design of population pharmacokinetic studies. *Journal of Pharmacokinetics and Biopharmaceutics*, 20, 279–294.

References

Wang, S.J. and Hung, H.M.J. (1997). Large sample tests for binary outcomes in fixed-dose combination drug studies. *Biometrics*, 53, 498–503.

Wang, Z. and Zhou, X.H. (2012). Random effects models for assessing diagnostic accuracy of traditional Chinese doctors in absence of a gold standard. *Statistics in Medicine*, 31, 661–671.

Wang, M., Robert-Jan, A.N., Lamers, R.A.N. et al. (2005). Metabolomics in the context of systems biology: Bridging traditional Chinese medicine and molecular pharmacology. *Phytotherapy Research*, 19, 173–182.

Ware, J.E. (1987). Standards for validating health measures definition and content. *Journal of Chronic Diseases*, 40, 473–480.

WHO (1996). Western Pacific Regional Office (WPRO). Communication with WHO Geneva, 16 April 1996.

WHO (1998). *Regulatory Situation of Herbal Medicine: A Worldwide*. World Health Organization. Geneva, Switzerland.

Williams, J.S. (1962). A confidence interval for variance components. *Biometrika*, 49, 278–281.

Williams, G.H. (1987). Quality of life and its impact on hypertensive patients. *American Journal of Medicine*, 82, 98–105.

Winkle, H.N. (2007). Implementing quality by design. PDA/FDA Joint Regulatory Conference—Evolution of the Global Regulatory Environment: A Practical Approach to Chang, Rockville, Maryland, September 24, 2007.

Wolfinger, R. (1993). Covariance structure selection in general mixed models. *Communication in Statistics, B*, 22, 1079–2006.

Woodcock, J. (2004). FDA's Critical Path Initiative. Available at http://www.fda.gov/oc/initiatives/criticalpath/woodcock0602/woodcock0602.html.

Woodcock, J., Griffin, J., Behrman, R. et al. (2007). The FDA's assessment of follow-on protein products: A historical perspective. *Nat. Rev. Drug Discov.*, 6, 437–442.

Wu, T., Zhan, S.Y. and Li, L.M. (2004). History of the development of epidemiology experimental study. *Chinese Journal of Epidemiology (Zhong Hua Liu Xing Bing Xue Za Zhi)*, 25, 633–636.

Xie, W. (1985). Treatment of progressive amyotrophic lateral sclerosis with modified Jian Bu Fu Zian Wan. *Shanghai Journal of Traditional Chinese Medicine*, 11, 32.

Xu, J.X. and Jiao, A.Q. (2005). The conception and syndromes of traditional Chinese medicine standardization research Chinese. *Zhong Guo Zhong Yi Ji Chu Yi Xue (Chin J Basic Med TCM)*, 11, 261–265.

Xu, L., Deng, D.H., Jiang, J.H., Yu, R.Q., Wu, X.M. and Zhao, Y. (2011). Developing novel and general descriptors for traditional Chinese medicine (TCM) formulas: A case study of quantitative formula-activity relationship (QFAR) model for hypertension prescriptions. *Chemometrics and Intelligent laboratory Systems*, 109, 186–191.

Yabe, T. (1985). The therapeutic experiences of Toukiinshi for pruritis. *Kanpo-Shinryo*, 4, 52–54.

Yakazu, D. (1985a). The descendent schools: The medical philosophy of Li and Zhu in the Qin and Yuan Dynasties. *Bulletin of the Oriental Healing Arts Institute*, 10 (4), 141–146.

Yakazu, D. (1985b). Myasthenia gravis. *Bulletin of the Oriental Healing Arts Institute*, 10 (6), 252–257.

Yan, B.J. and Qu, H.B. (2013). An approach to maximize the batch mixing process for improving the quality consistency of the products made from traditional Chinese medicines. *Journal of Zhejiang University Science B*, 14, 1041–1048.

Yan, B., Li, Y., Guo, Z. and Qu, H. (2014). Quality by design for herbal drugs: A feed-forward control strategy and an approach to define the acceptable ranges of critical quality attributes. *Phytochemical Analysis*, 25, 59–65.

Yang, P. (2007). Update on US FDA regulations on Chinese traditional medicine. *Trends in Bio/Pharmaceutical Industry*, 2, 21–32.

Yang, G.Y., Li, X., Li, X.L. et al. (2012). Traditional Chinese medicine in cancer care: A review of case series published in the Chinese literature. *Evidence-based Complementary and Alternative Medicine* 2012, 751046. Epub May 31, 2012.

Yang, X., Chongsuvivatwong, V., McNeil, E., Ye, J., Quyang, X., Yang, E. and Sriplung, H. (2013). Developing a diagnostic checklist of traditional Chinese medicine symptoms and signs of psoriasis: A Delphi study. *Chinese Medicine*, 8, 10. Available at http://www.cmjournal.org/content/8/1/10.

Yoder, L.H. (2005). Let's talk "cancer prevention." *Medsurg Nursing*, 14, 195–198.

Zhang, X. (1998). Regulatory situation of herbal medicines—A worldwide review. Traditional Medicine Programme, World Health Organization, WHO/TRM/98.1.

Zhang, L., Yan, B., Gong, X., Yu, L.X. and Qu, H. (2013). Application of quality by design to the process development of botanical drug products: A case study. *AAPS PharmSciTech*, 14, 277–286.

Zhou, X.H., Chen, B., Xie, Y.M., Liu, T.H. and Liang, X. (2012a). Variable selection using the optimal ROC curve: An application to a traditional Chinese medicine study on osteoporosis disease. *Statistics in Medicine*, 31, 628–635.

Zhou, X.H., Li, S.L., Tian, F. et al. (2012b). Building a disease risk model of osteoporosis based on traditional Chinese medicine symptoms and western medicine risk factors. *Statistics in Medicine*, 31, 643–652.

Zwinderman, A.H. (1990). The measurement of change of quality in clinical trials. *Statistics in Medicine*, 9, 931–942.

Index

Page numbers followed by f and t indicate figures and tables, respectively.

A

Abbreviated antibiotic drug application (AADA), 228
Abbreviated new drug application (ANDA), 219, 221t, 277
  for generic drugs, 35
Absorption, 30
Accelerated approval, 34t
Acceptance criteria
  for content uniformity testing, 79t
  for disintegration testing, 81
  for dissolution testing, 80
  quality control for consistency, 176; *see also* Statistical quality control for consistency
Acetonitrile, HPLC-grade, 333
Active control agent, 44
Acupuncture, 3; *see also* Traditional Chinese medicine (TCM)
  for stroke patients, 162
Acupuncture for diabetes treatment; *see also* Chinese herbal medicines, case studies of
  diagnosis and treatment, 350–351, 351t, 352t
  successful examples, 351–352
  TCM classification of diabetes, 350
Acute constipation, cure of, 339–340
Adaptive design methods in clinical trials, 41–42; *see also* Drug development
Adverse event, 70, 71, 94
Aggregated criteria for IBE assessment, 230
Alcohol soluble substances, 19
Allergies, alleviation of, 337–338
Allopathic medicine, 5

Alternative medicine, 5, 49
Amyotrophic lateral sclerosis (ALS), 356; *see also* Multiple sclerosis (MS), treatment of
Analysis of variance (ANOVA), 90, 161, 167t, 279, 281t
Analytical method, 29
Animal studies for TCM, 20–21
Animal studies for WM/TCM, 369–370; *see also* Traditional Chinese medicine (TCM) development, critical issues in
Anti-inflammatory Western drugs, 355
Approval pathway of biosimilars, 244–245; *see also* Follow-on biologics (FOB)
Area under plasma concentration-time curve (AUC), 220, 222, 236, 239–240, 287
Aristolochic acid, 68
Artificial imitations of TCM herbs, 52t
Asia-Pacific Economic Cooperation (APEC), 36
Association of American Retired People (AARP), 219
Association of Southeast Asian Nations (ASEAN), 36
Astringent, 76
Auscultation, 10, 152
Autocorrelation, 110, 115
Autoimmunity, 356
Autoregressive time series model, 109
Average bioequivalence (ABE)
  based on fasting studies, 278
  limitations of, 226; *see also* Bioequivalence assessment for generic approval
AVE test, 90

B

Balaam design, 284, 285t
Barthel index
  defined, 16
  for stroke, 17t
Basic matrix 2/3 on time design, 312, 313t
Batch-by-strength-by-package
      combinations, matrix on,
      314–315, 314t, 315t
Batches for stability testing, minimum
      number of, 300
Batch mixing optimization model,
      364–366; *see also* Raw materials
      (TCM), variation in
Batch sampling, 296–297; *see also* FDA
      stability guidelines
Bayesian approach, 260–261; *see also*
      Population pharmacokinetics
Bayesian methods, 225
Benign prostatic hyperplasia (BPH),
      treatment of, 95
Bias, 157
Binary responses, 321, 324
Bioavailability and bioequivalence
  bioequivalence assessment for
      generic approval
    blood sampling, 223–224
    IR product *vs.* CR product, 224
    limitations of average
      bioequivalence, 226
    sample size, 222–223, 222t
    statistical methods, 225
    study design, 224–225
    subject selection, 223
    washout, 223
  controversial issues
    fundamental bioequivalence
      assumption, 233–234
    log transformation, 235–238, 238t
    one-size-fits-all criterion, 234–235,
      235t
  defined, 220–221, 221t
  drug interchangeability
    about, 226, 227f
    drug prescribability/switchability,
      227
    FDA guidance on PBE/IBE,
      229–233

individual bioequivalence (IBE),
      227–229
    population bioequivalence (PBE),
      227
  follow-on biologics (FOB)
    approval pathway of biosimilars,
      244–245
    biosimilarity, 245
    fundamental differences, 243–244,
      243t
    interchangeability, 245
    scientific factors/practical issues,
      246
  frequently asked questions
    on AUC/C_{max} (maximum
      concentration), 239–240
    on failure of BE testing by small
      margin, 240
    on failure to meet bioequivalence
      criterion, 241
    on power/sample size calculation,
      241–242
    on raw data model/log-
      transformed data model,
      238–239
    on significant sequence effect,
      240–241
  for medical devices, 242–243
  multiplicity, adjustment for, 242
  overview, 219–220
  in vitro BE testing/*in vivo* BE
      testing/biosimilarity testing,
      comparison, 248t
Bioavailability of botanical drug, 67
Bioequivalence
  decomposition of, 225
  and generic drugs, 226
  test failure by small margin, 240
Bioequivalence assessment for
      generic approval; *see*
      also Bioavailability and
      bioequivalence
  blood sampling, 223–224
  generic drugs, 226
  IR product *vs.* CR product, 224
  limitations of average
      bioequivalence, 226
  sample size, 222–223, 222t
  statistical methods, 225

study design, 224–225
subject selection, 223
washout, 223
Biological product, defined in 1944
Biologics Act, 34
Biologics Price Competition and Innovation
(BPCI) Act, 245, 246
Biosimilarity
about, 245
testing, comparison with BE testing,
248t
Biosimilars; *see also* Follow-on biologics
(FOB)
approval pathway of, 244–245
and generic drugs, fundamental
differences, 243, 243t
Bivariate joint distribution, 125
Bivariate normal distribution, 192
Blinding, 342; *see also* Cancer care,
TCM in
Blood-Heat-Toxin, eczema by, 338
Blood sampling, 223–224; *see also*
Bioequivalence assessment for
generic approval
Bonferroni adjustment, 106
Bootstrap, 225, 252
Botanical drug products/substance, 4, 62;
see also Herbal products as drug
products in US; Traditional
Chinese medicine (TCM)
about, 61–62
CMC requirements for IND for, 63t
defined, 62
information for IND, 64f
investigational new drug (IND) for,
63t
marketing for, 66f
regulations on, 62–63, 63t, 64f
review process for, 63, 65, 66f
vs. chemical drugs
individualized treatments, 67
prior human experience, 68
priority, 68
purification and identification, 65
test and control, 65–67
toxicity, 68
Botanical review team (BRT), 65, 69
CDER, 374
Botanical substance for medical use, 204

Box-Behnken design for ethanol
precipitation, 334t
Box-Cox transformation, 239
Bridging study, 384
Bundesinstitut für Arzneimittel und
Medizinprodukte (BfArM), 58
Bureau of Pharmaceutical Affairs, 38
Buzhong Yiqi Tang, 358

C

Calibration, 117–118; *see also* Quality of
life (QOL)-like quantitative
instrument
of CDP, 156–157; *see also* Chinese
diagnostic procedures (CDP),
statistical validation of
of study endpoints, 371–372
Cancer care, TCM in; *see also* Chinese
herbal medicines, case studies
of
blinding, 342
outcome measurement, 342–343
overall conclusion/recommendation,
343
randomization, 342
remarks, 343–344
significant evidence, 343
study selection and data extraction,
341
TCM intervention, 341–342
Cancer clinical trials, 101
Capsules, 321
Case studies
of Chinese herbal medicines
acupuncture for diabetes
treatment, 350–352, 351t, 352t
in cancer care, 341–344
hypertension prescriptions,
modeling of, 344–350, 345t,
347t–348t
multiple sclerosis (MS), treatment
of, 353–359
nonclinical quality by design
QbD, case study of, 332–336, 333f,
334t, 335f, 336t
quality by design (QbD), concept
of, 328–329, 329t
statistical method for QbD, 329–332

TCM clinical cases, success of
  acute constipation, cure of, 339–340
  eczema/allergies/stress, alleviation of, 337–338
  power of Chinese herbal medicine, 336–337
  remarks on, 340
  upper respiratory infection with vertigo, 338–339
  for TCM development, overview, 327–328
Catechins, 69, 70
CDP, *see* Chinese diagnostic procedures (CDP)
Center for Biologics Evaluation and Research (CBER), 33, 35
Center for Devices and Radiological Health (CDRH), 33
Center for Drug Evaluation and Research (CDER), 33, 35, 62
Central composite design, 368, 369t; *see also* Component-to-component interactions
Chemical drugs *vs.* botanical products, *see* Botanical drug products
Chemistry, manufacturing, and control (CMC), 62
China Food and Drug Administration (CFDA), 25, 72, 372
Chinese diagnostic procedures, 1, 2t; *see also* Traditional Chinese medicine (TCM)
  about, 10–11
  objective *vs.* subjective criteria for evaluability, 11
Chinese diagnostic procedures (CDP), statistical validation of
  about CDP, 152–154
  calibration of, 156–157
  numerical example, 161–167, 163t–164t, 165t, 166f, 167t
  overview, 151–152
  study design, proposed, 154–155, 155f
  validation of
    reliability, 159–160
    ruggedness, 160–161
    validity of TCM instrument, 157–159

Chinese doctor's rating, 124–125, 128
Chinese herbal medicine, *see* Traditional Chinese medicine (TCM)
Chinese herbal medicines, case studies of
  acupuncture for diabetes treatment
    diagnosis and treatment, 350–351, 351t, 352t
    successful examples, 351–352
    TCM classification of diabetes, 350
  in cancer care
    blinding, 342
    outcome measurement, 342–343
    overall conclusion/ recommendation, 343
    randomization, 342
    remarks, 343–344
    significant evidence, 343
    study selection and data extraction, 341
    TCM intervention, 341–342
  hypertension prescriptions, modeling of
    example, 349–350
    herb properties and medical practice, 344, 345t
    least squares support vector machine, 346–349, 347t–348t
    remarks, 350
  multiple sclerosis (MS), treatment of
    amyotrophic lateral sclerosis, 356
    Chinese herbal therapy, 353–354
    diseases, 353
    multiple sclerosis clinical trial, 354–356
    myasthenia gravis, case study for, 358–359
    progressive spinal muscular atrophy studies, 356–358
    remarks, 359
Chinese herbal therapy, 353–354
Chinese massage, 4
Chinese Materia, 51
Chinese material medica, 73
Chinese *Materia Medica*, 3
Chinese medicinal herbal injections, 52t
Chinese Pharmacopoeia
  stability analysis of new drug, 319

Chinese Pharmacopoeia (CP), 21, 51, 72–74, 73t; *see also* Reference standards

Ching-hao and Scute Combination, 355

Chi-square distribution, 107, 159, 184

Cholesky-root parameterization, 271

Citizen petition, 234

Clinical development, pharmaceutical entity, 30–33

Clinical trials, regulations on TCM, 54–55

Clinical trials, TCM; *see also* Traditional Chinese medicine (TCM)
  clinical endpoint, 15–16, 17t
  matching placebo, 16–17
  sample size calculation, 18
  study design, 14
  validation of quantitative instrument, 14–15

Code of Federal Regulations (CFR), 31, 220

Cold patterns, signs, 351t

Combinational treatment, 44–45

Combination drug, global superiority of, 91–95, 91t, 92–97, 93t, 94t; *see also* Product characterization

Combination treatments
  for cancer, 87
  2×2 factorial design for, 87t
  multilevel factorial design for, 89t

Commission E, 21, 75

Committee on Herbal Medicinal Products, 57

Committee on Proprietary Medicinal Products (CPMP), 59

Common factor analysis, 132, 149–150

Common slope model, 307

Complementary and alternative medicine (CAM), 4–5; *see also* Traditional Chinese medicine (TCM)

Complete disintegration, defined, 81

Complexity of patent application, 363–364

Component-to-component interactions; *see also* Traditional Chinese medicine (TCM) development, critical issues in
  central composite design, 368, 369t

factorial design, 366–367, 367t
fractional factorial design, 367–368, 368t
remarks, 368

Composite health index, 384

Composite score, 142, 143t

Computer simulation, 275; *see also* Population pharmacokinetics

Concurrent validity, 106

Confidence interval approach, 225

Confidentiality protection by FDA, 376

Confirmatory approach to factor analysis, 133

Conjugated estrogens, 316, 324
  tablets, 277–278

Consistency, statistical test for, *see* Statistical test for consistency

Consistency assessment for QC/QA; *see also* Quality control/quality assurance (QC/QA)
  hypotheses testing, 197, 204, 205t–206t
  sample size determination, 195–197, 198t–200t, 201t–203t

Consistency index; *see also* Statistical test for consistency
  about, 172–175, 189
  critical values of proposed test for, 180t, 205t–206t
  defined, 19
  hypotheses testing of, 179
  of TCM, 192–193, 208
  theorem, 173–175

Consistency of new drug, 377

Constipation (acute), cure of, *see* Traditional Chinese medicine (TCM) clinical cases, successful

Container (closure) and drug product sampling, 297; *see also* FDA stability guidelines

Content uniformity testing, 79–80, 79t; *see also* Sampling plan and acceptance criteria

Controlled release (CR) product, 223, 224

Conventional medicine, 5

Correlation coefficient, 125, 127

Correlation matrix of QOL subscales, 145t
Covariance matrix, 125, 127
  factor analysis and, 133
  of QOL subscales, 144t
  of QOL subscales, PCA on, 146t
CQA, *see* Critical quality attributes (CQA)
Critical path opportunities list, 37–38
Critical quality attributes (CQA), 329, 330, 335f, 336t
Cronbach's α, 107
Crossover clinical trial, 14
Crossover designs
  higher-order, 224, 285t
CR product, *see* Controlled release (CR) product
Cupping, 4
Current good manufacturing practice (cGMP), 60, 380

D

Damp-heat syndrome, 354–355
Decoctions, 355, 357
Deficiency patterns, 351t
Degradation curve, 302
Deionized water, 333
Delphi method, 381–382
Delta's method, 211
Department of Health (DOH), 38
Dermatology life quality index (DLQI), 119, 121
Design of experiments (DOE), 330
Diabetes, TCM classification of, 350
Diabetes treatment, acupuncture for, *see* Acupuncture for diabetes treatment
Diagnostic checklist development; *see also* Traditional Chinese medicine (TCM), recent developments in
  criticisms of Chinese diagnostic procedures, 380–381
  objective diagnostic checklist, 381–382, 383t
  remarks, 382
Dietary Supplement and Health Education Act of 1994, 74

Dietary supplements, herbal products as (in US); *see also* Traditional Chinese medicine (TCM), regulations on
  quality issue, 60–61
  regulations for dietary supplements, 59–60
  remarks on, 61
  safety concern, 61
Dietary therapy, 4; *see also* Traditional Chinese medicine (TCM)
Disaggregated criteria for IBE assessment, 230
Disintegration testing, 80–81, 81t; *see also* Sampling plan and acceptance criteria
Disseminated sclerosis, 353
Dissolution curves of drug products, 290
Dissolution testing, 80, 80t; *see also* Sampling plan and acceptance criteria
DLQI, *see* Dermatology life quality index (DLQI)
Doctor of osteopathic medicine (DOM) degrees, 5
Documentation on prior human experience of botanical drug, 377
D-optimality criterion, 251, 263
Dosage determination, 54
Dose-effect information, 87, 89
Dose-effect relationship, 91, 92
Drug(s)
  absorption, 233–234
  categories, 52, 52t; *see also* Regulations on TCM in China
  classification of, 235t
  defined in FD&C Act (21 U.S.C. 321), 34
  discovery, 29
  expiration dating period, 29, 83
  made with commercially available crude extract, 379
  prescribability, defined, 227
  screening phase, 29
  switchability, defined, 227
  testing on animals/humans, 12
Drug Administration Law of the People's Republic of China, 49, 51–52

Index

Drug development; *see also* Global
  pharmaceutical development
  about, 37–38
  adaptive design methods in clinical
    trials, 41–42
  bridging studies, 40–41
  microdosing approach, 42–43
  remarks on, 42
Drug interchangeability; *see*
    also Bioavailability and
    bioequivalence
  about, 226, 227f
  drug prescribability/switchability,
    227
  FDA guidance on PBE/IBE, 229–233
  individual bioequivalence (IBE),
    227–229
  population bioequivalence (PBE), 227
Drug Price Competition and Patent Term
    Restoration Act, 219, 221
Drug product sampling, container
    (closure) and, 297; *see also* FDA
    stability guidelines
Drug products with multiple components,
    stability analysis for
  overview, 295
  regulatory requirements
    extension of shelf life, 301
    FDA stability guidelines, 296–297
    ICH guidelines for stability,
      297–299, 298t
    least protective packaging, 301
    least stable batch, 301
    minimum duration of stability
      testing, 299–300
    minimum number of batches for
      stability testing, 300
    remarks on, 299–302
    replicates, 301–302
    room temperature, definition of,
      300
    stability evaluation, general
      principles for, 302
  stability analysis
    basic concept, 316–317
    discussion, 320–321
    example, 319–320, 320t
    models/assumptions, 317–318
    shelf-life determination, 318–319

stability analysis with discrete
    responses
  about, 321–324
  remarks on, 324
stability designs
  basic matrix 2/3 on time design,
    312, 313t
  comparison of designs, 315–316
  matrix on batch-by-strength-by-
    package combinations, 314–315,
    314t, 315t
  matrix 1/3 on time design, 314, 314t
  matrix 2/3 on time design with
    multiple packages, 313, 313t
  matrix 2/3 on time design with
    multiple packages/multiple
    strengths, 313–314, 314t
  uniform matrix design, 315
statistical methods
  fixed batches approach, 303–304
  random batches approach,
    304–305
  remarks, 306
statistical model, 302–303
two-phase shelf-life estimation
  about, 306–307
  equal second phase slopes, case
    of, 309–310
  first-phase shelf life, 307–309
  single two-phase shelf-life label,
    determination of, 310–311
  unequal second-phase slopes,
    general case of, 311–312
Drug shelf-life
  determination of, 318–319; *see also*
    Stability analysis for drug
    products with multiple
    components
  extension of, 301; *see also*
    International Conference
    on Harmonization (ICH)
    guidelines for stability
Drug-to-drug interaction, *see*
    Component-to-component
    interactions
Dual design
  analysis of variance for, 281t
  bioequivalence in conjugated
    estrogen, 291

412
Index

Duration of stability testing, minimum, 299–300
Dynamic balance, 384

E

Eczema, alleviation of, 337–338
Effective dose, 30
Eigenvalues, 134, 135f, 136f
Eigenvectors, 139
Eight principles, 153, 350
  TCM function, 7t, 9
Electronic common technical document (eCTD) specifications, 36, 37
Emotional factors, 9t
Encephalomyelitis disseminate, 353
Envelope method, 342
Ephedrine, 358
Equal second phase slopes, 309–310; *see also* Two-phase shelf-life estimation
Equamax rotation, 134
Equilin sulfate, 278
Establishment license application (ELA), 34t, 35
Estrogen deficiency, 277
Estrone sulfate, 278
Ethanol precipitation
  Box-Behnken design for, 334t
  CQA of, 335f, 336t
  experiment of, 335
  objective of, 332
European Commission of European Union, 35
European Federation of Pharmaceutical Industries' Associations (EFPIA), 35
European Free Trade Area (EFTA), 36
European Health Authorities, 301
European Medicines Agency (EMA), 243, 244, 380
European Pharmacopoeia, 76–77; *see also* Reference standards
European scientific cooperative on phytotherapy (ESCOP), 59
European Union Directives, 76
Excess patterns, 351t
Exercise (*Qi Gong*), 3, 4, 6
Exogenous factors, 9t

Experience-based to evidence-based clinical practice, transition from, 372–373
Expiration dating period of drug product, 312, 318
Exploratory approach to factor analysis, 133
External Affairs and Industrial Liaison Working Group, CGCM, 23
Extraction process, 333
Extra-reference design, 225

F

Factor analysis; *see also* Principal component analysis (PCA); Quality of life (QOL) in hypertensive patients
  defined, 131–132
  example, 135–136, 135f, 136f, 137t, 138t
  goal of, 132–133
  number of factors, 134
  parameter estimation, 133–134
  QOL in hypertensive patients and, 146, 147t, 148t
  statistical model, 133
  types of, 132
Factorial design, 366–367, 367t; *see also* Component-to-component interactions
Factor loadings
  correlations among factors and, 136, 138t
  mixed outcome types, 138t
  under normality assumption, 135, 137t
  varimax rotation on, 147, 149t
Factor scores, 140, 141
FDA conjugated estrogen bioequivalence guidance, 290–292; *see also* Generic drug products with multiple components
FDA guidance on botanical drug products, questions/answers from; *see also* Traditional Chinese medicine (TCM), recent developments in; Traditional Chinese medicine (TCM) development, critical issues in

Index 413

commercial development program/
academic research project, 376
confidentiality protection by FDA, 376
consistency of new drug, 377
documentation on prior human
experience of botanical drug,
377
drug made with commercially
available crude extract, 379
GMP status of botanical raw
materials, 379–380
IND and lawfully marketed
botanical dietary supplement,
373–374
IND for botanical study, 374
individualized treatments, 377
level of priority, 380
NDA approval of botanical drug
products, 375
NDA requirements for botanical
drugs, 375–376
non-oral formulations for botanical
drug products, 376
phase 3 study of botanical product,
374–375
plants from native setting, 379
sponsors unfamiliar with new drug
development/regulatory
processes, 378–379
studies under IND/approval in
NDA, 378
toxic medicinal plants, 377–378
FDA guidance on PBE/IBE; *see also* Drug
interchangeability
about, 229–230
aggregated criteria *vs.* disaggregated
criteria, 230
masking effect, 231
outlier detection, 232–233
power/sample size determination, 231
replicated crossover design, 232
two-stage test procedure, 231–232
FDA guidance on population
pharmacokinetics; *see also*
Population pharmacokinetics
informative block randomized
approach, 263–264
missing data and outlier, 253
population PK analysis, 251

population PK model development/
validation, 252–253
study design, 252
timing for application, 253–254
FDA public hearings, 246
FDA stability guidelines; *see also*
Regulatory requirements for
stability testing
batch sampling consideration,
296–297
container (closure) and drug product
sampling, 297
purpose of, 296
sampling time considerations, 297
Feasible material space (FMS), 331, 332
Federal Food, Drug, and Cosmetic
(FD&C) Act, 33
Federal Institute for Drugs and Medical
Devices, 58
Federal Register, 224
Federal Trade Commission, 61
Feedforward control strategy, 329, 330
Fermentation products, 4
Fieller's theorem, 225
Fire-heat syndromes, 162, 163t–164t,
166f
First-order carryover effect, 279, 280, 281
First-order (FO) method for estimation,
250
First-phase shelf life, 307–309; *see also*
Two-phase shelf-life estimation
First-phase stability study, 306
Fisher information matrix, 250, 261,
262–263; *see also* Population
pharmacokinetics
Fitting information, pharmacokinetics
model, 270, 271t
Five elements, TCM, 7t, 8f
Five element theory, 153
Five Zang/six Fu in English/Chinese, 7t
Fixed batches approach to drug shelf
life, 303–304
Fixed-dose combination of drugs,
87–89, 87t; *see also* Product
characterization
Fixed dose of medicine, 45
Fixed dose *vs.* flexible dose, TCM, 12
Flaccidity syndrome, 359
Flexible doses in TCM, 45

Follow-on biologics (FOB); *see also* Bioavailability and bioequivalence
  approval pathway of biosimilars, 244–245
  biosimilarity, 245
  fundamental differences, 243–244, 243t
  interchangeability, 245
  scientific factors/practical issues, 246
Food and Drug Administration (FDA), 50
Formosa Cancer Foundation, 38
FORTRAN program, 257
Fractional factorial design, 301, 367–368, 368t; *see also* Component-to-component interactions
Frozen drug products, 306
Frozen study, 306–307
Fundamental Bioequivalence Assumption, 233–234, 248, 277; *see also* Bioavailability and bioequivalence

G

General Perceived Health (GPH), 147
Generic drug product and FDA regulation, 226
Generic drug products with multiple components
  FDA conjugated estrogen bioequivalence guidance, 290–292
  overview, 277–278
  in vivo drug release testing, 288–290
  in vivo single fasting bioequivalence study
    baseline adjustment, 287–288
    logarithmic transformation *vs.* significant first-order carryover effect, 288
    multiplicity of studies and ingredients, 286–287
    remarks on, 286
    sample size, 281–286, 285t
    study design, 279–281, 279t, 280t, 281t
Genomics, 27
Geometric mean ratio (GMR), 222

German regulations on herbal products; *see also* Herbal products in Europe, regulations on
  herbal medicines market, 57–58
  legal status, 58
  marketing authorizations for herbal remedies, 58–59
German Regulatory Authority, 21, 75
Ginseng and Astragalus Combination, 358
Global Cooperation Group (GCG), 36
Global drug development, *see* Global pharmaceutical development
Global dynamic balance among organs, 10
Global F test for testing additivity, 90
Globalization of Chinese Medicine (CGCM); *see also* Traditional Chinese medicine (TCM)
  consortium for, 22–23
  remarks on, 23–24
Global pharmaceutical development
  drug development
    about, 37–38
    adaptive design methods in clinical trials, 41–42
    bridging studies, 40–41
    microdosing approach, 42–43
    remarks on, 42
  modernization of TCM development
    about, 43–44
    combinational treatment, 44–45
    effective treatment, 45
    individualized treatment, 44
  multiregional clinical trials, 39–40
  overview, 27–28
  pharmaceutical development process
    about, 28–29
    clinical development, 30–33
    nonclinical development, 29–30
    preclinical development, 30
    probability of success for, 46t
  regulatory requirements
    International Conference on Harmonization (ICH), 35–36
    regulatory process in US, 33–35, 34t
    remarks on, 37
    role in pharmaceutical research, 38

Index

GMP status of botanical raw materials, 379–380

Good agricultural practice (GAP), 379

Good clinical practices (GCP), 343
defined, 37

Good collection practice, 379

Good Laboratory Practice (GLP), 78

Good manufacturing practice (GMP)
FDA's requirement for, 60

Good Statistics Practice (GSP), 36

Good Statistics Practice in drug
development, 36

Green tea, 69–70; *see also* Tea

Gruenwald, Joerg (botanist), 75

*Guidance for Industry-Botanical Drug
Products*, 5

*Guidance for Industry Immediate Release
Solid Oral Dosage Forms
Scale-Up and Post-Approval
Changes*, 291

Guidance for Statistical Procedures for
Bioequivalence Studies, 288

H

Hamilton-A (Hamilton scale for
anxiety), 101

Hamilton-D (Hamilton scale for
depression), 101

Hao Jin Qingtan Tang, 355

Health profile assessment, unified
approach for, 382–384

Health regulatory authority, 35

Heat patterns, signs, 351t

Hepatotoxicity, 68

Herba Epimedii (HE) extract, 181–182

Herbal medicines
manufacturing of, 55
market in German, 57–58

Herbal products as dietary supplements
in US; *see also* Traditional
Chinese medicine (TCM),
regulations on
quality issue, 60–61
regulations for dietary supplements,
59–60
remarks on, 61
safety concern, 61

Herbal products as drug products in
US; *see also* Traditional Chinese
medicine (TCM), regulations on
botanical drug products, 61–62
botanical products *vs*. chemical drugs
individualized treatments, 67
prior human experience, 68
priority, 68
purification and identification, 65
test and control, 65–67
toxicity, 68
regulations on botanical drug
products, 62–63, 63t, 64f
review process for botanical
products, 63, 65, 66f

Herbal products in EU, harmonization
on, 59

Herbal products in Europe, regulations
on; *see also* Traditional Chinese
medicine (TCM), regulations on
about, 56–57
German regulations
herbal medicines market, 57–58
legal status, 58
marketing authorizations for
herbal remedies, 58–59
harmonization on herbal products in
EU, 59

Herbal raw materials, 332–333

Herbal remedies, 5

Herb properties and medical practice,
344, 345t; *see also* Hypertension
prescriptions, modeling of

Herbs (with Chinese/English name), 74t

Higher-order crossover design, 224, 285t
defined, 224

High performance liquid
chromatography (HPLC), 335

Hu Qian Wan, 353–354, 355, 356

Hypertension, defined, 344

Hypertension prescriptions, modeling
of; *see also* Chinese herbal
medicines, case studies of
example, 349–350
herb properties and medical practice,
344, 345t
least squares support vector
machine, 346–349, 347t–348t
remarks, 350

Hypotheses testing for consistency index, 179, 197, 204, 205t–206t; *see also* Quality control/quality assurance (QC/QA)

I

IBE, *see* Individual bioequivalence (IBE)
ICH guidelines for stability, *see* International Conference on Harmonization (ICH) guidelines for stability
Immediate release (IR) product, 223, 224
Immunogenicity, 243t, 244, 246
Incomplete block design, 225
IND, *see* Investigational new drug (IND)
Individual bioequivalence (IBE), 227–229; *see also* Drug interchangeability
Individual bioequivalence criterion (IBC), 229
Individual difference ratio (IDR), defined, 229
Individual flexible dose, 12
Individualized medicine approach, 10
Individualized treatments, 44
  botanical products *vs.* chemical drugs and, 67
Individual therapeutic window (ITW), 235
IND Rewrite, 31
Informatics Working Group, CGCM, 23
Informative block randomized (IBR) approach, 251, 262, 263–264; *see also* Population pharmacokinetics
In-house product specifications, 81–82; *see also* Product specifications
Institut für Medizinische Statistik (IMS), 57
Integrative/integrated medicine, 5
Intellectual property (IP); *see also* Traditional Chinese medicine (TCM) development, critical issues in
  complexities of patent application, 363–364
  patentability requirements, 362–363

Interchangeability, 227, 245; *see also* Follow-on biologics (FOB)
International Conference on Harmonization (ICH), 27, 35–36; *see also* Global pharmaceutical development
International Conference on Harmonization (ICH) guidelines for stability; *see also* Regulatory requirements for stability testing
  about, 297–299, 298t
  extension of shelf life, 301
  general principles for, 302
  least protective packaging, 301
  least stable batch, 301
  minimum duration of stability testing, 299–300
  minimum number of batches required for stability testing, 300
  replicates, 301–302
  room temperature, definition of, 300
International Federation of Pharmaceutical Manufacturers Association (IFPMA), 36
Interrogation, 10, 152
Interstitial cystitis (IC), 135
Interstitial Cystitis Database (ICDB) study, 135
Intersubject variability, 253, 279
Interval hypotheses testing method, 225
Intraclass correlation coefficient (ICC), 382
Intrasubject PK model, 255–256
Intrasubject variability (ISV), 11, 171, 235, 253
Invariance principle, 173
Investigational Device Exemptions (IDE), 35
Investigational new drug (IND) application, 34t, 35, 42
  for botanical drug products, 63t
  for botanical study, 374
  clinical studies and, 67
  CMC requirements for, 63t
  and lawfully marketed botanical dietary supplement, 373–374
In vitro and *in vivo* correlation (IVIVC), 233

Index

In vitro BE testing/*in vivo* BE testing, 248t
In vitro dissolution testing, 289
In vitro drug release, 278, 291
In vivo and *in vitro* correlation (IVIVC), 277
In vivo bioequivalence testing, 277, 278, 289
In vivo drug release testing, 288–290;
    see also Generic drug products
    with multiple components
In vivo single fasting bioequivalence
    study; *see also* Generic drug
    products with multiple
    components
  baseline adjustment, 287–288
  logarithmic transformation *vs.*
    significant first-order carryover
    effect, 288
  multiplicity of studies and
    ingredients, 286–287
  remarks on, 286
  sample size, 281–286, 285t
  study design, 279–281, 279t, 280t, 281t
IR product, *see* Immediate release (IR)
    product
Ischemic stroke, Barthel index for, 16, 17t
Ischemic stroke, diagnostic criteria of, 162
Ishikawa diagram, 335f
Iterative two-stage method (ITS), 250

J

Japanese Ministry of Health, Labor and
    Welfare (MHLW), 35
Japanese Pharmaceutical Manufacturers
    Association (JPMA), 35
Jian Bu Hu Qian Wan, 357
Joint distribution, 125

K

Kaiser's criterion, 150
Karnofsky score, 343
Knowledge space, 332

L

Label, 22
  claim, 80
Lack-of-fit test, 157, 164t
Lagrangian multipliers, 348

Laplace's approximation, 259
Lawfully marketed botanical dietary
    supplement, 373–374
Lead optimization, 29
Least protective packaging, 301
Least squares estimator, 309, 318
Least squares support vector machine
    (LS-SVM), 346–349, 347t–348t;
    see also Hypertension
    prescriptions, modeling of
Least stable batch, 301
Left Restoring Pill, 354
Legal status, German regulations on
    herbal products, 58
Lifecycle management, 329t
Lifting, lowering, floating, and sinking
    (LLFS) properties, 344, 345t
Linear calibration curve, 117
Linear regression model, 156, 311, 315
Linear trend model, 307
Liu Junzi Tang, 354
Liver/kidney yin deficiency, 354
Logarithmic transformation, 288; *see*
    also In vivo single fasting
    bioequivalence study
Log-likelihood function, 262
Log transformation, 235–238, 238t;
    see also Bioavailability and
    bioequivalence
Log-transformed data model, 238–239
Lotus, medicinal parts of, 76
Lower bound (LB)
  content uniformity test, 85, 85t
  disintegration test, 86t
  dissolution testing, 86t
Lower product specification (LPS), 79, 82

M

Ma-huang, 358
Manual of Policies and Procedures
    (MAPP), 62
Marketing authorizations for herbal
    remedies in German, 58–59
Masking effect, 231, 241; *see also* FDA
    guidance on PBE/IBE
Matching placebo, 16–17; *see also* Clinical
    trials, TCM
  in clinical trials, 370–371

Matrix on batch-by-strength-by-package combinations, 314–315, 314t, 315t; *see also* Stability designs

Matrix 1/3 on time design, 314, 314t; *see also* Stability designs

Matrix 2/3 on time design; *see also* Stability designs
with multiple packages, 313, 313t
with multiple packages/multiple strengths, 313–314, 314t

Maximum concentration (C_{max}), 239–240

Maximum likelihood estimates, 257

Maximum likelihood estimator (MLE), 173, 193, 322

Maximum tolerable dose (MTD), 32, 33

Mean squared error (MSE), 157, 165t

Median effective dose, 30

Medical device, defined, 34
equivalence concept for, 242–243; *see also* Bioavailability and bioequivalence

Medical doctor (MD), 5

Medical practices of Asian countries, 37

Medical practice with TCM, 10

Medical theory and mechanism, 6–10, 7t, 8f, 8t, 9t; *see also* Traditional Chinese medicine (TCM)

Medicinal parts of herbs, 75–76

Medicines Act, 58

Microdose, defined, 42

Microdosing approach, 42–43; *see also* Global pharmaceutical development

Mili-Q academic water purification system, 333

Mind-body therapy, 4

Ministry of Health, Labor, and Welfare (MHLW) of Japan, 39, 40, 299, 300

Ministry of Public Health (MOPH), 51, 52

Minor Blue Dragon Combination, 358

Minor Bupleurum Combination (*Xiao Chaihu Tang*), 354, 355, 356

Mobilizing Powder (muscle-invigorating combination), 357

Monographs
in *Chinese Pharmacopoeia* 2010, 72, 73t
individual, 78, 79, 80
standards of, 78

Monotherapy, 92–94

Moxibustion, 4, 351

Multilevel factorial design, 97

Multiple-compartment model, 254

Multiple components, 12

Multiple-dose combinations of drugs, 87, 89–91, 89t; *see also* Product characterization

Multiple sclerosis, defined, 353

Multiple sclerosis (MS), treatment of; *see also* Chinese herbal medicines, case studies of
amyotrophic lateral sclerosis, 356
Chinese herbal therapy, 353–354
diseases, 353
multiple sclerosis clinical trial, 354–356
myasthenia gravis, case study for, 358–359
progressive spinal muscular atrophy studies, 356–358
remarks, 359

Multiple-stage sampling plan, 84

Multiple-trough sampling design, 265

Multiregional clinical trials, 39–40; *see also* Global pharmaceutical development

Multivariate analysis of variance (MANOVA), 188

Multivariate random effects model, 183–187, 186t; *see also* Tolerance region approach

Muscle-invigorating combination, 357

Myasthenia gravis, case study for, 358–359; *see also* Multiple sclerosis (MS), treatment of

N

National Center for Complementary and Alternative Medicine (NCCAM), 4

National Health Research Institutes (NHRI), 38

National Institute of Neurologic Disorder and Stroke (NINDS), 151

Natural painkillers, 3

NDA approval of botanical drug products, 375

Index

NDA requirements for botanical drugs, 375–376
Negative systematic error, 264
New Drug Application (NDA), 35, 50, 68, 301
New drugs, documentation for applications for, 52–53
New York Heart Association, 102
NIH Stroke Scale (NIHSS), 151
Nonclinical development, pharmaceutical entity, 29–30
Nonclinical quality by design; *see also* Case studies
  QbD, case study of, 332–336, 333f, 334t, 335f, 336t
  quality by design (QbD), concept of, 328–329, 329t
  statistical method for QbD, 329–332
Nonclinical safety assessment, 63t
Nonlinear mixed effects modeling approach; *see also* Population pharmacokinetics
  approximations, 159–160
  Bayesian approach, 260–261
  example, 257–259
  first-order method, 255–257
Nonlinear regression model, 255
Non-oral formulations for botanical drug products, 376
Nonparametric methods, 250
Nonrandomized (clinical) clinical studies (CCS), 341
Novelty test, 362–363
Nutraceutical, defined, 59–60

O

Office of Technology Assessment (OTA), 220
Olfaction, 10, 152
One-compartment model, 254
One-compartment open model, 257–258
One-size-fits-all criterion, for average bioequivalence, 234–235, 235t; *see also* Bioavailability and bioequivalence
One-way random model, 160
Order of the State Council of the People's Republic of China, 56

Ordinary least squares (OLS), 303
Orphan drugs, 35
Outliers
  detection in bioequivalence studies, 232–233; *see also* FDA guidance on PBE/IBE
  population PK and, 253
Over-the-counter (OTC) human drugs, 35

P

Pacify Relapse Decoction, 355
Package insert, 372
Palpation, 11
Pan American Network for Drug Regulatory Harmonization (PANDRH), 36
Parallel assessments of QOL-like instrument, 124–129, 128t, 129t; *see also* Quality of life (QOL)-like quantitative instrument
Parallel-group design clinical trial, 14
Parameterization in SAS, 273t
Parametric testing, 88
Partial least squares (PLS), 330
Patentability requirements, 362–363; *see also* Intellectual property (IP)
Patent application, complexities of, 363–364; *see also* Intellectual property (IP)
PBE, *see* Population bioequivalence (PBE)
PDR for herbal medicines, 74–76, 74t; *see also* Reference standards
Peak concentration (C_{max}), 287
Pearson's product moment correlation coefficient, 108
Peking University Clinical Research Institute (PUCRI), 344
Percutaneous nerve stimulation (PENS) therapy, 352
Performance characteristics of QOL-like instrument; *see also* Quality of life (QOL)-like quantitative instrument
  reliability, 106–108
  reproducibility, 108
  validity, 104–106

Personalized medicine approach, 10, 383

Pharmaceutical development, 329t
  defined, 28

Pharmaceutical development process; *see also* Global pharmaceutical development
  about, 28–29
  clinical development, 30–33
  nonclinical development, 29–30
  preclinical development, 30
  probability of success for, 46t

Pharmaceutical Research and Manufacturers of America (PhRMA), 35

Pharmacodynamic (PD) study, 274–275, 274f; *see also* Population pharmacokinetics

Pharmacokinetic (PK) parameter, 221, 222

Pharmacokinetics (PK)/pharmacodynamic (PD), relationship study, 274–275, 274f

Pharmacological requirements, TCM in China, 53–54

Pharmacopoeia, about, 73–74

Pharmacopoeia Commission, Ministry of Health, 72

Pharmacopoeia of the People's Republic of China, 51

Pharmacopoeia of the People's Republic of China (PPRC), 55; *see also* *Chinese Pharmacopoeia*

Phenolic acids, 333, 335

Pill of Tiger's Walk, 353

Ping Fu Tang, 355

Plant materials in botanical drug products, 66

Plasma concentration–time curve, 30

Polyphenon® E Ointment, 50

Population bioequivalence (PBE), 227, 228; *see also* Drug interchangeability

Population bioequivalence criterion (PBC), 228

Population covariance, 259

Population difference ratio (PDR), defined, 228

Population Fisher's information matrix (PFIM) approach, 262–263; *see also* Population pharmacokinetics

Population pharmacokinetics
  computer simulation, 275
  concerns and challenges, 273–274
  design of
    about, 261–262
    population Fisher's information matrix approach, 262–263
    remarks on, 264–265
  example, 265–273
  nonlinear mixed effects modeling approach
    approximations, 259–260
    Bayesian approach, 260–261
    example, 257–259
    first-order method, 255–257
  overview, 249–251
  pharmacokinetics (PK)/pharmacodynamic (PD), 274–275, 274f
  regulatory requirements
    informative block randomized approach, 263–264
    missing data and outlier, 253
    population PK analysis, 251
    population PK model development/validation, 252–253
    study design, 252
    timing for application, 253–254
  software applications, 275
  study protocol, 273
  traditional two-stage method, 254–255

Population PK, *see* Population pharmacokinetics

Positive systematic error, 264

Potency testing, 79, 82; *see also* Sampling plan and acceptance criteria

Power computation, 315

Power function for bioequivalence assessment, 231

Power index, 113–114; *see also* Quality of life (QOL)-like quantitative instrument

Power of Chinese herbal medicine, 336–337

Index

Precision index, 109, 111–113, 112; *see also* Quality of life (QOL)-like quantitative instrument

Preclinical development, pharmaceutical entity, 30

Premarin, 21, 316, 324

Premarket Approval (PMA), 242

Premarket Approval of Medical Devices (PMA), 35

Prescription *vs.* dietary supplement, 373

Principal component analysis (PCA); *see also* Factor analysis; Quality of life (QOL) in hypertensive patients

    on covariance matrix of QOL subscales, 146t

    interpretation of principal components, 140–141

    overview, 136, 137

    principal components, 139–140

    QOL in hypertensive patients and, 143, 146, 146t

    singular value decomposition, 139

Principal component(s)

    about, 139–140

    interpretation of, 140–141

Probability density function, 211

Process analytical technology (PAT), 329t

PROC NLMIXED procedure of SAS, 269t, 270t, 271t

Product characterization; *see also* Product specifications; Reference standards

    fixed-dose combination, 87–89, 87t

    global superiority of combination drug, 91–95, 91t, 93t, 94t

    multiple-dose combinations, 89–91, 89t

    overview, 87

    remarks on, 97–98

    response surface methodology, 96–97

Product license application (PLA), 34t, 35

Product specifications; *see also* Product characterization; Reference standards

    in-house specifications, 81–82

    overview, 77–78

    probability of passing USP tests, 84–86, 85t, 86t

    quality by design and, 329t

    release targets, 82–83

    remarks on, 83

    sampling plan and acceptance criteria

        about, 78–79

        content uniformity testing, 79–80, 79t

        disintegration testing, 80–81, 81t

        dissolution testing, 80, 80t

        potency testing, 79

    testing procedure, 78

Progressive spinal muscular atrophy studies, 356–358; *see also* Multiple sclerosis (MS), treatment of

Proprietary medicines, 53

Psoriasis, 381, 383t

Psychological distress (PSD), 147

Psychological well-being (PWB), 147

Pulse diagnosis, 153

Pulse taking, 11

Purification process for herbal drugs, 332

Q

QbD, *see* Quality by design (QbD)

QC/QA, *see* Quality control/quality assurance (QC/QA)

Qi and blood stasis syndrome, 354

Qi Gong (exercise), 3, 4, 6

QOL, *see* Quality of life (QOL)

Quadratic trend model, 308

Quality-adjusted life years, 117

Quality by design (QbD); *see also* Case studies

    case study of, 332–336, 333f, 334t, 335f, 336t

    concept of, 328–329, 329t

    statistical method for, 329–332

Quality control, TCM in China, 55–56

Quality control (QC) method, 19

Quality control/quality assurance (QC/QA)

    consistency assessment for hypotheses testing, 197, 204, 205t–206t

    sample size determination, 195–197, 198t–200t, 201t–203t

    discussion, 208–209

example, 204, 207–208, 207t
overview, 191–192
statistical model, 192–195
theorem, proof of, 209–217
Quality control working group, CGCM, 23
Quality matching placebo, 371
Quality of life (QOL) in hypertensive patients; *see also* Factor analysis; Principal component analysis (PCA)
   analysis results, 147, 149, 149t
   background, 142
   development of QOL instrument
      about, 142–143, 143t, 144t, 145t
      correlation matrix of QOL subscales, 145t
      covariance matrix of QOL subscales, 144t
      factor analysis, 146, 147t, 148t
      principal component analysis, 143, 146, 146t
      QOL composite scores, 143t
      QOL subscales, 143t
Quality of life (QOL)-like quantitative instrument
   calibration, 117–118
   overview, 101–102
   parallel assessments, 124–129, 128t, 129t
   performance characteristics
      reliability of QOL instrument, 106–108
      reproducibility, 108
      validity of QOL instrument, 104–106
   QOL assessment, 102–104
   responsiveness/sensitivity of QOL instrument
      about, 108–109
      power index, 113–114
      precision index, 111–113
      sample size determination, 114–116
      statistical model, 109–111
   for TCM evaluation, 118–124, 119t–120t, 122t–123t
   utility analysis, 116–117
Quantitative formula–activity relationship (QFAR), 344, 346

Quantitative instrument, validation of, 14–15; *see also* Clinical trials, TCM
Quarimax rotation, 134
Questionnaire
   DLQI-based, 118
   QOL-like, for assessment of Chinese herbal medicine, 119t–120t

R

Rand Health Insurance Experiment, 103
Random batches approach to drug shelf life, 304–305
Randomization method, 342; *see also* Cancer care, TCM in
Randomized controlled trials (RCT), 341, 370
Randomized placebo-control crossover clinical trial, 14
Rater-to-rater variability, 161
Rating scale, 116
Raw data model, 238–239
Raw materials, botanical products, 55, 66
Raw materials (TCM), variation in
   batch mixing optimization model, 364–366
   remarks, 366
   utilization ratio of extract (URE), 364
Receiver operating characteristics (ROC) curve, 106
Reference standards; *see also* Product characterization; Product specifications
   Chinese Pharmacopoeia (CP), 72–74, 73t
   European Pharmacopoeia, 76–77, 77t
   PDR for herbal medicines, 74–76, 74t
   remarks on, 77
Regulations on TCM in China; *see also* Traditional Chinese medicine (TCM), regulations on
   about, 51
   clinical trials, 54–55
   documentation for applications for new drugs, 52–53
   drug categories, 52, 52t
   manufacturing, 55

pharmacological requirements, 53–54
quality control, 55–56
raw materials, 55
regulatory approval process, 51–52
remarks on, 56, 56t
Regulatory approval process, 51–52
Regulatory process for pharmaceutical
    entity in US, 33–35, 34t; *see
    also* Global pharmaceutical
    development
Regulatory requirements, TCM, 21
Regulatory requirements for stability
    testing; *see also* Drug products
    with multiple components,
    stability analysis for
  FDA stability guidelines
    batch sampling consideration,
        296–297
    container (closure) and drug
        product sampling, 297
    sampling time considerations, 297
  ICH guidelines for stability
    about, 297–299, 298t
    extension of shelf life, 301
    general principles for, 302
    least protective packaging, 301
    least stable batch, 301
    minimum duration of stability
        testing, 299–300
    minimum number of batches
        required for stability testing, 300
    replicates, 301–302
    room temperature, definition of,
        300
Release targets, 82–83; *see also* Product
    specifications
Reliability; *see also* Chinese diagnostic
    procedures (CDP), statistical
    validation of
  of QOL instrument, 106–108; *see also*
    Performance characteristics of
    QOL-like instrument
  validation of CDP and, 159–160
Replicated crossover design, 232; *see also*
    FDA guidance on PBE/IBE
Replications, 301–302; *see also*
    International Conference
    on Harmonization (ICH)
    guidelines for stability

Reproducibility; *see also* Performance
    characteristics of QOL-like
    instrument
  assessment of, 108
  defined, 108
  inter-rater, 108
Residual effect, 279
Response surface methodology,
    96–97; *see also* Product
    characterization
Responsiveness of QOL instrument; *see
    also* Quality of life (QOL)-like
    quantitative instrument
  about, 108–109
  power index, 113–114
  precision index, 111–113
  sample size determination, 114–116
  statistical model, 109–111
Retest period, defined, 299
Rheumatoid arthritis, treatment of, 319
Robust analysis, 280
Room temperature, definition of, 300
Ruggedness, 160–161; *see also* Chinese
    diagnostic procedures (CDP),
    statistical validation of

S

Sample size determination, 114–116; *see
    also* Quality of life (QOL)-like
    quantitative instrument
  for bioequivalence assessment, 231
  consistency assessment for QC/
    QA and, 195–197, 198t–200t,
    201t–203t
  statistical QC for consistency, 176
Sample size in TCM clinical trials, 18
Sampling plan and acceptance criteria;
    see also Product specifications
  about, 78–79
  content uniformity testing, 79–80, 79t
  disintegration testing, 80–81, 81t
  dissolution testing, 80, 80t
  potency testing, 79
Sampling time, 297; *see also* FDA
    stability guidelines
Satterthwaite approximation, 186
Satterwaite's method, 281
Scaled average bioequivalence (SABE), 226

424 *Index*

Scale-up program, 29–30
Schuirmann's test procedure, 283
Score function, 127
Second-order carryover effects, 280
Second-phase stability study, 306
Sensitivity
    defined, 109
    of QOL instrument, *see*
        Responsiveness of QOL
        instrument
Serious adverse event (SAE) reporting, 37
Serum concentrations of theophylline,
    265, 266t–269t
Seven emotional factors, 9, 9t
Sexual functioning (SEX), 146, 147
Shapiro-Wilk's method, 236
Shelf-life of drugs, 20, 29, 83
Shengji Yisui Tang, 357
Shosikoto, 61
Sickness Impact Profile, 103
Significance test, 157
Significant first-order carryover effect,
    288; *see also In vivo* single
    fasting bioequivalence study
Significant sequence effect and
    bioequivalence assessment,
    240–241
Similar biological drug product (SBDP),
    243
Simulated power, 197, 201t–203t
Single active ingredient *vs.* multiple
    components, TCM, 12
Single-dosage form drugs, 87
Single dose combination, 97
Single-dose toxicity, 42
Single herbs, principal actions of,
    347t–348t
Single two-phase shelf-life label,
    determination of, 310–311;
    see also Two-phase shelf-life
    estimation
Singular value decomposition
    (SVD), 139; *see also* Principal
    component analysis (PCA)
Six exogenous factors, 9, 9t
Six Herbs Combination (*Liu Junzi Tang*),
    354
Skin diseases, QLQI/VAS/AQ
    assessment for, 122t–123t

Slutsky theorem, 195, 212
Small-molecule drug products,
    243–244
Software applications for population PK
    studies, 275
Solid oral dosage forms, 321
Southern African Development
    Community (SADC), 36
Spleen deficiency, 358
Spleen-stomach weakness, 354
Squared loadings, 141
Stability analysis, TCM, 20
Stability analysis for drug products
    with multiple components
    basic concept, 316–317
    discussion, 320–321
    example, 319–320, 320t
    models/assumptions, 317–318
    shelf-life determination, 318–319
Stability analysis with discrete
    responses
    about, 321–324
    remarks on, 324
Stability designs; *see also* Drug products
    with multiple components,
    stability analysis for
    basic matrix 2/3 on time design, 312,
    313t
    comparison of designs, 315–316
    matrix on batch-by-strength-by-
    package combinations, 314–315,
    314t, 315t
    matrix 1/3 on time design, 314, 314t
    matrix 2/3 on time design with
    multiple packages, 313, 313t
    matrix 2/3 on time design with
    multiple packages/multiple
    strengths, 313–314, 314t
    uniform matrix design, 315
Stability testing; *see also* International
    Conference on Harmonization
    (ICH) guidelines for stability
    minimum duration of, 299–300
    minimum number of batches
    required for, 300
    for thawed study, 307
Standard curve, 156, 159, 165
Standard normal distribution, 85, 108,
    112, 114

Index

Standard two-stage method (STS), 250
Standard two-treatment crossover
 design, 288
Statistical analysis software (SAS), 315
Statistical approaches to establishing
 bioequivalence, 229
Statistical methods, 41; *see also* Drug
 products with multiple
 components, stability analysis
 for
 for bioequivalence assessment, 225
 fixed batches approach, 303–304
 random batches approach, 304–305
 remarks, 306
Statistical model, 109–111; *see also*
 Quality of life (QOL)-like
 quantitative instrument
 for drug products with multiple
 components, 302–303
 for factor analysis, 133
 for QC/QA, 192–195; *see also* Quality
 control/quality assurance (QC/
 QA)
Statistical quality control (QC) for
 consistency
 about, 175
 acceptance criteria, 176
 example, 181–183, 182t, 183t
 sampling plan, 176–177, 178t
 strategy for statistical quality control,
 179–181
 testing procedure, 179, 180t
Statistical test for consistency
 consistency index, 172–175
 overview, 171–172
 statistical quality control for
 consistency
 about, 175
 acceptance criteria, 176
 example, 181–183, 182t, 183t
 sampling plan, 176–177, 178t
 strategy for statistical quality
 control, 179–181
 testing procedure, 179, 180t
 tolerance region approach
 example, 187–188, 187t, 188f
 multivariate random effects
 model, 183–187, 186t
Sterile needles, use of, 3

Storage conditions for drug, 298–299
Strength-stress relationship, 192
Stress, alleviation of, 337–338
Stroke
 acupuncture for patients, 162
 aspirin for patients, 162
 CDP for, 151
Strychnos, 357–358
Study endpoint, 371–372
Subjective Chinese diagnostic
 procedure, 11
Subjective Chinese quantitative
 instrument, 16
Subscales; *see also* Quality of life (QOL)
 in hypertensive patients
 partial correlations between, 148t
 QOL, 142, 143t
Subsequent entered biologics (SEB), 243
Summary of product characteristics
 (SPC), 59
Sum of squared residuals (SSR), 305
Supine diastolic blood pressure, 93t
Support vector machine (SVM)
 classifier, 346
Systems biology, 384; *see also* Traditional
 Chinese medicine (TCM),
 recent developments in

T

Tablets, 321
Tai Chi, 152
Taiwanese regulatory authority, 38
Taiwan Food and Drug Administration
 (TFDA), 25, 372
Taiwan Intellectual Property Office
 (TIPO) Guidelines for Patent
 Examination, 363
Taiwan Patent Law, 363
Tangniao-bing (sugar urine illness), 350
Taylor series expansion, 259
TCM, *see* Traditional Chinese medicine
 (TCM)
Tea
 benefits of, 69–70
 overdose of, 70
 side effects of, 70
Test for consistency, TCM, 19–20
Thawed study, 306

Theophylline concentration data, 266t–269t
Therapeutic exercise, *see Qi Gong* (exercise)
Time tradeoff technique, 116–117
Titration process, 96
Tolerance factor, defined, 187t
Tolerance region approach; *see also* Statistical test for consistency
   example, 187–188, 187t, 188f
   multivariate random effects model, 183–187, 186t
Tonification, 359
Toxic degradation product detection, 321
Toxicity
   botanical products *vs.* chemical drugs, 68
   of herb, 345, 345t
Toxic medicinal plants, 377–378
Traditional Chinese medicine (TCM)
   acupuncture, 3
   botanical drug product, 4
   Chinese diagnostic procedure
     about, 10–11
     objective *vs.* subjective criteria for evaluability, 11
   Chinese herbal medicine, 3
   clinical trials
     clinical endpoint, 15–16, 17t
     matching placebo, 16–17
     sample size calculation, 18
     study design, 14
     validation of quantitative instrument, 14–15
   complementary and alternative medicine (CAM), 4–5
   consistency index of, 192–193, 208
   defined, 3
   development of
     about, 18–19
     animal studies, 20–21
     indication and label, 22
     regulatory requirements, 21
     stability analysis, 20
     test for consistency, 19–20
   diabetes, classification of, 350
   dietary therapy, 4
   formulation, 182t

Globalization of Chinese Medicine (CGCM)
   consortium for, 22–23
   remarks on, 23–24
   medical practice, 10
   medical theory and mechanism, 6–10, 7t, 8f, 8t, 9t
   modernization of, 24
   with multiple components, 131
   prescribed by Chinese doctor, 171
   quality control (QC) required for, 191
   stability data of, 320t
   tolerance region, 188f
   treatment
     about, 11
     fixed dose *vs.* flexible dose, 12
     rheumatoid arthritis (example), 181–183
     single active ingredient *vs.* multiple components, 12
   and western medicine (WM), differences, 6, 6t
Traditional Chinese medicine (TCM), recent developments in
   diagnostic checklist development
   criticisms of Chinese diagnostic procedures, 380–381
   objective diagnostic checklist, 381–382, 383t
   remarks, 382
   systems biology, 384
   unified approach for health profile assessment, 382–384
Traditional Chinese medicine (TCM), regulations on
   background, in China, 51
   herbal products as dietary supplements in US
     quality issue, 60–61
     regulations for dietary supplements, 59–60
     remarks on, 61
     safety concern, 61
   herbal products as drug products in US
     botanical drug products, 61–62
     botanical products *vs.* chemical drugs, 65–68

Index

regulations on botanical drug
products, 62–63, 63t, 64f
review process for botanical
products, 63, 65, 66f
herbal products in Europe,
regulations on
about, 56–57
German regulations, 57–59
harmonization on herbal products
in EU, 59
overview, 49–50
regulations
about, 51
clinical trials, 54–55
documentation for applications
for new drugs, 52–53
drug categories, 52, 52t
manufacturing, 55
pharmacological requirements,
53–54
quality control, 55–56
raw materials, 55
regulatory approval process,
51–52
remarks on, 56, 56t
Traditional Chinese medicine (TCM)
clinical cases, successful; *see
also* Case studies
acute constipation, cure of, 339–340
eczema/allergies/stress, alleviation
of, 337–338
power of Chinese herbal medicine,
336–337
remarks on, 340
upper respiratory infection with
vertigo, 338–339
Traditional Chinese medicine (TCM)
development, critical issues
in; *see also* FDA guidance
on botanical drug products,
questions/answers from;
Traditional Chinese medicine
(TCM), recent developments in
animal studies, 369–370
calibration of study endpoints,
371–372
component-to-component
interactions
central composite design, 368, 369t

factorial design, 366–367, 367t
fractional factorial design,
367–368, 368t
remarks, 368
experience-based to evidence-based
clinical practice, transition
from, 372–373
intellectual property
complexities of patent application,
363–364
patentability requirements,
362–363
matching placebo in clinical trials,
370–371
package insert, 372
prescription *vs.* dietary supplement,
373
raw materials, variation in
batch mixing optimization model,
364–366
remarks, 366
utilization ratio of extracts, 364
Traditional Chinese medicine (TCM)
development, modernization
of; *see also* Global
pharmaceutical development
about, 28, 43–44
combinational treatment, 44–45
effective treatment, 45
individualized treatment, 44
Traditional two-stage method for
population PK modeling,
254–255; *see also* Population
pharmacokinetics
Translational medicine research,
38
Treatment with TCM; *see also* Global
pharmaceutical development;
Traditional Chinese medicine
(TCM)
about, 11
combinational, 44–45
effective, 45
fixed dose *vs.* flexible dose, 12
individualized, 44
single active ingredient *vs.* multiple
components, 12
Trifluoroacetic acid, HPLC-grade, 333
Tsu Chung, 151

Two-phase shelf-life estimation; *see also* Drug products with multiple components, stability analysis for
  about, 306–307
  equal second phase slopes, case of, 309–310
  first-phase shelf life, 307–309
  single two-phase shelf-life label, determination of, 310–311
  unequal second-phase slopes, general case of, 311–312
Type I error probability, 88
Type 2 diabetes, 10

U

Unconjugated equilin, 278
Unconjugated estrone, 278
Unequal second-phase slopes, 311–312; *see also* Two-phase shelf-life estimation
Unified approach for health profile assessment, 382–384; *see also* Traditional Chinese medicine (TCM), recent developments in
Uniform matrix design, 315; *see also* Stability designs
Upper product specification (UPS), 79, 82
Upper respiratory infection with vertigo, 338–339; *see also* Traditional Chinese medicine (TCM) clinical cases, successful
US Food, Drug, and Cosmetic Act (FD&C), 244
US Food and Drug Administration (FDA), 21
  regulations, 4
US Pharmacopeia/National Formulary (USP/NF) standards, 29
  for drug products, 77–79, 81
  room temperature, definition of, 300
USP tests, probability of passing, 84–86, 85t, 86t; *see also* Product specifications

US Public Health Service Act (PHS), 244
Utility analysis, health state, 116–117; *see also* Quality of life (QOL)-like quantitative instrument
Utilization ratio of extract (URE), 364; *see also* Raw materials (TCM), variation in

V

Validation of a population PK model, 252
Validity of QOL instrument; *see also* Performance characteristics of QOL-like instrument
  in clinical trials, 104–106
  defined, 104
Validity of TCM instrument, 157–159; *see also* Chinese diagnostic procedures (CDP), statistical validation of
Variability
  batch-to-batch, 181
  intersubject, 116
  within-subject, 116
Variance-covariance matrix, 270
Varimax rotation, 134
  on factor loadings, 147, 149t
Veregen™, 50, 70
Visual analog scale (VAS), 118, 121, 122t–123t

W

Wanfang Database, 370
Washout, 223; *see also* Bioequivalence assessment for generic approval
Water-soluble substances, 19
Wei syndrome, 353
Western clinician's rating, 124–125
Western drug discovery process, 363
Westernization of TCM, 1, 2
Western medicine (WM)
  about, 1
  animal studies for, 369–370
  for cancer, 342
  clinical endpoint for, 156, 157

practiced by MD/DOM, 5
single active ingredient in, 151
for specific organ, 49
and TCM, comparison, 361
and TCM, differences, 6, 6t
Westlake's symmetric confidence
interval approach, 225
Wilcoxon-Mann-Whitney two one-sided
tests procedure, 225
Williams' design, 225
Williams-Tukey interval, 161, 167
WinBUGS interface, 261
Wind, effects on body, 339
Wind syndrome, 162, 163t–164t, 166f
Wishart distributions, 186, 187
Within-subject variability, 171
Working Group for Herbal Resources,
CGCM, 23
Working Group for Intellectual
Property, CGCM, 23
Working Group for Regulatory Affairs,
23
World Health Organization (WHO), 102

X

Xenografts, 370
Xiao Chaihu Tang, 354
Xiao-ke (wasting and thirsting), 350

Y

Yang, 350, 352t
Yang and Yin, examples, 8t
Yang organs, 9
Yang people, 153
Yin, 350, 352t
    deficiency fire, 357
Yin people, 153

Z

Zang Fu organ, 9, 153
Zang organs, 9
Zheng composition, 381
Zhu Danxi, 354, 356
Zuo Gui Wan, 354